Medical Education for the 21st Century

Edited by Michael S. Firstenberg and Stanislaw P. Stawicki

Published in London, United Kingdom

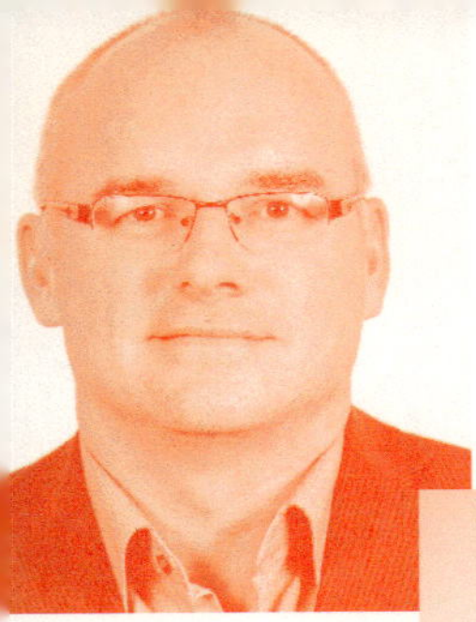
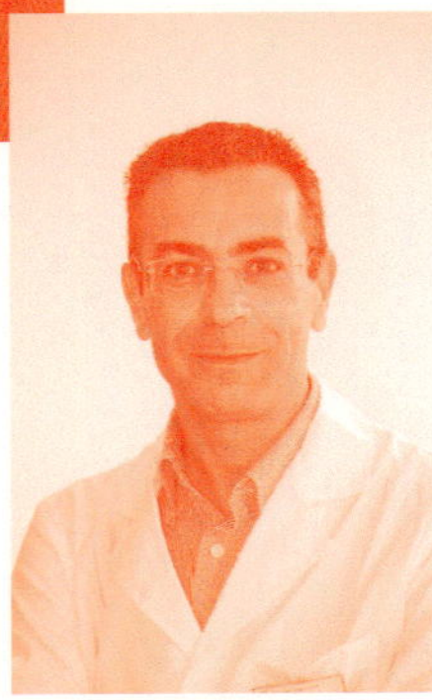
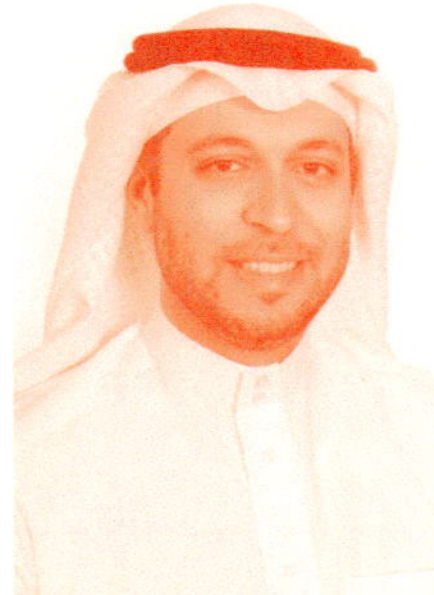
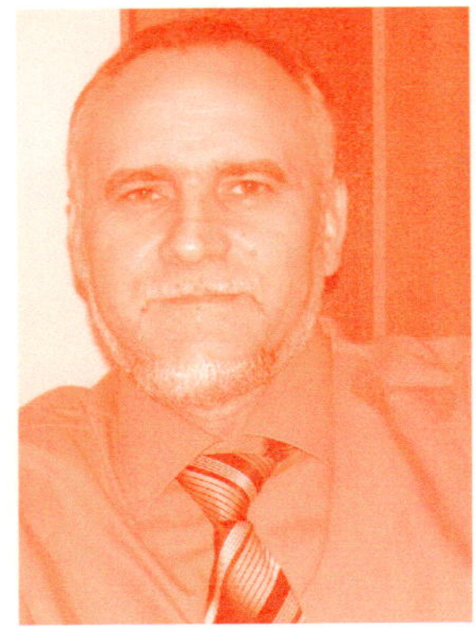
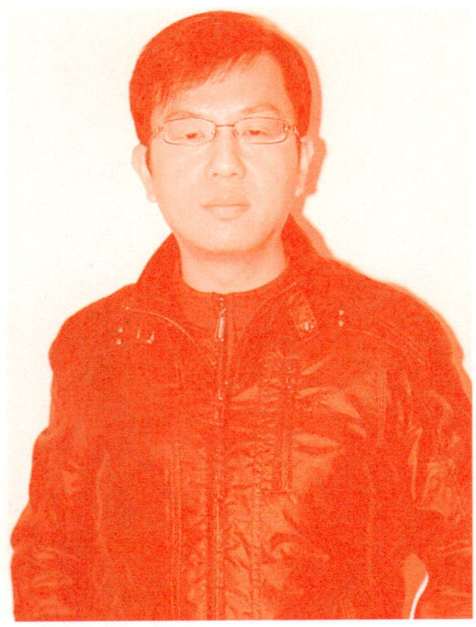
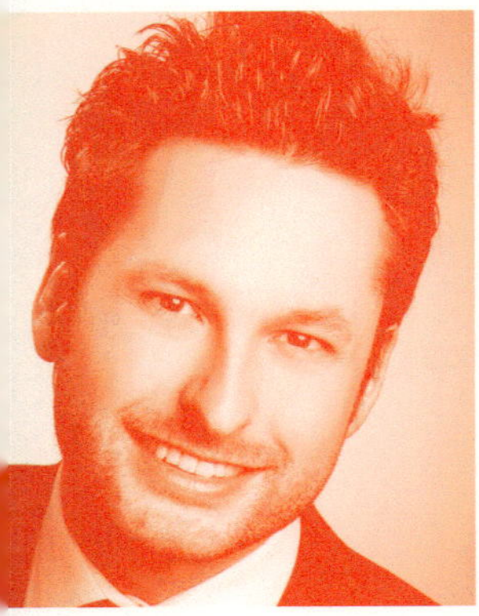
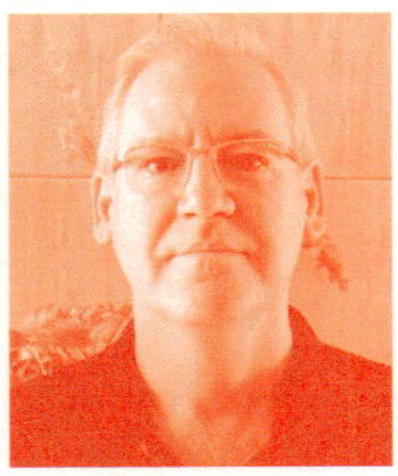

IntechOpen

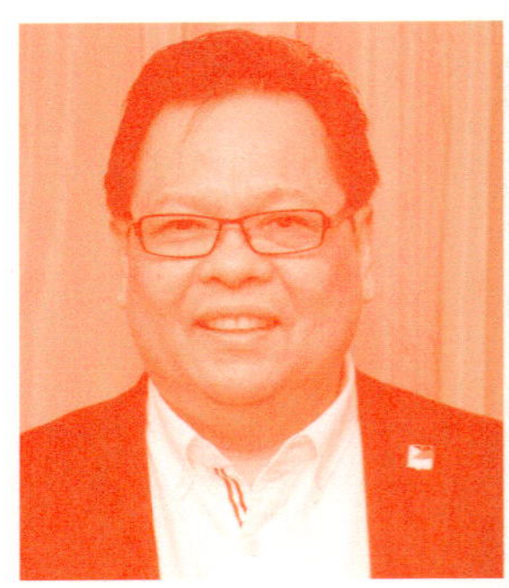
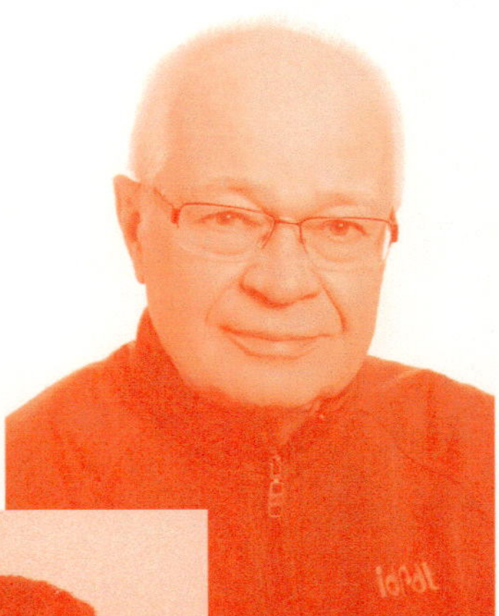
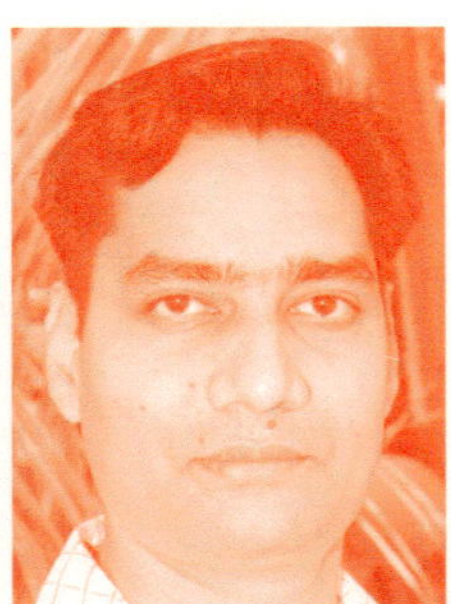
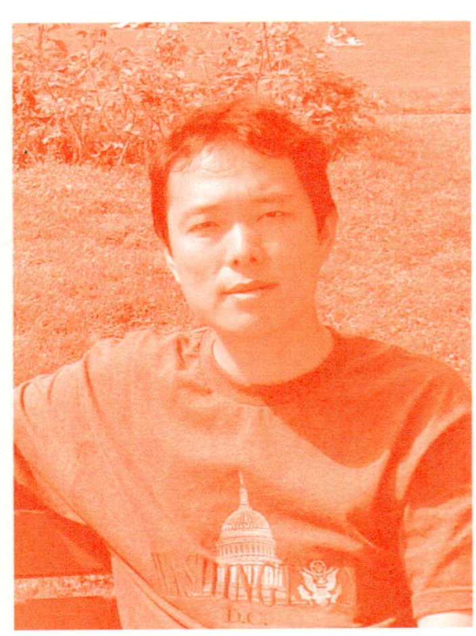
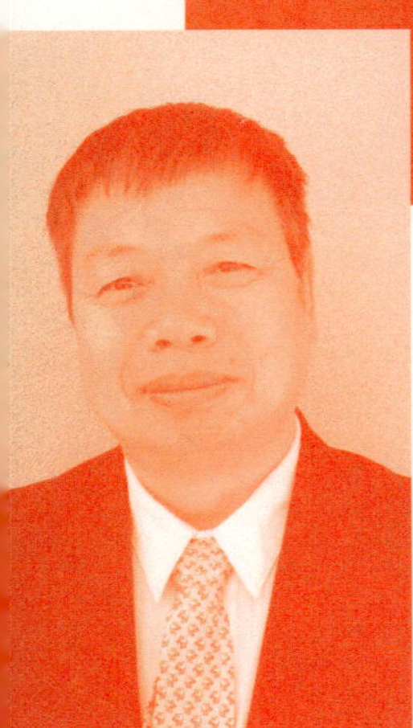
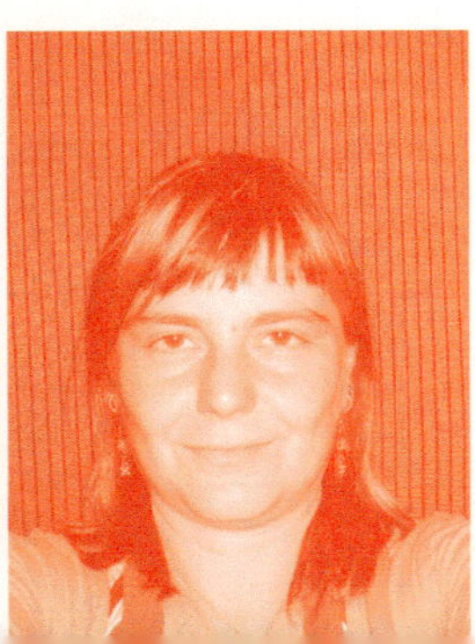

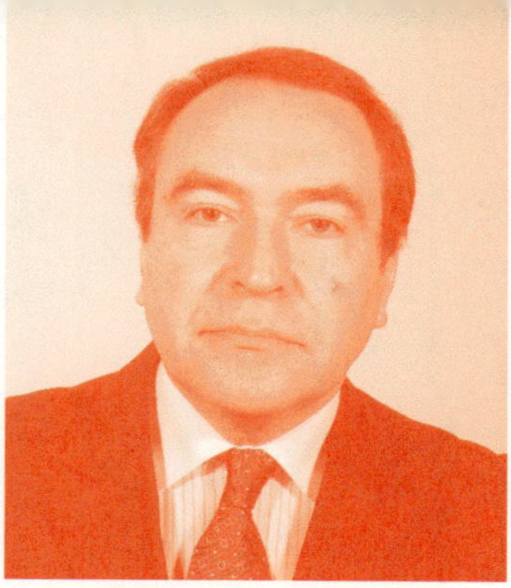
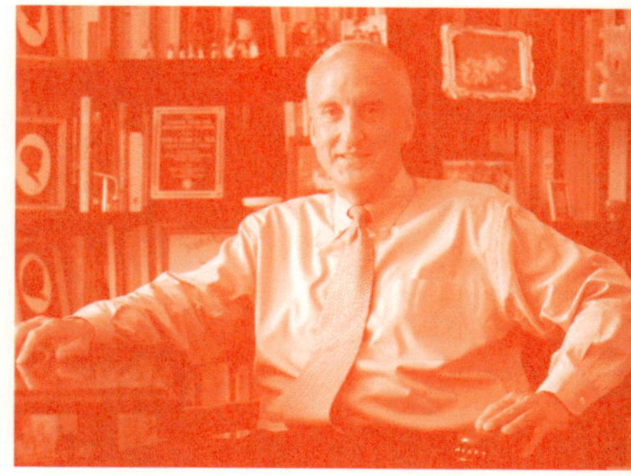
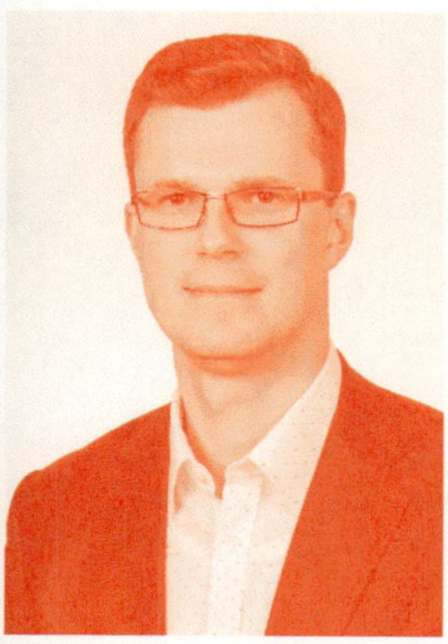
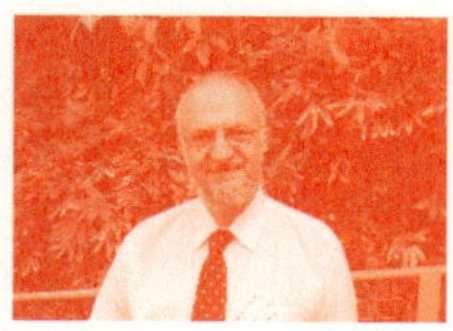
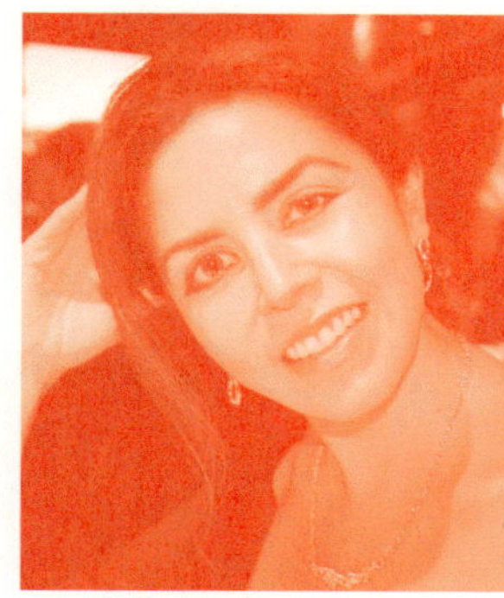

Supporting open minds since 2005

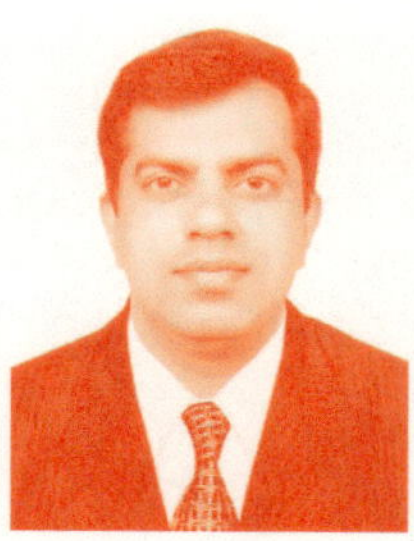
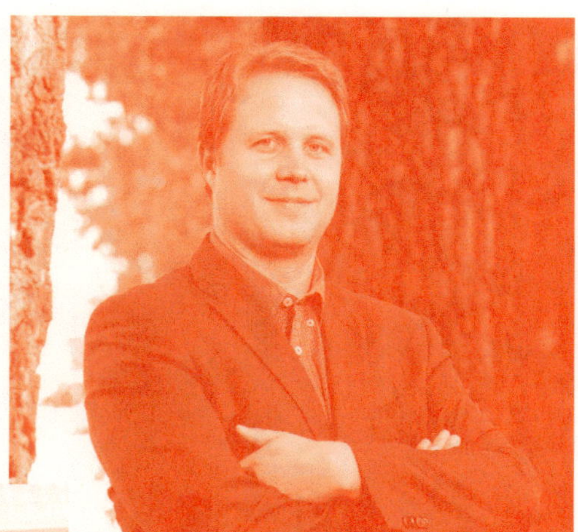
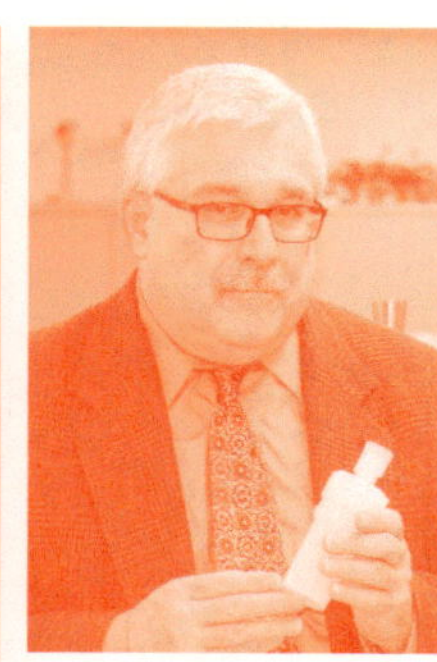
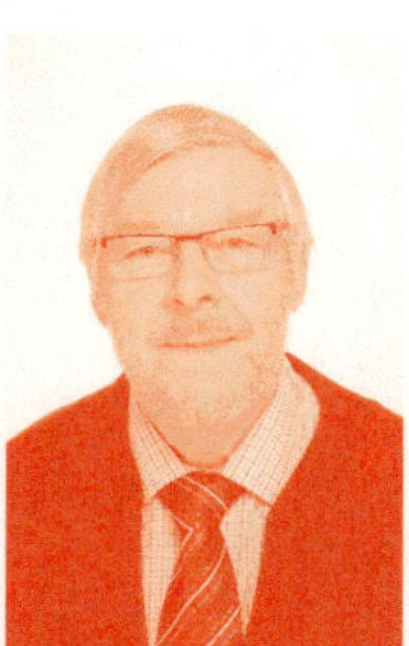
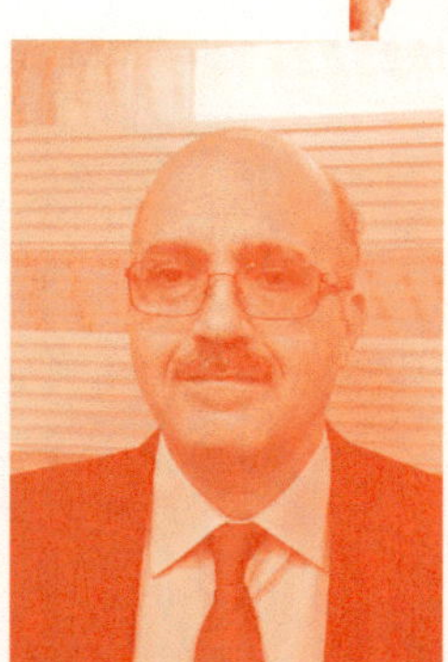
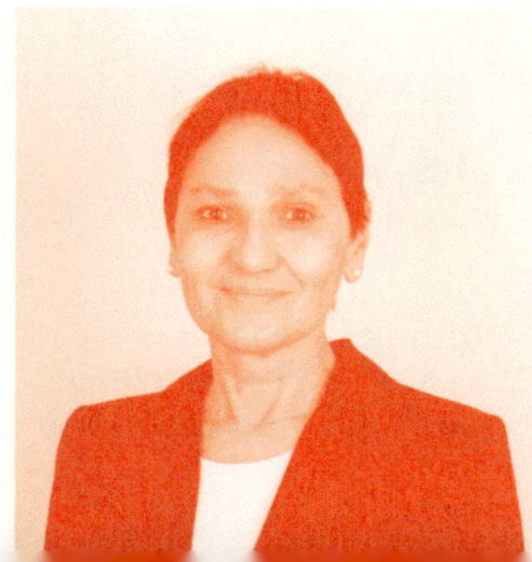
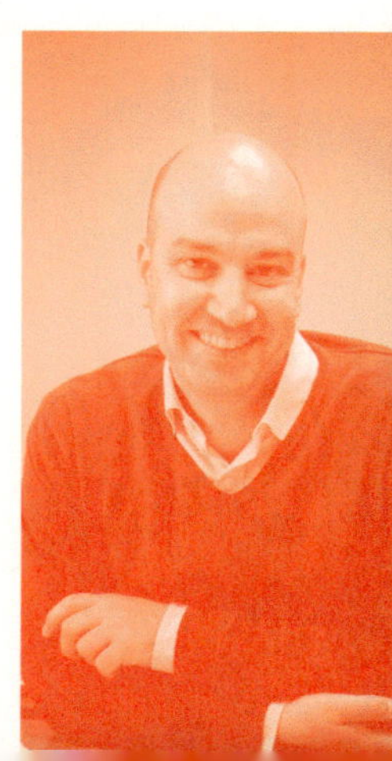

Medical Education for the 21st Century
http://dx.doi.org/10.5772/intechopen.95701
Edited by Michael S. Firstenberg and Stanislaw P. Stawicki

Contributors
Ssassi Boughizane, Badra Bannour, Imen Bannour, Marwa Masmoudi, Feten Hachani, Jalel Boughizane, Sabri Youssef, Melita Peršolja, Priyadarshini Dattathreya, Lior Naamati-Schneider, Adaya Meirovich, Louis Maximilian Buja, Graziela Moreto, Pablo González Blasco, Maria Auxiliadora C. Craice De Benedetto, Marcelo Levites, Samhaa Abd Elmoneim, Assad Ali Rezigalla, Anant Mahaveer Khot, Vincenza Ferrara, Thomas Robert Wojda, Seul Jee Ha, Sridhar Reddy Patlolla, Niva Dolev, Paul-Eric Dossou, Luiza Foreste, Eric Misumi, Vaikunthan Rajaratnam, Norana Abdul Rahman, Chaoyan Dong, Hannah Jia Hui Ng, Reema R Safadi, Lubna Abushaikha, Roderick M. Quiros, Anthony P. Allsbrook, Michael S. Firstenberg, Stanislaw P. Stawicki

First published in London, United Kingdom, 2022 by IntechOpen
IntechOpen is the global imprint of INTECHOPEN LIMITED, registered in England and Wales, registration number: 11086078, 5 Princes Gate Court, London, SW7 2QJ, United Kingdom
Printed in Croatia

British Library Cataloguing-in-Publication Data
A catalogue record for this book is available from the British Library

Additional hard and PDF copies can be obtained from orders@intechopen.com

Medical Education for the 21st Century
Edited by Michael S. Firstenberg and Stanislaw P. Stawicki
p. cm.
Print ISBN 978-1-83969-731-9
Online ISBN 978-1-83969-732-6
eBook (PDF) ISBN 978-1-83969-733-3

For EU product safety concerns:
IN TECH d.o.o., Prolaz Marije Krucifikse Kozulić 3, 51000 Rijeka, Croatia, info@intechopen.com or visit our website at intechopen.com.

Meet the editors

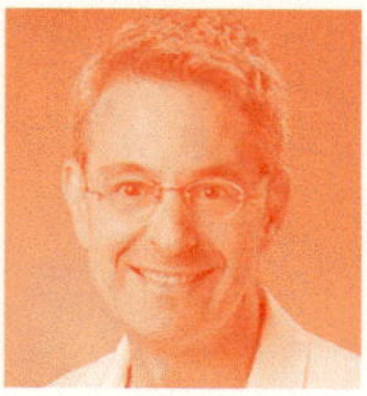

Dr. Michael S. Firstenberg is a thoracic surgeon at the St. Elizabeth Medical Center (Ascension), Appleton, Wisconsin. He attended Case Western Reserve University Medical School, Cleveland, OH, received his general surgery training at University Hospitals in Cleveland, and completed thoracic surgery fellowships at The Ohio State University and the Cleveland Clinic. He is an active member of the Society of Thoracic Surgeons (STS), American Association of Thoracic Surgeons (AATS), American College of Cardiology (ACC), and American College of Academic International Medicine (ACAIM), for which he served as president in 2021–2022. He has authored more than 250 peer-reviewed manuscripts, abstracts, and book chapters and has edited several textbooks and lectured worldwide on topics ranging from medical leadership, COVID-19, endocarditis, and extra-corporeal membrane oxygenation (ECMO).

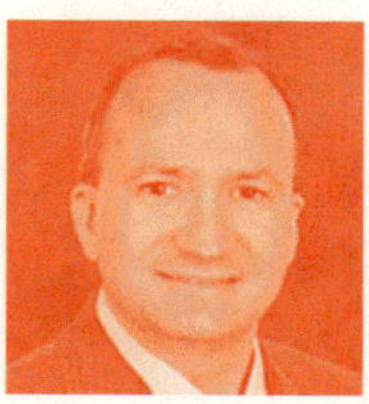

Dr. Stanislaw P. Stawicki is a Professor of Surgery and chair of the Department of Research and Innovation, St. Luke's University Health Network, Bethlehem, Pennsylvania. A specialist in general surgery, surgical critical care, and neurocritical care, he has co-authored more than 650 scholarly works, including more than 20 books. In addition to local, national, and international medical leadership roles, Dr. Stawicki is a member of numerous editorial boards. His areas of expertise are diverse and include health security, medical information security, blockchain technology, patient safety, academic leadership, mentorship and leadership development, traumatology, surgical critical care, and sonography.

Contents

Preface

As with many, if not all aspects of twenty-first-century society, contemporary medical education (ME) is evolving at a tremendous rate with the traditional models of education—learning and teaching—being challenged in the process. In the past, the roles and responsibilities of teachers and students were well defined, as the content and curriculum, at least in the context of ME, was based upon mastering the core topics of basic science, followed by the introduction of clinical curricula focusing on various medical and surgical specialties and subspecialties. While this basic paradigm still exists as a foundation for learning "facts" about diseases and their treatments, it is becoming clear that the topic of ME is much broader and more complex. The search continues for better tools and techniques aimed at teaching and objectively testing core knowledge, its application to patient care, and the early integration of basic and clinical sciences as the ME system continues to evolve. Furthermore, the key principles that described the "art of medicine" as historically lectured, tested, and applied are still emphasized, but the education of a contemporary physician is much more complex and will continue to get more so.

Traditionally, the physician is often viewed as the leader of the healthcare team. In a manner that was often viewed as absolute and without question, he (as most were males) directed the care of patients by generating hypotheses and ordering various diagnostic tests and procedures, and coordinating care with consultants and colleagues. As the role of the physician evolved, especially in the context of leadership, the focus moved toward healthcare team integration with the role often viewed as more of a politician who negotiates an agenda for care in which 'best practices' are often the subject of intense debate. The concept of effective teamwork, regardless of how defined, is a crucial component of being a successful physician. Consequently, physicians are now expected to learn how to lead, manage, and navigate a full spectrum of healthcare challenges, in addition to overseeing the overall care of an individual patient. Examples of multidisciplinary teams include Cancer Tumor Boards, Heart Teams, Trauma Teams, as well as various Critical Care and Emergency Specialty (e.g., Emergency Medicine, Stroke, High-risk Obstetrics, etc.) teams and, more and more, subsets of such teams for disease or therapy-specific situation. The physician is expected to develop, champion, and run such teams, recognizing and leveraging the unique value that each team member brings to the table. There is also a rapidly growing profession of non-physician providers such as physician assistants, doctors of nursing, and advanced nurse practitioners who are becoming critical members of the overall healthcare team. In addition to disease or organ-specific specialization, such individuals are often serving as de facto team leaders, champions, and coordinators or, as commonly described, navigators. As such, the current ME initiatives must provide the foundation that allows trainees to understand and appreciate the need for mutual respect, professionalism, and division of roles, expertise, and responsibilities that everyone brings to the bedside regardless of educational background or titles.

It is clear, as emphasized in this text, that the traditional approaches toward teaching (and learning) medicine have changed significantly over the past two decades, and even more so as we continue on in this digital information age.

In the past, lecture halls were filled with students taking notes while listening to a lecturer, never-ending group sessions debating papers and standard textbooks, various hands-on experiences in an anatomy lab, and even early bedside training experiences, all have changed to incorporate evolving ideas and theories of how teachers can best "teach" and how students can best "learn." Novel approaches incorporate the need for simulation labs and the integration/analysis of content from multiple sources. Modern sources of information include non-traditional media platforms, and the overwhelming amount of scientific content – some peer-reviewed, some non-peer-reviewed. Evolving content sources, and often the content itself, all require a great deal of critical thinking and the ability to detect various biases, and agendas, and to reconcile often conflicting points of view. A strong ME system will help the student decide how to use such content and, just as importantly, how not to use it, as the concept of a critical review is much more complex and difficult than in the past as statistical techniques, study purpose, and even patient selection and site investigators must be approached with the same inherent skepticism as one would challenge the methods and result of the study itself.

We must acknowledge that modern medicine is a "big business," and that health care in general (across the world) constitutes an increasing proportion of the global economy. This trend is inescapable, especially when both global development and changing demographics are considered. The financial implications, resource limitations, conflicting personal biases, and employment models all impact how care is delivered. While most medical students are familiar with the financial costs associated with ME in general, few understand the very complex issues that pertain to the different compensation, reimbursement, and practice models that currently exist. Even navigating local and regional politics and potentially questionable agendas can be more difficult than actual patient care and hence must be understood. There is an ongoing evolution of fee-for-service toward pay-for-performance, and a broad-based understanding of these issues, along with how employment models are structured and function, is critical. More and more, "being a good doctor" is no longer just about caring, compassion, and medical knowledge, but also about being a good steward in the setting of limited resources. An understanding of the challenges in caring for the uninsured, underinsured, and financially disadvantaged in the context of the tremendous costs associated with providing health care, in general, must be understood and integrated into a systems-based approach to resource management.

As the modern educational process is better understood, which also includes more refined theories and their applications, there must be a critical awareness of the importance of diversity, equity, and inclusion (DEI). DEI initiatives run parallel and typically complement the much-needed reforms that focused on optimization of outcomes while providing highly individualized approaches and emphasis on "building on one's strengths." These concepts are extremely important as physicians must recognize that respect for others (and not just patients, but all the members of patient-care teams) is a cornerstone for being a good doctor and that learning and appreciating various cultural dynamics in a rapidly changing world is a critical component of being a modern healthcare provider. Consequently, our ME systems must instill at the very beginning of the educational process that even minor or subtle appearances of biased communications and/or behaviors may cause emotional harm, are unacceptable, and should not be tolerated. Even in the most innocent and well-meaning of circumstances, the perceptions of any form of bias can have substantial negative implications. ME systems must acknowledge that many students, as a function of their own limited individual experiences and exposures, will require and benefit from a broader and more standardized curriculum that must consider participant age, maturity, and a variety of geo-social, cultural, and economic factors.

This test is designed to provide a solid and useful foundation and resource for all of those interested in and involved in ME, regardless of their role. After all, another aspect of ME is a realization that the lines that separate educators, students, and administrators are sometimes overlapping and poorly defined, as we are all lifelong learners. This text considers the full spectrum of topics such as curriculum building, student-guided learning, nursing staff integration into teaching programs, surgical education, and learning through art. Other equally important topics included in this text address the importance of the creation of learner support structures and systems, the need for mentorship, and a balance between emotional intelligence, work-life integration, and empathy.

The rapid changes that are occurring in modern ME are happening near or potentially at the levels at which real-time integration is no longer possible. Nevertheless, it is important that everyone involved at all levels of ME recognize their role in being active – not passive – participants in this evolutionary period of transformation and growth. It is also important to recall that the very tools that are used to assist us during this never-ending journey are themselves evolving continuously. This is a concept that can be both positive (such as the immediate availability of knowledge to a global community) and negative (biased, conflicting agendas, non-peer-reviewed, political/cultural censorship) and must be mastered. The challenges that the current generation of medical students face may seem overwhelming to the students of the past, but the opportunities and tools for success – as reviewed in this text – when used properly are aimed toward assisting the educational systems to be as effective and efficient in ways that were never possible or available in the past. In conclusion, now is a great and exciting time to be a medical student!

Stanislaw P. Stawicki
Department of Research and Innovation,
St. Luke's University Health Network,
Bethlehem, Pennsylvania, USA

Michael S. Firstenberg
Department of Cardiothoracic Surgery,
St. Elizabeth Medical Center,
Appleton, Wisconsin, USA

Chapter 1

Introductory Chapter: Medical Education at the Crossroads - Things Are Not How They Used to Be, Things Are Not as They Seem

Michael S. Firstenberg and Stanislaw P. Stawicki

"When you come to a fork in the road, take it!"
Yogi Berra

1. Introduction

Contemporary medical education (ME) is transforming rapidly. The old paradigms are being re-shaped, stakeholder expectations are being re-formulated, and the view of ME morphing into a truly life-long pursuit is becoming increasingly dominant [1–3]. The historical models of medical education were based on learning the core topics that related to various basic sciences – physiology, immunology, biochemistry, anatomy, pharmacology, pathophysiology, etc. – and how they apply to different disease states with regard to the diagnosis and management of clinical problems [4]. Students were provided with a foundation that subsequently served

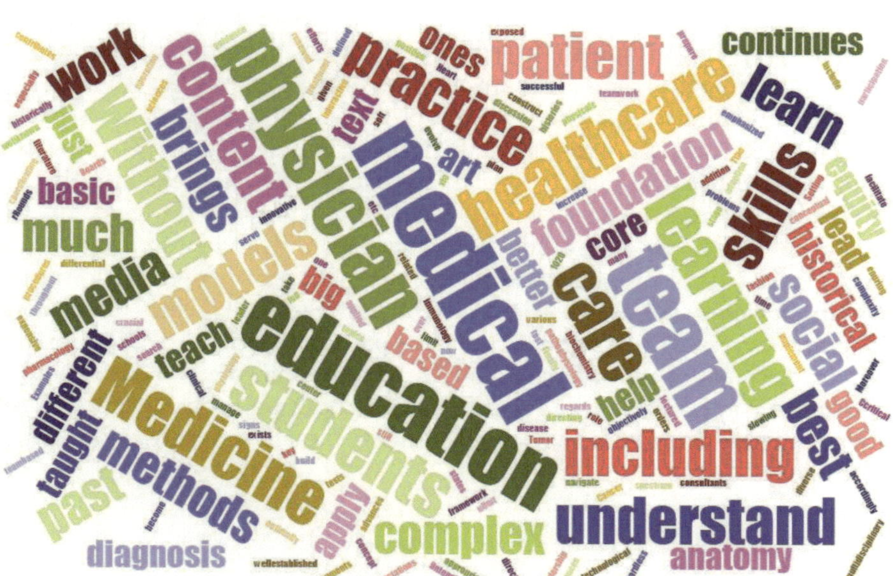

Figure 1.
Word cloud representing key concepts related to the content of this chapter and the current book.

as a springboard to build upon as their skills evolved into the art and practice of "histories and physicals." Finally, students learned to construct a "differential diagnosis" and implement a treatment plan based upon the best available literature, in an evidence-based fashion.

While such a basic foundation still exists, contemporary medical schools are continuing to search for better, more innovative methods to teach and objectively test core knowledge, including its application(s) to patient care [5, 6]. Without a doubt the evolution of ME, as emphasized throughout this text, continues to take center stage, with an increasing focus on evidence-based methods, adoption of technological advances and interactive simulation, social media platforms, and renewed emphasis on "soft skills" such as emotional and coping intelligence [7–11]. In addition to the key conceptual framework of the "art of medicine" as historically lectured, taught, and applied, the education of a contemporary physician is much more complex (and substantially more expensive) than at any other time in the past. Moreover, the overall complexity of the ME process continues to increase, without any signs of slowing. See **Figure 1** for key concepts featured in this chapter as well as throughout the current book.

2. Emotional intelligence in the context of healthcare team structure and function

In the past, the physician was often viewed as the leader of the healthcare team – directing the care of patients via providing guidance, orders, tests, procedures, and coordinating care with consultants and colleagues. However, more and more the role of a physician, especially in a leadership position, is to facilitate healthcare team integration and operation [12]. The concept of teamwork is a crucial component of being a successful physician (regardless of how defined) [13, 14]. Physicians must now learn how to lead, manage, and navigate a full spectrum of healthcare provider interactions, within diverse teams, ensuring that each team member contributes optimally to the overall care of a given patient.

Medical students are increasingly exposed to this complex environment. The ability to establish appropriate expectations, along with directed educational efforts that prepare one for team-based participation, will become critical within the evolving ME environment. Examples of team-based approaches are many, so we will limit our discussion here to some of the better-known instances. Such well-established team approaches include "Cancer/Tumor Boards", "Cardiovascular Taskforces", and "Critical Care/Intensive Care Unit Teams." In such multi-disciplinary environments, the physician is expected to not only help develop, but also champion, and run – often on a daily basis – such team(s) and recognize the unique value that each participating member contributes. The growing population of non-physician providers such as Physician Assistants and Advanced Nurse Practitioners is becoming increasingly recognized as valued participants in the health care team. Thus, current medical educational initiatives must provide the foundation for understanding, appreciation, and mutual respect, with a continued focus on professionalism, division of roles, and responsibilities that each team participant brings to the bedside [15, 16].

3. Work-life integration/balance and burnout

The practice of medicine can be both highly demanding and unforgiving to healthcare providers. Moreover, such demands can be both physical and emotional [17, 18]. Healthcare systems are fundamentally and primarily set up to provide services to our patients, and within such a framework it is easy for the individual provider to "forget" about his or her own well-being. Consequently, it is becoming more appreciated that endless work, without the opportunities to step away from the bedside – again, both emotionally and physically – can lead to burn-out and imbalances in work-life integration [19]. The unhealthy consequences on both the physician and the patient are certainly of big concern, and while the topic is far beyond the scope of the current text, the ability to understand, appreciate, and integrate these concepts will be critical to the long-term professional and personal success and fulfillment that a career in medicine brings. Learning appropriate coping techniques and related skills early in one's training can be invaluable, but must also be balanced with the respect for other stakeholders (including work partners, colleagues, various team members, and most importantly – the patients) and hospital administration. The ability to draw boundaries and function within a system that respects such boundaries may be very important "first steps," but the life skills needed to prevent burnout must be viewed as a component of continuing medical education as the techniques and adaptive traits learned early in a medical career might not effectively apply later on, as roles and responsibilities also evolve and change [20, 21].

4. Modern didactics: increasing quantity and accretion knowledge

Without a doubt, the traditional methods of teaching and learning medicine have changed substantially over the past 10–20 years, particularly since the beginning of the digital age [22, 23]. The historical models of a lecture hall filled with students taking notes while listening to a professor, endless reading of papers and textbooks, the hands-on experiences of an anatomy lab, and even the early bedside training experiences have transitioned toward evolving concepts of how to best "teach" and how to best "learn" – including the need for simulation labs, being able to integrate and analyze content from multiple (and sometimes unreliable, inaccurate, or outdated) sources, non-traditional media (i.e. social media platforms, online content, curated videos, computer-based applications, and learning tools) and the endless peer-reviewed, non-peer-reviewed, biased, for-profit, industry-sponsored content that is ubiquitously available to all. One emerging term utilized to describe this transformation is "connectivism" – it reflects well the blend of key components of the modern educational information flow ecosystem [23]. A strong foundation established early during the ME process will help the student decide how to use such content and, just as importantly, how not to.

5. Managing conflicting practice management structure, function, and economics

To ensure its long-term viability and sustainability, medicine is a business. In fact, it is a very big, multi-sectoral business, constituting a substantial proportion of the national gross domestic product (regardless of the country or region of the globe). Various contributors to the overall "business of medicine" include pharmaceutical manufacturers, research and development, clinics and hospitals, integrated health networks, outpatient/home services, and insurance providers [24–28]. While most students are familiar with the debt component of their medical education – few understand the very complex issues that pertain to the different compensation, reimbursement, and practice models that exist. Of importance, there is a gradual evolution from fee-for-service to pay-for-performance models. A broad-based understanding of related concepts and issues, along with how modern employment models are structured and/or function, is critical. In other words, being a competent doctor is no longer just about being a caring and compassionate individual, who is well-versed in the healing arts. An entire new skill set of an effective healthcare provider now requires one to be a well-informed and shrewd business person (or at least possess the awareness of the "business issues" involved in healthcare and the need for appropriate expertise within the greater healthcare team).

6. Diversity, equity, and inclusion

Along with a better understanding of the educational process, including more refined theories and their practical implementations, increasing awareness of the importance of diversity, equity, and inclusion (DEI) brought much-needed reforms that focused on optimization of outcomes while providing highly individualized approaches and emphasis on "building on one's strengths" [29–32]. Such concepts are becoming more and more important as physicians need to understand, appreciate, and converse with an extremely broad range of demographics and individual identities. Respect for others is a cornerstone of being a good doctor, but learning and appreciating the cultural dynamics in a rapidly changing social milieu is especially important in that inadvertent missteps might not be understood, could be taken out of context, and in some cases may not be tolerated (including various hardwired disciplinary policies and procedures) [33–35]. There is no room in society for racism, disrespect for gender or cultural identities that might be different from one's own, or biases that might impact the ability of the physician to be a leader in championing the health and overall wellbeing of a team, a community, and of society as a whole. Such foundations must be emphasized in medical school, especially when it is still common for students to have only a limited amount of exposure to meaningful diversity and inclusion initiatives. In addition, the overall complexity of the issue is further compounded by variables such as medical student age, maturity, and geo-social, cultural, and economic upbringing.

7. Strong foundation

The current book is designed to provide both a strong foundation and a helpful resource for those interested in exploring ME from diverse perspectives – as educators, students, and administrators. Topics discussed are diverse, including curriculum building, nursing staff integration into teaching programs, student-guided learning, surgical education, learning through art, creation of learner support structures, the importance of mentorship, emotional intelligence, and empathy, as well as many other topics and concepts.

8. Synthesis and conclusion

The rate of change in modern ME continues to increase, and the corresponding rate of evolution within the ME system is approaching levels that exceed our ability to meaningfully adapt. Nonetheless, we must strive to be active – not passive – participants in this evolutionary process of growth and transformation. We must remember that the tools available to help with this process are in constant evolution – a concept that can be both good (immediate availability of knowledge to all) and bad (biased, conflicting agendas, non-peer-reviewed content) – and therefore significant level of mastery is required. Furthermore, comprehensive medical education is no longer limited to learning about the normal and abnormal structure and function of the human body and how to treat disease, but also the complex social challenges that patients face, how to effectively function in a healthcare environment and team, and the importance of a solid foundation in various business aspects of healthcare. The challenges facing the current generation of students may seem overwhelming to medical students of the past, but the tools and opportunities for success – as outlined in this text – when used properly are all geared towards facilitating the educational process to be more efficient and effective in ways that were never available in the past. In brief, now is a great time to be a medical student – and probably more so than ever before!

Author details

Michael S. Firstenberg[1] and Stanislaw P. Stawicki[2]*

1 Department of Cardiothoracic and Vascular Surgery, Ascension St. Elizabeth Medical Center, Appleton, Wisconsin, USA

2 Department of Research and Innovation, St. Luke's University Health Network, Bethlehem, Pennsylvania, USA

*Address all correspondence to: stawicki.ace@gmail.com

References

[1] Sood R, Singh T. Assessment in medical education: Evolving perspectives and contemporary trends. National Medical Journal of India. 2012;**25**(6):357-364

[2] Neame R et al. Universities without walls: Evolving paradigms in medical education. BMJ. 1999;**319**(7220):1296

[3] Stawicki S. Changes I experienced as a resident. Current Surgery. 2004;**1**(61):98-99

[4] Rangachari P. Basic sciences in an integrated medical curriculum: The case of pharmacology. Advances in Health Sciences Education. 1997;**2**(2):163-171

[5] Shumway JM, Harden RM. AMEE guide No. 25: The assessment of learning outcomes for the competent and reflective physician. Medical Teacher. 2003;**25**(6):569-584

[6] Bereiter C and Scardamalia M, Learning to Work Creatively with Knowledge. Powerful Learning Environments: Unravelling Basic Components and Dimensions. EARLI Advances in Learning and Instruction Series. 2003. p. 55-68

[7] Strosberg DS et al. Medical simulation and the surgical resident: Creating synergies through focus on education and morbidity reduction in general laparoscopy. International Journal of Academic Medicine. 2017;**3**(1):90

[8] Stawicki TT et al. From "pearls" to "tweets:" how social media and web-based applications are revolutionizing medical education. International Journal of Academic Medicine. 2018;**4**(2):93

[9] Uchino R et al. Focus on emotional intelligence in medical education: From problem awareness to system-based solutions. International journal of academic medicine. 2015;**1**(1):9

[10] Taylor N, Kelley KC, Firstenberg MS, Davido HT, Papadimos TJ, McCallister DE, et al. Facing adversity during graduate medical training: The concept of 'coping intelligence'. In: Stawicki SP, Firstenberg MS, Orlando JP, Papadimos TJ, editors. Contemporary topics in graduate medical education - Volume 2 [Working Title] [Internet]. London: IntechOpen; 2021 [cited 2022 Apr 20]. Available from: https://www.intechopen.com/online-first/78405. DOI: 10.5772/intechopen.99698

[11] Hafferty FW, Castellani B. The hidden curriculum: A theory of medical education. In: Handbook of the Sociology of Medical Education. New York, New York, USA: Routledge; 2009. pp. 29-49

[12] Stawicki, S and Firstenberg MS, Fundamentals of Leadership for Healthcare Professionals. Hauppauge, New York, USA: NOVA Science Publishers; 2018

[13] Firstenberg MS, Stawicki SP. Teamwork in Healthcare. London, England, UK: IntechOpen; 2021

[14] Taylor N et al. Introductory chapter: Teams in healthcare-a voyage from 'Nice to Have'to 'the way to go'. In: Teamwork in Healthcare. London, UK: IntechOpen; 2021

[15] Torbeck LJ et al. Optimizing the integration of advanced practitioners in a department of surgery: An operational improvement model. The American Journal of Surgery. 2019;**217**(4):597-604

[16] Clark CJ et al. Supervisor, colleague, or assistant: General surgery resident perceptions of advanced practitioners. The American Surgeon. 2018;**84**(2):294-299

[17] DeCaporale-Ryan L et al. The undiagnosed pandemic: Burnout and

depression within the surgical community. Current Problems in Surgery. 2017;**54**(9):453-502

[18] Stawicki SP. Short timer's syndrome among medical trainees: Beyond burnout. International Journal of Academic Medicine. 2017;**3**(3):150

[19] Tolentino JC et al. What's new in academic medicine: Can we effectively address the burnout epidemic in healthcare? International Journal of Academic Medicine. 2017;**3**(3):1

[20] Eckleberry-Hunt J, Kirkpatrick H, Barbera T. The problems with burnout research. Academic Medicine. 2018;**93**(3):367-370

[21] Squiers JJ et al. Physician burnout: Are we treating the symptoms instead of the disease? The Annals of Thoracic Surgery. 2017;**104**(4):1117-1122

[22] Cullen MW et al. Reinvigorating continuing medical education: Meeting the challenges of the digital age. In: Mayo Clinic Proceedings. New York, New York, USA: Elsevier; 2019

[23] Goldie JGS. Connectivism: A knowledge learning theory for the digital age? Medical Teacher. 2016;**38**(10):1064-1069

[24] Toma S-G, Catana S. Big Pharma, Big Business. Ovidius University Annals, Economic Sciences Series. 2021;**21**(1):677-683

[25] Blockmans W, Engwall L, Weaire D. Science as big business. Wenner-Gren International series. 2014;**87**:143-150

[26] Burns LR, Burns LR. The Business of Healthcare Innovation. New York, New York, USA: Cambridge University Press; 2012

[27] Jones WJ. The "business"—Or "public service"—Of healthcare. Journal of Healthcare Management. 2000;**45**(5):290-293

[28] Sapolsky HM. Empire and the business of health insurance. Journal of Health Politics, Policy and Law. 1991;**16**(4):747-760

[29] Gonzalez P et al. Changing teaching practice: The evolving purpose of the teacher in higher education. Journal of University Teaching & Learning Practice; 2021;**18**(6):1-11

[30] van Buuren A et al. Later is too late: Exploring student experiences of diversity and inclusion in medical school orientation. Medical Teacher. 2021;**43**(5):538-545

[31] Mullett TA et al. Description of a novel curriculum on equity, diversity and inclusion for pediatric residents. Journal of the National Medical Association. 2022 Jan 1;**113**(6):616-625

[32] Fuentes MA, Zelaya DG, Madsen JW. Rethinking the course syllabus: Considerations for promoting equity, diversity, and inclusion. Teaching of Psychology. 2021;**48**(1): 769-79

[33] Johnson PR, Indvik J. Rebels, criticizers, backstabbers, and busybodies: Anger and aggression at work. Public Personnel Management. 2000;**29**(2):165-174

[34] Tatebe L, Swaroop M. Disruptive physicians: How behavior can undermine patient safety. Vignettes in Patient Safety. 2018;**2**:273

[35] Ensor K, Swaroop M, Tatebe L. Dealing with disruptive team members: Correcting "bad behaviors" while avoiding disruptions. In: Fundamentals of Leadership for Healthcare Professionals. Hauppauge, New York, USA: Nova Science Publishers, Inc.; 2018. pp. 183-199

Chapter 2

Surgical Education in the 21st Century

Anthony P. Allsbrook and Roderick M. Quiros

Abstract

Surgical education has evolved drastically since the 19th century. Previously education of surgical residents was limited to on job clinical training following the "see one, do one, teach one" model with knowledge gleaned from textbooks and journals. Presently a growing emphasis has been placed on both patient safety and resident well-being leading to a development of novel training paradigms. The textbook, while remaining a core source of knowledge, is now only one of many resources available to residents. Many residencies have their libraries online, making learning possible almost anywhere, even without physical books in hand. Most programs now incorporate education days where a structured curriculum allows for standardized education; this makes it less likely that residents miss out on mandatory concepts. The 2020 Covid-19 pandemic has led to further evolution of this model, making the classroom virtual yet interactive. Technology has allowed for residents to train on surgical simulators, so that laparoscopic and robotic skills may be practiced before application on a live patient. Altogether residents are afforded multiple ways to learn due to greater availability of time, structured educational modules, and technology.

Keywords: Surgical education, residency, training, curriculum, simulation

1. Introduction

Surgical education has evolved drastically over the centuries. Before the 19th century, the main model of surgical training and education was centered around apprenticeship, when instruction was garnered through direct observation from a mentor. There were no formalized standards on age or length of training; however, typical training would begin at the age of 12–13 and would last 5–7 years [1–3]. It was not until the end of the 19th century that Dr. William Halstead made the shift to a standardized training model.

In the late 1800s, Dr. Halstead pioneered a new era for surgical education in the United States. Using principles from the German philosophy of surgical education, he set forth to create a formalized, structured surgical curriculum. Incorporating Sir William Osler's bedside teaching and integration of basic science into surgical education, he developed a training model [1, 4]. Halstead's concept of surgical training was based on the following: First, the trainee must have repetitive opportunities to take care of surgical patients under the supervision of an experienced surgical teacher. Second, the trainee must understand the scientific basis of surgical disease. Lastly, the trainee obtains graded enhanced responsibility in patient care until independence [1]. The maxim, "see one, do one, teach one" was developed, allowing surgeons to pass down operative techniques from one generation to the next. Using this principle, one was able to accept increasing responsibility in the operating room and eventually progress to surgical independence [1, 3].

Surgical training in the 21st century has been affected by challenges not identified in previous eras. In 1999, a paper published by the Institute of Medicine reported that preventable medical errors kill between 44,000–98,000 patients per year [3]. In 2003, the Accreditation Council for Graduate Medical Education (ACGME) instituted an 80-hour work week to prevent unfavorable outcomes secondary to resident fatigue. This focus on restricting the amount of work hours has been seen not only in the United States, but throughout the world. For example, the new European working time directive restricted work hours to 48 hours per week [5]. Globally, this has caused surgical residency programs to reform past curriculums to fulfill this new training requirement [3]. Programs began incorporating part of their training outside of the operating room to accommodate these new restrictions. Curricula were now refocused to prioritize quality over quantity of education. There has now been a spotlight on the well-being of trainees as a crucial element to the benefit of their own health as well as that to their patients [6].

Simulation-based training in surgical education has rapidly developed during the 21st century. While some aspects of training occur outside of the operating room and trainees are working less clinical hours, surgical residents are still expected to reach the same technical proficiency as their predecessors [1, 3]. With patient safety in mind, the development of simulation has become a cornerstone of today's surgical training. Simulation training provides an opportunity to develop both open and minimally invasive surgical techniques on artificial platforms before utilizing them on a live patient [3].

Lastly the 2020 COVID-19 pandemic has not only impacted millions of lives on a personal level but has also significantly affected medical education. Surgical training has been uniquely impacted both operatively and nonoperatively. Residents had to quickly adapt to a 'new normal' as many elective surgeries were canceled, resident lectures and conferences were moved to online platforms, and rotations were canceled or shortened to redistribute the workforce [7, 8]. This pandemic has demonstrated that surgical education needs to adapt to train tomorrow's surgeons.

2. Surgical requirements and education during the 21st century

Prior models of surgical education emphasized an acquisition of technical and practical knowledge as paramount, even at potential personal cost to the trainee. Surgical education has taken on a more holistic approach with a focus on developing a well-rounded physician both inside and outside the operating room. The American Board of Surgery (ABS) reports that the purpose of graduate surgical education is, "to acquire a broad understanding of human biology as it relates to surgical disorders, and the technical knowledge and skills appropriate to be applied by a surgical specialist" [9]. In some regards surgical education is still influenced by the previous Halsteadian model in which the resident gradually assumes increased levels of responsibility until the final stage of training when he or she handles complete patient management [3]. However, education today is equally focused on resident well-being and education. In the United States, now work a maximum of 80 hours per week, with allotted time set aside for protected, uninterrupted education time. Didactics, journal clubs, and weekly conferences are also incorporated into current residency training programs.

Previous eras were not guided by standards in terms of length of training or what information/skills needed to be taught [1]. The ABS has since developed a set of standards and minimum requirements for individual trainees and their residency programs. As of 2021, in the United States, training requirements include:

1. A minimum of 60 months in a progressive residency program with at least 48 weeks of full-time clinical activity each year. At least 54 of these months must be dedicated to clinical surgical experience.

2. No more than 6 months of nonclinical or nonsurgical disciplines during years 1–3

3. Completion of Fundamentals of Laparoscopic Surgery (FLS)

4. Completion of the ABS Endoscopy Curriculum and the Fundamentals of Endoscopic Surgery (FES)-residents are required to perform 50 colonoscopies and 35 upper endoscopies.

5. The entire chief resident experience is in content areas of general surgery [9].

In addition to training, minimum requirements for the operative experience have been set forth by the ABS. This includes a minimum of 850 operative procedures over 5 years with at least 200 occurring during the chief resident year. Residents are also required to perform 25 teaching assistant cases in which a senior resident guide another through an operative procedure. Lastly, 40 surgical critical care cases are required prior to graduation [9].

Didactics and lectures make up an important component of surgical training. In the early 2000's there was push among resident education leaders to develop a standardized national curriculum. In response the Surgical Counsel on Resident Education (SCORE) was developed in 2004 with the mission to improve resident education in general surgery. SCORE developed a curriculum which lists the topics that should be covered in a five-year general surgery residency training program. The curriculum was developed in agreement with the six core competencies defined by the ACGME. The competencies expected from a graduating resident include: patient care, medical knowledge, professionalism, interpersonal and communication skills, practice-based learning, and systems-based practice [10, 11].

In addition to the curriculum, SCORE developed an online "Portal" to provide residents and residency training programs with educational materials and a structured learning schedule. Today, most surgical programs in the United States utilize this resource for resident education. The Portal provides over 800 topics, a topic of the week program, over 13 surgical textbooks, 2,000+ multiple choice questions, and 200+ narrated operative videos. The portal provides a weekly structured program which repeats over two-year cycle. This program specifically dives into the SCORE curriculum, providing a methodical way for residents and programs to learn material expected of a practicing general surgeon [11].

3. Simulation-based training

Simulation training has quickly become a standard among surgical residents in the 21st century. The first roots of simulation training were set by the aviation industry in the early 1900s. With many accidents attributed to novice aviators and a high demand for pilots secondary to World War I, there was a push to develop better, cheaper, and safer approaches to training. The first wildly used flight simulator was created by Edwin Link in 1928 [12]. The medical community was slower to utilize simulation and the first examples were not seen until the late 1950s where the Laerdal Company developed Resusi-Anne. This was a full-sized mannequin helped trainees practice a variety of clinical scenarios including management of obstructed airways and administration of chest compressions [12]. The field of anesthesia was one of the earliest adopters of simulation in the medical community; in the 1960s anesthesiologists utilized simulators that were able to replicate some basic human physiology and respond to medications [12]. From the basic models to teach CPR to sophisticated virtual reality simulators that can replicate the most complex human physiology, simulation training is now at the forefront of medical education.

Surgical training today has moved away from the traditional apprenticeship model where skills are developed solely in the operating room. In an era where minimizing healthcare expenditure is at the forefront; operating room time is too valuable for the development of basic surgical skills [13]. In a 2018 article published in JAMA, every minute in the operating room costs between $36 to $37 dollars [14]. Bridges et al. found that increased operative times related to resident training cost approximately $53 million dollars per year [15]. Surgical simulation has provided opportunities for residents to develop competence with surgical skills, increase deftness, and become more comfortable using a variety of instruments [1]. Montbrun et al. argues the ethical basis for incorporating stimulation into surgical education. He states that it ensures that at least some practice has taken place prior to operating on a patient [13]. Lastly, simulators help combat the work hour restriction as simulators are always available to be used during a resident's free time. There are a variety of different simulators that residents use today.

Bench top models are an example of one of the oldest and most effective tools in surgical simulation. These models use synthetic or animal tissue to replicate a variety of surgical procedures. Different specialties have developed unique bench top models to replicate real life procedures. Montbrun et al. describe benchtop models in surgical education as inexpensive, allowing familiarity to equipment along with unlimited practice opportunities, which translates well to operative skills on live patients [13].

Skill acquisition is the goal of bench top models and has been supported by a variety of studies. Lauscher et al. performed a randomized control trial comparing the Berlin Operation Trainer (BOPT), a benchtop model, to conventional training methods. Results demonstrated significant improvements in speed and performance score among the BOPT group [16]. Anastakis et al. demonstrated improved performance among surgical interns in multiple open surgical procedures like fascial closure and bowel anastomosis [17]. Multiple studies have also demonstrated that the skills obtained from bench top models can be translated to improved performance on a live patient [13]. For example, Palter et al. demonstrated that learning abdominal fascial closure on a benchtop model correlated to improved operating room performance among surgical novices [18]. Furthermore, Datta et al. demonstrated that assessment of skills on a benchtop model correlates well to performance on a live patient. The authors argue that use of benchtop work can also be used in the assessment of surgical skills [19].

Laparoscopic surgery advanced quickly in all surgical specialties since the first laparoscopic cholecystectomy was performed in 1988 by J. Barry McKernan and William Sayer [20]. Because of the early learning curve, there was a push to introduce simulation into laparoscopic surgery [10]. Compared to open surgery, laparoscopy forced the surgeon to work in a two-dimensional space with minimal tactile feedback. The ABS noticed the effectiveness of simulation in assessing laparoscopic skills and developed the Fundamentals of Laparoscopic Surgery (FLS) and introduced it into their graduation curriculum in 2008 [9, 13].

There are a variety of laparoscopic trainers used today by surgical residents, but the most well-known is the McGill Inanimate System for Training and Evaluation of Laparoscopic Skills (MISTELS) [13]. The MISTELS trainer is used to evaluate precision and speed during FLS. This low fidelity system is a simple box trainer that uses a variety of laparoscopic instruments and a laparoscope [13]. This system evaluates basic laparoscopic skills including peg transfer, intra- and extracorporeal knot tying, pattern cutting, and ligating loop placement [13, 21]. The benefit of the MISTELS system has been demonstrated in multiple studies. McCluney et al. performed a prospective study which demonstrated that FLS simulator scores independently predicted intraoperative laparoscopic performance [22]. Sroka et al. established in a randomized control trial, residents who underwent FLS training with MISTELS had significant improvement in elective laparoscopic cholecystectomies [23]. In addition to the low fidelity trainers such as MISTELS, some surgical programs incorporate virtual reality laparoscopic trainers into surgical education. These virtual reality simulators include full procedure models in which a variety of different surgical procedures can be performed [13].

Robotic surgery has quickly developed a niche among the surgical community. Sheetz et al. demonstrated that robotic surgery accounted for 15.1% of all surgeries in 2018, up from 1.8% in 2012 [24]. The rapid implementation of robotic surgery has led to specific robotic curriculums among training programs. Just as with laparoscopic surgery, robotics offers the opportunity for the trainee to become proficient prior to use in the operating room. Current robotic curriculums follow a stepwise progression for trainees, starting with observation, then providing bedside assistance, then performing with supervision, and lastly practicing independently [24].

Robotic surgical curriculums first start with patient side training. During this phase, the trainee is not personally at the console performing the operation but aiding the surgeon at bedside. Besides the obvious benefit of observing and learning the steps to the operative procedure, the trainee also develops a variety of necessary skills, including patient positioning, robot docking, and port placement. While assisting at bedside the resident learns how to help the procedure run more efficiently [25].

The second phase of the robotic curriculum includes console training. The console is a distinct area where the surgeon gets a 3D image of the patient's anatomy and where the surgeon performs the operation. The robot converts the operator's hand and finger motion into simultaneous movement of the surgical instruments [26]. Console training begins with online computer modules which include basic information on the robot, the parts of the system, and trouble shooting. After obtaining this certification, training begins on the console [25]. Similar to laparoscopic training, there are variety of different tools with which the resident can become proficient prior to operating on patients. Current techniques used for console competency include virtual reality simulators along with dry and wet lab training [25].

Just as with laparoscopic surgery, virtual reality simulators are essential for robotic procedures. This often serves as the first step in developing basic to advanced robotic skills. There are variety of robotic simulators in use today which have been shown to be effective in the development of robotic skills. These simulators all enhance the trainee's skill set through task which incorporate needle control, suturing, clutching, energy use, and dissection. Dry skills lab is another area utilized in robotic surgical training. This is a cost-effective method in which the surgical trainee sits at the actual daVinci robot. Here utilizing the console, the trainee will use the actual robotic instruments on material mimicking human tissue. This allows development of advanced robotic skills in real time with no patient risk. The last form of console training is wet skills lab training. This method allows one to perform full surgical procedures utilizing the robot on both live animal as well as human cadaveric models [25].

4. Resident education during COVID

The 2020 COVID-19 pandemic has had an impact on all aspects of general surgery training. Residency conferences and didactics moved to online platforms, rotations were canceled to reduce viral exposure, and non-urgent elective cases were delayed or rescheduled [7, 8, 27]. A concern for skills decay with the decrease in opportunities for procedural training emerged as a result.

There has been a significant reduction in surgical case volumes among all surgical specialties throughout the COVID 19 pandemic. For example, Aziz et al. found a significant reduction in operative case volume among 1,102 general surgery trainees in the United States [8]. Reduction in case volume has caused concern among both residents and directors as minimum case requirements are increasingly difficult to obtain. Rosen et al. demonstrated these results among the urological community as 60% of urology program directors were concerned that residents would not reach required operative volumes secondary to the COVID pandemic [28]. Similarly, there has been a shift to nonoperative management among previously emergent presentations like appendicitis [27]. The pandemic has shed light on an evident shift in surgical management that has been occurring over the past 50 years. Even before the emergence of COVID-19, the introduction of new data and technologies for certain disease processes, that were managed with complex surgical procedures in the past, has led to treatment with less invasive methods. For example, in surgical oncology the advent of the sentinel lymph node biopsy has drastically decreased the amount of completion lymph node dissections for melanoma and breast cancer [29, 30]. The advent of endovascular surgical techniques in vascular and cardiothoracic surgery has decreased trainee's exposure to a variety of open surgical cases. Smith et al. demonstrated a significant decrease in the amount of open abdominal aortic aneurysm repairs. Over a five-year study period from 2010 to 2014 trainees demonstrated a 38% decrease in open repairs, with one half of trainees in 2014 having exposure to less than five open repairs [31].

The obvious concern among surgical residents is inadequate operative skills secondary to decreased case volumes. Simulation training is now as important as ever to develop surgical skills among trainees. Doulias et al. argues that to prevent deterioration of operative skills, programs need to expand simulation training [32]. To improve surgical skills, online video conferencing platforms are now used to provide real time feedback from experts to surgical trainees undergoing laparoscopic and robotic training.

Despite many negative impacts from COVID on training Hope et al. argues for some positive implications. The authors argue that the adaptation of online learning has allowed greater access to educational material. Electronic-learning has now become a staple within surgical education [27]. Focus has shifted from in person lectures to a variety on online tools like podcasts, social media, YouTube videos, virtual peer reviewed libraries, and video conferencing platforms. Video conference platforms like Microsoft Teams and Zoom have provided an outlet for remote didactics, conferences, and virtual rounding [32]. Future studies will investigate the effectiveness of these new learning modalities on surgical education, but they will likely continue to have an impact in the post COVID era.

5. Conclusion

Surgical education over the last 50 years has proven to be a constantly evolving process. No longer is the Hasteadian "see one, do one, teach one" the sole maxim in training. With a growing emphasis on both patient safety and resident well-being, there has been a development of novel training paradigms. Greater emphasis has been placed on surgical simulation as a means for increasing operative skills. Training today also places an emphasis on didactics, conferences, and research as protected time is set aside for during the 80-hour work week for residents to develop their skills outside of the operating room. The lasting effects of the COVID-19 pandemic on surgical education are unknown, but the use of simulation and online training will likely continue to increase throughout the remainder of the 21st century to ensure stable and consistent training.

Author details

Anthony P. Allsbrook[1,2] and Roderick M. Quiros[1,2]*

1 Department of Surgery, St. Luke's University Health Network, Bethlehem, Pennsylvania, USA

2 Department of Research and Innovation, St. Luke's University Health Network, Bethlehem, Pennsylvania, USA

*Address all correspondence to: roderick.quiros@sluhn.org

References

[1] Polvarapu V, Harsha MD; Kulayat N. Afif, MD, MSC; Sun, Susie MD; Hamed, Osama MD. *100 years of surgical education: The past, present, and future.* Bulletin of the American College of Surgeons. 2013. Available from: https:// bulletin.facs.org/2013/07/100-years-of-surgical-education/

[2] Dobson J, Walker RM. *Barbers and Barber-Surgeons of London: A History of the Barbers' and Barber-Surgeons Companies*. Oxford: Blackwell Scientific Publications for the Worshipful Company of Barbers;1979:171.

[3] Khan MR, Begum S. Apprenticeship to simulation - The metamorphosis of surgical training. J Pak Med Assoc. 2021 Jan;71(Suppl 1)(1):S72-S76. PMID: 33582727.

[4] Grillo HC. To impart this art: The development of graduate surgical education in the United States. Surgery. 1999;125(1):1-14.

[5] Drossard S. Structured surgical residency training in Germany: an overview of existing training programs in 10 surgical subspecialties. *Innov Surg Sci*. 2019;4(1):15-24. Published 2019 May 10. doi:10.1515/iss-2018-0033

[6] Quiros RM, Black E. "Wellness in Residency: A Paradigm Shift." [online] IntechOpen, DOI:10.5772/intechopen. 82343. Available from:https://www. intechopen.com/online-first/wellness-in-residency-a-pardigm-shift.

[7] Imai TA, Soukiasian HJ, Truong A, Chau V, Amersi F. The lasting footprint of COVID-19 on surgical education: A resident and attending perspective on the global pandemic. Am J Surg. 2020 Dec 30:S0002-9610(20)30824-2. doi: 10.1016/j.amjsurg.2020.12.046.

[8] Aziz H., James T., Remulla D. Effect of COVID-19 on surgical training across the United States: a national survey of general surgery residents [published online ahead of print, 2020 Jul 30] J Surg Educ. 2020 doi: 10.1016/j. jsurg.2020.07.037. S1931-7204(20) 30271-30273

[9] *Booklet of Information Surgery.* American Board of Surgery Inc. 2020. Philadelpha, PA. Available from: https:// www.absurgery.org/xfer/BookletofInfo-Surgery.pdf

[10] SCORE-Surgical Council on Resident Education. The American Board of Surgery. Available from: https://www.absurgery.org/default. jsp?aboutscre

[11] SCORE. About Score. Available from: https://www.surgicalcore.org/ public/aboutscore

[12] Drews FA, Bakdash JZ. Simulation Training in Health Care. Reviews of Human Factors and Ergonomics. 2013;8(1):191-234. doi:10.1177/ 1557234X13492977

[13] de Montbrun SL, Macrae H. Simulation in surgical education. Clin Colon Rectal Surg. 2012;25(3):156-165. doi:10.1055/s-0032-1322553

[14] Childers CP, Maggard-Gibbons M. Understanding Costs of Care in the Operating Room. JAMA Surg. 2018;153(4):e176233. doi:10.1001/ jamasurg.2017.6233

[15] Bridges M, Diamond D L. The financial impact of teaching surgical residents in the operating room. Am J Surg. 1999;177(1):28-32.

[16] Lauscher J C, Ritz J-P, Stroux A, Buhr H J, Gröne J. A new surgical trainer (BOPT) improves skill transfer for anastomotic techniques in gastrointestinal surgery into the operating room: a prospective

randomized trial. World J Surg. 2010;34(9):2017-2025

[17] Anastakis D J, Regehr G, Reznick R K. et al. Assessment of technical skills transfer from the bench training model to the human model. Am J Surg. 1999;177(2):167-170.

[18] Palter V N, Grantcharov T, Harvey A, Macrae H M. Ex vivo technical skills training transfers to the operating room and enhances cognitive learning: a randomized controlled trial. Ann Surg. 2011;253(5):886-889.

[19] Datta V, Bann S, Beard J, Mandalia M, Darzi A. Comparison of bench test evaluations of surgical skill with live operating performance assessments. J Am Coll Surg. 2004;199(4):603-606.

[20] Reynolds W Jr. The first laparoscopic cholecystectomy. JSLS. 2001;5(1):89-94.

[21] Derossis A M, Fried G M, Abrahamowicz M, Sigman H H, Barkun J S, Meakins J L. Development of a model for training and evaluation of laparoscopic skills. Am J Surg. 1998;175(6):482-487.

[22] McCluney A L, Vassiliou M C, Kaneva P A. et al. FLS simulator performance predicts intraoperative laparoscopic skill. Surg Endosc. 2007;21(11):1991-1995.

[23] Sroka G, Feldman L S, Vassiliou M C, Kaneva P A, Fayez R, Fried G M. Fundamentals of laparoscopic surgery simulator training to proficiency improves laparoscopic performance in the operating room-a randomized controlled trial. Am J Surg. 2010;199(1):115-120.

[24] Sheetz KH, Claflin J, Dimick JB. Trends in the Adoption of Robotic Surgery for Common Surgical Procedures. JAMA Netw Open. 2020;3(1):e1918911. doi:10.1001/jamanetworkopen.2019.18911

[25] Sridhar AN, Briggs TP, Kelly JD, Nathan S. Training in Robotic Surgery-an Overview. Curr Urol Rep. 2017;18(8):58. doi:10.1007/s11934-017-0710-y

[26] The da Vinci Surgical System. Da Vinci Surgical Community. 2014. Available at: https://www.davincisurgerycommunity.com/systems_i_a#:~:text=Surgeon%20Console,to%20his%20or%20her%20eyes.

[27] Hope C, Reilly JJ, Griffiths G, Lund J, Humes D. The impact of COVID-19 on surgical training: a systematic review. Tech Coloproctol. 2021;25(5):505-520. doi:10.1007/s10151-020-02404-5

[28] Rosen GH, Murray KS, Greene KL, Pruthi RS, Richstone L, Mirza M. Effect of COVID-19 on Urology Residency Training: A Nationwide Survey of Program Directors by the Society of Academic Urologists. J Urol. 2020;204(5):1039-1045. doi: 10.1097/JU.0000000000001155.

[29] Faries MB, Thompson JF, Cochran AJ, Andtbacka RH, Mozzillo N, Zager JS, Jahkola T, Bowles TL, Testori A, Beitsch PD, Hoekstra HJ, Moncrieff M, Ingvar C, Wouters MWJM, Sabel MS, Levine EA, Agnese D, Henderson M, Dummer R, Rossi CR, Neves RI, Trocha SD, Wright F, Byrd DR, Matter M, Hsueh E, MacKenzie-Ross A, Johnson DB, Terheyden P, Berger AC, Huston TL, Wayne JD, Smithers BM, Neuman HB, Schneebaum S, Gershenwald JE, Ariyan CE, Desai DC, Jacobs L, McMasters KM, Gesierich A, Hersey P, Bines SD, Kane JM, Barth RJ, McKinnon G, Farma JM, Schultz E, Vidal-Sicart S, Hoefer RA, Lewis JM, Scheri R, Kelley MC, Nieweg OE, Noyes RD, Hoon DSB, Wang HJ,

Elashoff DA, Elashoff RM. Completion Dissection or Observation for Sentinel-Node Metastasis in Melanoma. N Engl J Med. 2017 Jun 8;376(23):2211-2222. doi: 10.1056/NEJMoa1613210

[30] Giuliano AE, Ballman KV, McCall L, Beitsch PD, Brennan MB, Kelemen PR, Ollila DW, Hansen NM, Whitworth PW, Blumencranz PW, Leitch AM, Saha S, Hunt KK, Morrow M. Effect of Axillary Dissection vs No Axillary Dissection on 10-Year Overall Survival Among Women With Invasive Breast Cancer and Sentinel Node Metastasis: The ACOSOG Z0011 (Alliance) Randomized Clinical Trial. JAMA. 2017 Sep 12;318(10):918-926. doi: 10.1001/jama.2017.11470.

[31] Smith ME, Andraska EA, Sutzko DC, Boniakowski AM, Coleman DM, Osborne NH. The decline of open abdominal aortic aneurysm surgery among individual training programs and vascular surgery trainees. J Vasc Surg. 2020 Apr;71(4):1371-1377. doi: 10.1016/j.jvs.2019.06.204.

[32] Triantafyllos Doulias, Gaetano Gallo, Ines Rubio-Perez, Stephanie O. Breukink & Dieter Hahnloser (2020) Doing More with Less: Surgical Training in the COVID-19 Era, Journal of Investigative Surgery, DOI: 10.1080/08941939.2020.1824250

Chapter 3

Reflections in Medical Education: Empathy, Emotions, and Possible Pedagogical Resources for the Emotional Education of Medical Students

Graziela Moreto, Pablo González Blasco,
Maria Auxiliadora C. De Benedetto
and Marcelo Rozenfeld Levites

Abstract

Outcomes, guidelines, and clinical trials are at the forefront of the current medical training. However, we observe well-trained technological physicians with a reduced humanistic perspective which leads to attitudes that lack ethics and professionalism. There is a growing concern about the human dimension of the future physician and how it can be taught or reinforced in the educational environment allowing to integrate technical science with the humanism. Empathy could bridge the gap between patient-centered medicine and evidence-based medicine. Role modeling and caring carefully for the emotional dimension of medical students are possible resources for preventing the erosion of empathy. Humanities and arts help in building a humanistic perspective of doctoring because they enable doctors to understand patients in their whole context. The inclusion of humanities in the curriculum occasions deep rethinking of what it means to be sick and what it means to take care of the sick.

Keywords: medical humanism, empathy, humanities

1. Introduction

1.1 Technology and humanism: finding a new balance

We live in an era in which outcomes, guidelines and clinical trials are at the forefront of medical training. We observe well-trained technological physicians with a reduced humanistic perspective which leads to attitudes that lack ethics and professionalism. It is necessary to overcome the dichotomy that scientific knowledge is objective, while everything that is subjective - of the subject, of the patient - is second-class information. This statement is not only false, but also an obstacle to alleviating suffering [1].

The vocation of doctors is to care for patients. Nevertheless, the frequent dissatisfaction of patients points more to the human deficiencies of medical professionals than to their technical shortcomings. Complexity comes mostly from patients, not from diseases. While technical knowledge helps in solving disease-based problems, the patient affected by these diseases remains a real challenge for the practicing doctor.

There is a growing concern about the human dimension of the future physician and how it can be taught or reinforced in the educational environment [2]. Medical students - often young people learning to be doctors as they develop as human beings- could have their attention captivated by emerging technology. It is up to educators to be attentive to overcome this challenge and facilitate a balance in student's education, using humanities and culture in general. It is well known that while technical dimension and knowledge grow through training and study, improving attitudes, developing virtues and incorporating values require reflection.

Researchers on this subject [3] comment on the balance that always existed in medicine, between the two inseparable facets that compose it: medicine as science and medicine as an art. The vertiginous scientific advances would require, to maintain that balance, an extension of the scope of humanism, that is, a humanism at the height of scientific progress. And it would be this expansion of humanism, adapted to the current days, in a modern version.

When this humanist update is missing, it falls into a disproportion that is reflected in technically trained professions but with serious human deficiencies. Deformed professionals, with hypertrophy, without balance, who naturally do not conquer the confidence of the patient who expects a balanced doctor. It would be, therefore, a function of the University and the academic institutions, to expand the humanist concept in modern molds, without the aroma of mothballs, knowing how to open horizons and new perspectives. For achieving this goal methodology, systematics, and relearning to do things are required; specially when these things are too many, wrapped in high technology, and commanded by the scientific progress that advances for seconds [4].

The French thinker Gustave Thibon [5] brings together in a volume a set of essays, to which he gives the title "Balance and Harmony." The balance is the composition of opposing forces, compromise solution, resulting from vectors that cancel each other out. Harmony is the perfect fit of the parts into a whole, so that they collaborate for the same purpose. And, quoting Victor Hugo, he comments: "Above balance is harmony, above the balance is the harp".

When we look at the actions that seek to humanization - without achieving it - we realize that the mistake is, perhaps, in seeking balance and not harmony. The balance assumes that the forces are antagonistic, that modern science supported by evidence has to be seasoned with humanitarian attitudes such as, for example, hearing the patient's history with love and feeling compassion. We recognize that this is already enormous progress and an advance on what, unfortunately, we contemplate daily, where the patient is a mere adjuvant that often disturbs the doctor's practicing. But that balance is insufficient, it lacks consistency. They are still two attitudes that do not mix, like water and oil. The clear water of the evidence, and the comforting oil. But each of them with its density and applied each to its time and in its moment. This "medical performance schizophrenia" is unsustainable in itself, it lasts for a short time, and when the doctor gets tired, he will pay attention to one to the detriment of the other.

Medical science, cutting edge medicine, demands a new humanism [6]. A position that knows how to place liver function and neurological sequelae in the same reasoning, with the meaning of life; transaminases and albumin combined with humiliation, suffering and loss. A science that is an art and therefore manages to place in the same equation dimensions so different, that apparently do not mix. In truth, they are completely mixed in life: prothrombin and discouragement, neurotransmitters and tiredness of living, hepatocytes and indignation.

This seems to be the time to invoke the construction of harmony, and know how to play, with different strings to get the perfect chord. Balance is to assume a monotonic composition, or science, or art, a bit of albumin and measured doses of affection. Harmony is to put each competence in its place and have the soul of an artist to know how to play in the harp of life - of that person who is unique - the strings of different shades. These are the chords that allow the doctor to travel the path between the sick person and the meaning that the disease has for the patient, which is a way of being in life. A way of life that has its own language and must find, in the sensitive physician, the receiver necessary to properly decode the meanings. This implies for the doctor to have an attitude of active anthropology: Humanism and anthropology are possibilities of his self-demand, challenges to his rational thought, levels of knowledge in style and ascending aspiration of nonconformity [7].

Humanism is thus a source of knowledge that the doctor uses for his profession [8]. Knowledge is as important as those acquired by other paths that help you in the desire to take care of the human being who is sick. Humanism in medicine is not a temperamental question, an individual taste, not even an interesting complement. All that would lead to place "humanist attitudes" on the scale, to compensate for the excesses of science. Humanism as harmony, as musical virtuosity is, for the doctor, a true work tool, not a cultural appendix. It is a scientific attitude, weighting, the result of a conscious effort of learning and methodology [9, 10].

The doctor's inspiration will often come from the cord of compassion that vibrates easily in a heart willing to help. That will be the note that will give the tonality for the further development of its performance, for the harmonic chords of clinical reasoning. Gregorio Marañón, a humanist doctor and a profound connoisseur of this harmonic symbiosis, warns: "The doctor, whose humanity must always be alert within the scientific spirit, must first count on individual pain; and although he is full of enthusiasm for science, he must be willing to adopt the paradoxical position of defending the individual, whose health is entrusted to him, against his own scientific progress" [11].

In this context, the narratives and life stories, now complete and harmonious - transaminases and distresses, albumin and heartbreak - have their true space and function: to approach the human being who suffers and awaits our care. Once more Marañón gives us a reflection in the perfect chord: "On several occasions I noted to those who work by my side, that a pure diagnostic system, deduced exclusively from analytical data, dehumanized, independent of the direct and endearing observation of the patient, it implies the fundamental error of forgetting the personality, which is so important in the etiologies and to stipulate the prognosis of the patient and teach us doctors what we can do to alleviate their sufferings" [11]. We know well from our own experience how difficult this harmony of action is: how to govern technique and humanism with expertise so we can offer a true symphony of health care [6].

The first step that the doctor must take if he wants to humanize medicine is admitting that he must humanize himself first. And for this, he cannot give up his efforts to reflect, to look for solutions and find resources that allow him to integrate technical science - which grows every second - with the humanism that medical practice requires [12].

Hans Jonas, with his ethics of responsibility [13], points out that what distinguishes human beings from animals is a tripod constituted by the tool, the image and the tumulus. The tool is the technique, and in this there is no doubt that we distinguish ourselves from animals, because when we are born, we quickly incorporate all the techniques accumulated in the history that precedes us. Animals lack a scientific heritage, and each one has to be built from scratch, without taking advantage of the experiences of the ancestors of their species. We can evoke Ortega [14] when he says that the current tiger is the same tiger of thousands of years ago, and that only the human being is born on a history that precedes him, the history that sets together with the technique and the corresponding progress.

The second element that distinguishes us from animals is the image, which includes the ability that mankind has to represent reality through art. Art and humanities are ways to better know the reality in which the human being is immersed and to know himself, in his bodily and spiritual dimension. Finally, the third leg of the tripod is represented by the tumulus. Only the human being has an awareness of transcendence, and the representation of death is what puts him in contact with a dimension that extends beyond his own being.

It is not difficult to conclude that if, as far as technique and progress are concerned, being noticeable the distance between mankind and animals, the other two elements of the tripod have been atrophied; and if not for that reason we necessarily become animalized, there is no doubt that the human equilibrium presents itself with dangerous instability. The man – the doctor, in the case at hand – stops frequenting the arts and humanities and deprives himself of ways of knowing the world; loses the ability to admire and feel that most of the phenomena that surround him are independent of him. And, not least, he loses the sense of transcendence, the spiritual dimension, the sense of eternity and the duration of time around him and his own. The consequences are alarming, because of not frequenting "the tumulus, door of transcendence" it becomes difficult to maintain the sense of mission, and the need to feel useful in this world, as part of the happiness we pursue. This reflection opens the way to the next point: the necessary contingency of the human being, surrounded by suffering and death.

2. Meeting patients' needs through empathy: an educational challenge

Empathy, a Greek word that implies understanding the feelings of another, came to the English language to designate the perception that someone has when contemplating a work of art. Only later, from 1918 onwards, Southard incorporates it into the scenario of the doctor-patient relationship as a tool that facilitates diagnosis and treatment [15]. Empathy has to do with deeply understanding the other and is a path to bridge scientific knowledge with compassion for better caring.

Empathy, one of the most studied humanistic attitudes today, is the cornerstone of ethical and humanized behavior and medical professionalism. Empathy has also been considered an essential element in any humanization strategy [16]. It is a personal quality necessary for understanding the inner experiences and feelings of patients. It represents the essence of the doctor-patient relationship. Developing meaningful interpersonal relationships between patients and physicians is important even for improving clinical outcomes [17].

Before entering the concept of empathy in the context of the patient- physician relationship, it is worth pausing to understand the term from a philosophical point of view. In this field, we cannot fail to cite the work developed by Edith Stein (1891 – 1942), a philosopher who developed his doctoral thesis on empathy. Macintyre [18] in his book on the philosophical action of Edith Stein comments that an essential feature of empathic awareness is the awareness of the feelings of others. The relationship we have with the feelings of others is analogous to the relationship we have with our own past feelings. We may notice what the other is feeling, but we do not have to feel the same as him/her. The same is true when we remember our own feelings - even clearly - does not mean that we will feel the same way we have in the past. A deep understanding, real understanding, but no need to incorporate it. We can fully understand what we feel on one occasion, but we do not have to feel it equally at this time.

It takes caution to state that "I am putting myself in another's shoes." Yes, it is possible to do so, but with our own patterns (our feelings, our reactivity, our understanding of vital reality, our own biographical history) and not his own, so that I cannot truly understand. It is not enough to put ourselves hypothetically in the other's place and continue to be ourselves experiencing this place in which I place myself. One must also be detached from one's own standards to arrive at empathic knowledge. Regarding this perspective, Stein reminds us that empathy is not simply intuition, but an attitude that requires reflection, to turn back and again on ourselves and others, a course that enriches one's own and others' knowledge. It is not a spasm of knowledge, but something worked.

In the context of medical education, the concept of empathy has a broad and varied spectrum. Some authors consider empathy to be a predominantly cognitive quality: it would encompass an understanding of the patient's experiences and concerns combined with communication skills [19]. Irving and Dickson [20] define it as an attitude that contemplates behavioral ability along with the cognitive and affective dimensions.

Most authors place empathy on the affective dimension, giving it the ability to experience the other person's experiences and feelings. In this case, it can be deduced that the ability to be empathic implies a spontaneous feeling of identification with the suffering person, a process in which emotion is involved.

Most of the authors with an affective-oriented approach presuppose that, during the empathic event, there is something that can be characterized as a partial identification of the observer with the observed. This aspect also becomes clear especially in Carl Rogers' definition, which describes empathy as being the ability "to sense the client's private world as if it were your own, but without losing the 'as if' quality". According to this definition, the differentiation between one's own experience and the experience of another is the decisive criterion for defining effective empathy [21].

It is necessary to distinguish empathy from sympathy [22] because this distinction, which is not just semantic, has important consequences in the doctor- patient relationship. The patient's emotions, which must be addressed, cannot become an obstacle to care. On the other hand, a sympathetic doctor may lack objectivity and professionalism. Empathy leads the physician to consider the quality of the patient's emotional experience, while simple solidarity focuses more on the intensity and quantity of suffering. Researchers conclude that empathy does not need limits, while sympathy does need to be moderated [23].

It is not easy to separate the emotional from the cognitive components that make up empathy. Even so, two conclusions can be drawn from this difficult navigation in the definitions and components of empathy. The first is that an excessive preoccupation with oneself (of the subject who intends to act empathically) is an obstacle to helping others [24]. It is necessary to detach from the image itself to understand the other and understand him as "another me". The second conclusion is that empathy could be an element of this necessary bridge to unite evidence-based medicine with patient-centered medicine. A personalization resource with broad diagnostic and therapeutic potential.

The question that arises at this point is whether it is possible to teach empathy, and what would be the teaching-learning process of this attitude [25, 26].

2.1 Teaching the non-teachable issues

It is worth remembering a classic study [27] designed to help choose candidates for medical schools, which emphasizes that those who have the potential to be good doctors, and not simply good students, should be chosen. In this way, 87 characteristics of a good doctor were classified, and classified according to the importance and ease of teaching-developing this characteristic. In this way, what the authors call the NTII was arrived at, an index that combines these two variables.

Thus, important and necessary characteristics for an excellent doctor are pointed out, which are very difficult to teach in medical school, or in further training. At the top of the list -important and difficult to teach characteristics- appear factors related to empathy: understanding of people, concern for others, idealism and compassion, service capacity, ability to persevere in difficulties with resilience, learning to establish priorities in care. All of these factors are important, but very difficult to teach - at least with the resources employed today in medical education.

Some neurophysiological studies provide some clues [28, 29] to resolve the dilemma of how to teach something that is difficult to teach. This is the case of empathy that can be fostered through examples. The so-called mirror neurons in the brain are involved in certain actions related to behavior and emotions. Contemplating another's attitudes, mirror neurons somehow evoke those same attitudes and emotions [30]. It is the simple case of children who, without having a clear perception of their own emotions, end up mirroring the emotions they contemplate in their parents. In this way, the example -of the teacher, the doctor preceptor- is a resource to provoke empathy in the student. Something is known, but now it has a neurophysiological basis [31, 32]. The mechanism of functioning of mirror neurons can be considered a prerequisite for empathy [33].

Several questions arise here: would not "imitated" empathy be something artificial that the patient perceives as such? Wouldn't this attitude end up being summarized in a checklist of routines that a physician must follow to build an empathetic attitude? The student's own experiences -which are even more powerful than a simple example- would be a condition for growing in empathy. In other words: is it necessary for a physician to go through personal and family suffering to be empathetic with the patient's suffering?

The experiences and biographical experiences are an important resource in medical education, when well used. Also, the example that promotes reflection and the construction of attitudes. Thus, establishing an educational setting where examples and experiences have space to be assimilated through reflection and facilitated discussion, seems to be a favorable resource to foster empathy. This model, which is classic -seeing doing, seeing acting, incorporating the example- is what is called Tag Along. A resource that has always been used, and that now, with modern communication tools, runs the risk of falling into oblivion. It must be rescued with a modern perspective. Along with this example-learning model, the experiences can be amplified through the arts. Humanistic education, cultural foundation, is necessary to promote those characteristics difficult to teach by traditional pedagogical methods. Literature, poetry, music, cinema bring resources that evoke experiences in students and allow for reflection [34].

Beside tag-alongs, some authors emphasize the importance of art, literature, cinema and reflecting over one's own life in developing empathy [35]. To give an example, it is worth quoting a literary classic about a rural doctor, (A Fortunate Man) [36] where empathy is magnificently described under the name of recognition: "The task of the doctor is to recognize the man. (..) I am fully aware that I am here using the word recognition to cover whole complicated techniques of psychotherapy, but essentially these techniques are precisely tools for furthering the process of recognition. (..) To treat the illness fully, the doctor must first recognize the patient as a person. Good general diagnosticians are rare, not because most doctors lack medical knowledge, but because most are incapable of taking in all the possible relevant facts – emotional, historical, environmental as well as physical. They are searching for specific conditions instead of the truth about a patient which may then suggest various conditions. (..) A good doctor is acknowledged because he meets the deep but unformulated expectation of the sick for a sense of fraternity. He recognizes them. Sometimes he fails, but there is about him the constant will of a man trying to recognize".

Role modeling, giving the right example to follow, caring carefully for the emotional dimension of medical students and for that using arts and humanities are possible resources for preventing the erosion of empathy. Because, at the end, is not just about to teach how to be empathetic -people that enter in a medical school already have quite a degree of empathy- but, mainly, to prevent of losing empathy through the so-called educational process that in many cases lacks this perspective [37, 38].

While teaching ethics requires establishing rules, guidelines and rational decisions, creativity and recognizing the role that emotions play in decision-making are also required. The educator has, therefore, to go beyond protocols and to have the creativity for bringing together objective guidelines, prudence, and wisdom, as well as incorporating the affective dimension. It is not possible to ignore emotions because they get involved in the decisions that ethical dilemmas imply. Furthermore emotions, when properly handled, become an essential tool. Therefore, opening space to share emotions in an environment with pedagogical support is to pave the way for a true education of affectivity that will transform into better patient care [39, 40].

Fostering reflection is a permanent objective for educators who intend to go beyond the simple transmission of knowledge. Creating favorable environments for joint reflection allows us to get to know the students better, personalize teaching by adapting it to each one, and implement the pedagogical excellence that knows how to unite intellectual creation with the art of teaching. Art is necessary for dealing with the student's unexpected questions. The humanities help to polish this artistic dimension of medical education [41].

3. Why do we need humanities for educating patient-centered doctors?

3.1 Humanities in medical education: from emotions to ethical attitudes

To care implies comprehending the human being and the human condition and for this endeavor, humanities and arts help in building a humanistic perspective of doctoring. Humanities must be included in medical education, not as a simple appendix or a dilettantism, but with the same emphasis as teaching internal medicine, differential diagnosis, or complex case discussions. They are a tool that educates physicians, understanding the patient as a whole -as the person's own unit- to provide the best care for that specific patient [42].

A doctor without humanism would be nothing more than a mechanic of people. To provide effective care, it is essential to incorporate the human dimension into medical practice [43]. This is the role of the humanities that bring the necessary balance to the reductionism related to positive science. Approaching the patient only with "technical objectives" resources will possibly lead to inefficiency in care. Technical progress requires constructing a new, modern, updated medical humanism to provide the necessary balance [44].

When incorporated into medical education, the arts and humanities allow us to approach human emotions, both patient and physician. The humanities make us think about the human being, about illness, about terminality, about transcendence. They lead us to reflect on the attitudes necessary to build professionalism and ethics in medical practice. The wide variety of issues raised with pieces of art, film clips, songs, and music, intuitively help in the decision that involves complex moral choices. As a well-known researcher put it, "the humanities are like the midwife who helps in the birth of human experience, with its mysteries and its certainties". When cinema, poetry, music is used, student's emotions arise easily, and teachers can take advantage of this scenario to broaden perspectives and educate affectivity. The characters that appear in the performing arts, and the values they carry, impact as an example, they are a learning path. Being attentive to the awakening of emotions in students is an expression of affection and love from the teacher, which strengthens learning more than a theoretical model [45].

Typically, students' emotions precede concept construction. Affective intuition precedes emotion. First, the heart gets involved, then the rational process helps to build learning. This is the normal path, in medical education and in life, to assimilate sustainable concepts and values. But this does not mean that teaching should be limited to simple emotions [46]. Students, who are usually immersed in a culture where feelings and visual impact prevail, awaken to learning that, later, will be solidly leveraged, through the necessary reflection. Emotions are thus the gateway to learning processes, a shortcut, a runway for higher educational flights [47].

The arts and humanities, impregnated with narratives, arouse emotions, and prepare the ground for the transmission of concepts. Using students' empathetic language, moving in the familiar terrain of the emotions that the student feels, acts as a facilitator that allows to provoke reflection and suggest attitudes. The teacher's role is that of a catalyst for the process that takes the student from emotions, through reflection, to incorporate attitudes and values.

The teacher's role is to identify emotions and then stimulate reflection. Based on this experience of reflected emotion, it is possible to generate attitudes that modulate behavior [48]. Through an environment that allows for reflection, the development of qualities that will enrich personal development becomes possible.

On the other hand, teachers also use emotions - although little time and space are left to discuss them. When this reflective environment is provided among teachers -a faculty development scenario-, joint reflection leads to improving teaching methods and understanding with the students themselves [49]. Teacher meetings are often monopolized by addressing problems, and problematic students. Little time remains to reflect and help each other, and thus build resources for better teaching performance. Here, too, the medical humanities are an effective resource. After all, any process that aims to humanize medical education must include reflection at all levels, both among professors and students, in addition to facilitating the environment and making time for this reflection to be regular and fruitful [50].

3.2 Narrative medicine: reloading a millenary resource for caring

A predominantly biomedical focus attributed to teaching and practice in health sciences contributes to a dehumanization process. Any strategy that intends to address the issue depends on the presence of well-educated health professionals from both the technical and humanistic points of view. The greatest deficits concern humanistic education. Research about the effectiveness of using narratives as a didactic resource in humanistic education points out issues related to the concealed curriculum and the importance of medical students' exposure to a patient-centered teaching model that gives priority to ethical reflections [51].

It is true that narratives are an important educational topic in the context of Medicine. Narrations, life stories, allow us to contemplate the patient's world, meet him as a person, so that we can take care of him in a competent manner. There is also a tendency to think that the narrations are just a complement to positive science, which is not possible to measure with laboratory results. Thus, it would be just a methodology that broadens a way of aiming to reach out to the person, and focus on her care, without deterring the illness that affects her. That perspective takes the risk of being "complementary", that is, the soft edge of what really matters. The dissociation between science and art remains, as two forces that act synergistically, but in parallel, and therefore never found themselves. The medical action that would fall would be condemned to these complementary positions, in which competency and compassion never meet.

Medicine as Art recognizes that each patient is unique. Not only from the perspective of the disease that attacks him/her, but in the way that pathology "becomes incarnate and concretized": this is an illness, being sick [52]. The disease is always personalized, installed in someone who will become sick "in their own way", according to their personal being. A bifocal perspective is necessary, which manages to unite in artistic symbiosis the attention to the disease - with all the technical evolution - and to the patient who feels sick – with the vital understanding that entails. This is a person-centered medical performance, simultaneous exercise of science and art [53].

Listening carefully is a skill that the doctor needs to heal [54]. This requires the rescue of the ancient resources of medical art [55]. Patients show subtle clues about their experience with the condition, but doctors often ignore them because we hear only "the voice of medicine" and have trained us to ignore the emotional side, that is, the "voice of the patient's life." [56].

Already in the middle of the twentieth century, Gregorio Marañón [11]– paradigm of art and science – warned of the danger of using purely technical tools without knowing the patient, without listening carefully, without really caring about him: "It must be admitted that ordinary medicine is usually reduced, or to problems that are easy to solve, or completely insoluble for the most gifted man of wisdom. The fundamental thing in any case is that the doctor be with his five senses in what he is, and not thinking about other things." When the doctor sits and listens to the patient, he is communicating a humanistic attitude for excellence. Today we have sophisticated technology - important - but we are losing the pleasure of sitting down and hearing narratives of life. We lack chairs or, perhaps, patience to sit and listen.

A well-known researcher in medical humanities quotes: "we are midwifing a medicine that makes contact with the mysteries of human experience along with its certainties—a medicine that appreciates the deep beauty of health, the silence of health, the wisdom of the body, and the grace of its genius. It is an arch to far times and places, a site for all the living and the dying that go on; it is a link to what it means to be human" [57].

Teaching through humanities includes several modalities in which art is involved [58]. Literature and theater [59], poetry [60], opera [61] are all useful tools when the goal is to promote learner reflection and construct what has been called the professional philosophic exercise [62]. Teaching with movies is also an innovative method for promoting the sort of engaged learning that education requires today [63, 64]. For dealing with emotions and attitudes, while promoting reflection, life stories derived from movies fit well with the learners' context and expectations. Teaching with films engages the emotions and could serve as a great launching point for discussions of both the emotions and ethical scenarios [65–67]. The crucial role of teaching is to help frame these discussions in such a way as to foster reflective practice among clinicians and clinicians-in-training.

4. Teaching with movies to foster reflective practice

A film is the favored medium in our current culture, teaching with cinema is particularly well-suited to the learning environment of medical education. Cinema is the audiovisual version of the narrative, framed in emotions and images. A reality very close to the language of the student who is inserted in this emotional and visual culture and which makes it easier for him to enter the world of his interlocutor: the patient, with all the circumstances that surround him.

We know of the pedagogical power of narratives, something secular that comes from classical Greece, where stories were resources to teach ethics and values [68]. Cinema, illustrating stories in a modern way, helps to expand life experiences, to get to know the human being. On the other hand, film stories act as a catharsis of emotions - something that Aristotle already warned with stories in Greek education. Emotions are revealed, brought out, and capable of being sorted, educated, through reflection. This is the core of the use of cinema in the education of affectivity.

Cinema provides a fast and straightforward teaching setting [69]. The scenes suggest important issues, emotions appear, students can better understand the universe of affection, which is often tumultuous. It is common for them to transport the projected scene to their own reality, to their own lives, because they act as an emotional wake-up call that evokes daily realities, not only from the medical learning environment, but from life itself. And in the same way, the experiences they have in the pedagogical environment with cinema are then taken to their daily lives, as a resource that helps to remember all that learning. Cinema, therefore, works as an emotional alarm that facilitates the student's posture in analogous situations they face in their daily lives.

For teaching ethics, we can follow the rational method, approaching the theoretical basis to refine attitudes, acquire virtues and incorporate values. But this classic method of medical deontology classes finds an alternative path when using films. In cinema, the examples are accompanied by a strong emotional charge, leading the viewer to accept or reject that attitude presented. Reflection also accompanies this experience; and from reflection comes the desire to incorporate an attitude, not just intellectually, but beginning from emotions as a starting point. When individual reflections are amplified by facilitated discussion, the motivations, and incentives in the construction of ethics also grow in the group of students.

This learning scenario stimulates learner reflection. In life, important attitudes, values, and actions are taught using role modeling, a process that impacts the learner's emotions. Since feelings exist before concepts, the affective path is a critical shortcut to the rational process of learning. While technical knowledge and skills can be acquired through training with a little reflection, reflection is required to refine attitudes and incorporate values. As already explained, this methodology with the cinema does not intend only to provide "sentimental, emotional education", but to provoke reflection that leads to incorporating attitudes. Reflection is, without a doubt, the bridge that allows the transition from emotions to attitudes. This universe is not limited to the solution of purely medical issues, but it reaches out to life, awakens desires for integrity. Education with cinema does not intend to offer results - something like the moral of the fable, to show the right way to behave - but rather to provoke the reflection that leads to lasting attitudes [70]. To foster reflection is the main goal in this cinematic teaching set. The purpose is not to show the audience how to incorporate a particular attitude, but rather to promote their reflection and to provide a forum for discussion. And this works for any kind of audience, despite cultural background or language [71].

This is possible when reflection and discussion are allowed in the pedagogical environment where cinema is instituted. Doubts and dilemmas often emerge about the professional role, ethical attitudes, reporting of good examples – and some that are not edifying- for which the student usually does not have space in the curriculum. It is precisely this attitude, thinking and reflecting relentlessly, and not giving in to mediocrity, that Hannah Arendt suggested as prevention so as not to fall into the banality of evil [72].

Film education is also useful for continuing training with doctors, so that they learn to deal with their own emotions. Little attention is paid -both in the undergraduate and graduate curriculum space- to the education of emotions. When emotions -especially negative ones- are not ventilated and dealt with, the most common is to assume an attitude of emotional closure with the patient, a distance that leads to a lack of competence in care and destroys professionalism [73].

Cinema offers a wide range of possibilities for learning to deal with negative attitudes and values. Without necessarily solving dilemmas, it offers the opportunity to reflect calmly, with emotional detachment. The film allows us to go beyond illustrations of theories and principles so that we can develop a range of emotional and interpretive skills, including habits of the heart. Discussions among colleagues are exciting and enriching that make us reflect on who we are and who we want to be [74].

In this sense, film, like art, can affect the root of our being. Using film clips in a structured way allows for new opportunities in ethics education. Here comes the specific methodology using movie clips.

4.1 The movie clip methodology: using wisely short time teaching

Which movies are useful for teaching this or that point? This is a common question people ask. The answer could be something like this: "What you get out of a film often depends upon what you bring to it". Useful movies for teaching whatever you want, are those that are valuable to you, those that touched you and lead you to reflect. I can share what movies touched me and why, but I am not able to say what will impress you and be part of your life. When a movie seems remarkable for the educator, we always find a way to incorporate our teaching set. So, you need to build your own experience before sharing it with your audience. Keep in mind what you want to teach, the specific ethical dilemma.

Although, in education with cinema some use medical films-as a case discussion- it is not the usual pedagogical resource that we are discussing here [75], Our goal is to go beyond the medical scene to immerse into the human reality, where attitudes, emotions and responses emerge. Therefore, it is not medical-themed films that we have used the most in our pedagogical scenario. However, the "translation" of human problems to the medical environment is done with enormous facilities by students.

Do you use a whole movie or just some scenes? Here comes another usual question. The answer depends on what you want to point out, the time you have at your disposal, and the outcomes you expect. Our experience affirms the effectiveness of using the movie-clip methodology in which multiple movie clips are shown in rapid sequence, along with facilitator comments while the clips were going on [76]. Using clips with scenes from different movies is, in our experience, more profitable than projecting entire movies. Besides, the time available is not always a lot. With a few minutes, it is possible to raise many questions, all saturated with emotions, when the clips are used with agility. The facilitator's comments enhance the reflection, amplifying it. They are not an obstacle to following the scenes presented, but, in our experience, they function as a resource that facilitates shifting the reflection from the clip's report to life itself. As someone in the audience once commented: "the comments are not about the film, nor about the teacher's experience… It's something that goes in between and touches our lives".

The comments are not sought for student agreement, but only intended to provoke individual reflection. In essence, the facilitator's comments are their own reflections made aloud.

The most used resource in our experience are scenes from different films, with varied themes, which when presented together provoke a real flood of emotions. They are not projected according to a thematic background, but varied, showing a wide spectrum of attitudes. The joint reflection and discussion about this collection of scenes are what causes the real learning. Several previous publications have covered the methodology in detail, and the appendix of many of them contains a list of films, with suggested scenes to be used and comments [77].

Proving the effectiveness of this methodology is something that often arises in the academic community, especially in international congresses and various presentations. It should be remembered that excellent education does not imply measuring -with the usual metrics- all pedagogical tools. It is known that many of the so-called "intangible themes" are difficult to assess, although it is possible to see the results. Thus, themes such as empathy, ethics, compassion, and commitment -which are factors of professionalism- can be pointed out and promoted with the resource of education with cinema. Without a doubt, esthetic education -this is the core of the humanities- necessarily completes the education of physicians. They are, in Pascal's words, "the reasons of the heart, which reason is not capable of understanding".

In cinema education, the educational outcomes do not materialize simply from watching movies. People attend cinema all the time and see the same scenes, and while they might have similar emotions, the reflective process is lacking. This is where the competence and the teaching skills of the facilitator come into play, that is by putting all the scenes together and fostering reflection through comments and personal thoughts, even as unanswered open questions are introduced. That is the teacher's role.

There is still a remaining question. Does this movie teaching methodology depend on the charisma of the presenter or can it be well developed by anyone? There is no definitive answer. All we can say is: if you love movies, if you like to teach deep from your heart you deserve to try this. Try it and wait for the surprises!

Author details

Graziela Moreto*, Pablo González Blasco, Maria Auxiliadora C. De Benedetto and Marcelo Rozenfeld Levites
SOBRAMFA - Medical Education and Humanism, São Paulo, Brazil

*Address all correspondence to: graziela@sobramfa.com.br

References

[1] Cassell EJ. Diagnosing suffering: a perspective. Ann.Int. Med. 1999;**131**:531-534

[2] Moyer C, Arnold L, Quaintance J, Braddock C, Spickard A, Wilson D, et al. What Factors Create a Humanistic Doctor? A Nationwide Survey of Fourth-Year Medical Students. Academic Medicine. 2010;**85**:1800-1807

[3] Robb D. Ciência, Humanismo e Medicina. Rasegna. 1985;**3**:21-32

[4] Blasco PG, Benedetto MAC, Reginato V. Humanismo em Medicina. Vol. 100. São Paulo: SOBRAMFA-Educação Médica e Humanismo; 2015. p. 437

[5] Thibon G. El equilibrio y la armonía. Belacqua: Barcelona; 2005

[6] Blasco PG, Janaudis MA, Levites MR. Un nuevo humanismo médico: la armonía de los cuidados. Atención Primaria. 2006;**38**(4):225-229

[7] Monasterio F. Planteamiento del Humanismo Médico. Humanismo y Medicina. Murcia: II Encuentro Cultural de la Sociedad Española de Médicos Escritores; 1982

[8] Correa FJL, Blasco PG. (organz). La Humanización de la Salud y el Humanismo Médico en Latinoamérica. Santiago de Chile: FELAIBE, SOBRAMFA y Facultad de Ciencias de la Salud de la Universidad Central de Chile; 2018. p. 253

[9] Roncoletta AFT, Moreto G, Levites MR, Janaudis MA, Blasco PG, Leoto RF. Princípios da Medicina de Família. São Paulo: Sobramfa; 2003

[10] Blasco PG. De los principios científicos para la acción: el idealismo práctico de la Medicina de Familia. Atencion Primaria. 2004;**34**(6):313-317

[11] Marañón G. La medicina y nuestro tiempo. Madrid: Espasa; 1954

[12] Levites MR, Blasco PG. Competencia y Humanismo: La Medicina Familiar en Busca de la Excelencia. Archivos de Medicina Familiar y General. 2009;**6**:2-9

[13] Jonas H. El Principio de Responsabilidad: ensayo de una ética para la civilización tecnológica. Barcelona: Herder; 1995

[14] Ortega y Gasset J. La rebelión de las masas. Madrid: Revista de Occidente; 1930. pp. 38-39

[15] Hojat M. Empathy in Patient Care. In: Antecedents, Development, Measurement, and Outcomes. New York: Springer; 2007

[16] Costa SC, Figueiredo MRB, Schaurich D. Humanization within adult intensive care units (ICUs): Comprehension among the nursing team. Interface (Botucatu). 2009;**13**(1):571-580

[17] Hojat M, Gonnella JS, Mangione S, Nasca TJ, Veloski JJ, Erdmann JB, et al. Empathy in medical students as related to academic performance, clinical competence and gender. Medical Education. 2002;**36**:522-527

[18] Mac IA, Stein E. Un prólogo filosófico. Ed Nuevo Inicio: Granada; 2008

[19] Hojat M, Vergare MJ, Maxwell K, Brainard G, Herrine SK, Isenberg GA, et al. The Devil is in the Third Year: A Longitudinal Study of Erosion of Empathy in Medical School. Academic Medicine. 2009;**84**:1182-1191

[20] Irving P, Dickson D. Empathy: Towards a conceptual framework for health professionals. International Journal of Health Care Quality Assurance Incorporating Leadership in Health Services. 2004;**17**:212-220

[21] Neumann M, Bensing J, Mercer J, Ernstmann N, Ommen O, Pfaff H. Analyzing the "nature" and "specific effectiveness" of clinical empathy: A theoretical overview and contribution towards a theory-based research agenda. Patient Education and Counseling. 2009;**74**:339-346

[22] Stephan WG, Finlay KA. The role of empathy in improving inter-group relations. Journal of Social Issues. 1999;**55**:729-743

[23] Hojat M, Gonnella JS, Nasca TJ, Mangione S, Vergare M, Magee M. Physician empathy: Definition, components, measurement, and relationship to gender and specialty. The American Journal of Psychiatry. 2002;**159**:1563-1569

[24] Aderman D, Berkowitz L. Self-concern and the unwillingness to be helpful. Social Psychology Quarterly. 1983;**46**:293-301

[25] Bayne HB. Training medical students in empathic communication. J Spec Group Work. 2011;**36**:316-329

[26] Moreto G, González-Blasco P, De Benedetto MAC. Reflexiones sobre la enseñanza de la empatía y la educación médica. Aten Fam. 2014;**21**(3):94-97

[27] Sade R, Stroud M, Levine J, Fleming G. Criteria for Selection of Future Physicians. Annals of Surgery. 1985;**201**:225-230

[28] Decety J, Jackson P. A social-neurosience perspective on empathy. Current Directions in Psychological Science. 2006;**15**:54-58

[29] Gallese V. The roots of empathy: the shared manifold hypothesis and the neural basis of intersubjectivity. Psychopathology. 2003;**36**:17180

[30] Rizzolatti G, Sinigaglia C. So quell che fai: il cervello che agisce e I neuroni specchio. R Cortina Ed.: Milano; 2006

[31] Decety J, Jackson P. The functional architecture of human empathy. Behavioral and Cognitive Neuroscience Reviews. 2004;**3**:71-100

[32] Wicker B, Keysers C, Plailly J, Royet JP, Gallese V, Rizzolatti G. Both of us are disgusted in my insula: The common neural basis of seeing and seeking disgust. Neuron. 2003;**40**: 644-655

[33] Bauer J. Warum ich fühle, was Du fühlst. Intuitive Kommunikation und das Geheimnis der Spiegelneurone (Why I feel what you feel. Intuitive communication and the mystery of the mirror neurons). Hoffmann und Campe: Hamburg; 2005

[34] Blasco PG, Roncoletta AFT, Moreto G, Levites MR, Janaudis MA. Accompanying physicians in their family practice: A primary care model for medical students' Learning in Brazil. Family Medicine. 2006;**38**(9):619-621

[35] Larson EB, Yao X. Clinical empathy as emotional labor in patient-physician relationship. Journal of the American Medical Association. 2005;**293**(9): 1100-1106

[36] Berger J, Mohr J. A Fortunate Man. In: The story of a country doctor. New York: Vintage; 1997

[37] Moreto G, Santos I, Blasco PG, Pessini L, Lotufo PA. Assessing empathy among medical students: A comparative analysis using two different scales in a Brazilian medical school. Educación Médica (Ed. impresa). 2018;**19**:162-170

[38] Moreto G. Avaliação da empatia de estudantes de medicina em uma universidade na cidade de São Paulo utilizando dois instrumentos (thesis). Biblioteca Digital USP. Teses e dissertações; 2015. Available from: http://www.teses.usp.br/teses/disponiveis/5/5169/tde-19062015-154448/pt-br.php

[39] Christianson CE, McBride RB, Vari RC, Olson L, Wilson HD. From traditional to patient-centered learning: Curriculum change as an intervention for changing institutional culture and promoting professionalism in undergraduate medical education. Academic Medicine. 2007;**82**:1079-1088

[40] Marcus ER. Empathy, humanism, and the professionalism of medical education. Academic Medicine. 1999;**74**:1211-1215

[41] Bain K. What the Best College Teachers Do. Cambridge, MA: Harvard University Press; 2004

[42] Mullangi S. The synergy of medicine and art in the curriculum. Academic Medicine. 2013;**88**:921-923

[43] Blay PC. Como evaluar el desarrollo profesional continúo. Evaluación de la competencia: métodos y reflexiones. Jano. 2006;**V. Extra**:36-42

[44] Belling C. Sharper Instruments: On Defending the Humanities in Undergraduate Medical Education. Academic Medicine. 2010;**85**:938-940

[45] Pulchrum R-RA. Reflexiones Sobre La Belleza. Madrid: Rialp; 1999

[46] Ferres J. Educar en una cultura del espectáculo. Paidós: Barcelona; 2000

[47] Blasco PG, Alexander M. Ethics and human values. In: Alexander M, Lenahan P, Pavlov A, editors. Cinemeducation: A Comprehensive Guide to Using Film in Medical Education. Oxford, UK: Radcliffe Publishing; 2005. pp. 141-145

[48] Blasco PG, Moreto G, Janaudis MA, Benedetto MAC, Altisent R, Delgado-Marroquin MT. Educar las emociones para promover la formación ética. Persona y Bioética. 2013;**17**:28-48

[49] Palmer PJ. The Courage to Teach. San Francisco: Jossey-Bass; 1998

[50] Blasco PG, Moreto G, González-Blasco M, Levites MR, Janaudis MA. 2015. Education through movies: Improving teaching skills and fostering reflection among students and teachers. 2015;**11**:145-160

[51] De Benedetto MAC. O Papel das Narrativas como Recurso Didático na Formação Humanística dos Estudantes de Medicina e Enfermagem (thesis). São Paulo: Universidade Federal de São Paulo (UNIFESP); 2017. Available from: http://repositorio.unifesp.br/handle/11600/41856;jsessionid=98F4DC608499AB2DF69BE2A2364A7BB9

[52] Kleinman A, Eisenberg L, Good B. Culture, Illness, and Care. Clinical Lessons from Anthropologic and Cross-Cultural Research. Ann Int Med. 1978;**88**:251-258

[53] Roncoletta AFT, Moreto G, Levites MR, Janaudis MA, Blasco PG, Leoto RF. Princípios da Medicina de Família. Sobramfa: São Paulo; 2003

[54] Greenhalgh T. Narrative based-medicine: Why study narrative? BMJ. 1999;**318**:48-50

[55] Greenhalgh T. Narrative based-medicine in an evidence-based world. BMJ. 1999;**318**:323-325

[56] Brown. The first component: exploring both the disease and the illness experience. In: Stewart M, Brown JB, Weston WW, Mc Wninney R, Mc William CL, Freeman TR, editors. Pacient-centered medicine. Transforming the Clinical Method. 2ª ed. Abingdon U.K: Radcliffe Med Press; 2003. pp. 3-52

[57] Charon R. Calculating the Contributions of Humanities to Medical Practice Motives, Methods and Metrics. Academic Medicine. 2010;**85**:935-937

[58] Ousager J, Johannessen H. Humanities in Undergraduate Medical

Education: A Literature Review. Academic Medicine. 2010;**85**:988-998

[59] Shapiro J. Literature and the arts in medical education. Family Medicine. 2000;**32**(3):157-158

[60] Whitman N. A poet confronts his own mortality: What a poet can teach medical students and teachers. Family Medicine. 2000;**32**(10):673-674

[61] Blasco PG, Moreto G, Levites MR. Teaching humanities through opera: Leading medical students to reflective attitudes. Family Medicine. 2005;**37**(1): 18-20

[62] Decourt LV. William Osler- a Intimidade de seu Pensamento in A Didática Humanista do Professor. Ed. Atheneu, São Paulo; 2005. pp. 135-141

[63] Baños JE, Bosch F. Using feature films as a teaching tool in medical schools El empleo de películas comerciales en las facultades de medicina. Educación Médica. 2015;**16**(4):206-211

[64] Self DJ, Baldwin DC. Teaching medical humanities through film discussions. The Journal of Medical Humanities. 1990;**11**(1):23-29

[65] Colt H, Quadrelli S, Friedman L. The Picture of Health: Medical Ethics and the Movies. New York: Oxford University Press; 2011

[66] Self DJ, Baldwin DC, Olivarez M. Teaching medical ethics to first-year students by using film discussion to develop their moral reasoning. Academic Medicine. 1993;**68**(5): 383-385

[67] Searight HR, Allmayer S. The use of feature film to teach medical ethics: overview and assessment. International Journal of Modern Education Forum (IJMEF). 2014;**3**(1):1-6

[68] McIntyre AC. After Virtue. A Study in Moral Theory. Notre Dame: Notre Dame Press; 1984

[69] Blasco PG. Humanizando a Medicina: Uma Metodologia com o Cinema. São Paulo: Centro Universitário São Camilo; 2011

[70] Blasco PG, Benedetto MAC, Garcia DSO, Moreto G, Roncoletta AFT, Troll T. Cinema for educating global doctors: From emotions to reflection, approaching the complexity of the Human Being. Primary Care. 2010;**10**:45-47

[71] Blasco PG, Mônaco CF, Benedetto MAC, Moreto G, Levites MR. Teaching through movies in a multicultural scenario: overcoming cultural barriers through emotions and reflection. Family Medicine. 2010;**42**(1): 22-24

[72] Blasco PG. Commentary on Hannah Arendt. Academic Medicine. 2016;**91**:675

[73] Shapiro J. Does medical education promote professional alexithymia? A call for attending to the emotions of patients and self in medical training. Academic Medicine. 2011;**86**:326-332

[74] Blasco PG. Review of Henri Colt, Silvia Quadrelli, and Lester Friedman (eds), The Picture of Health: Medical Ethics and the Movies: Getting Familiar with the Cinema Education Methodology. American Journal of Bioethics. 2011;**11**:9-41

[75] Blasco PG. Medical Education, Family Medicine and Humanism: Medical students' expectations, dilemmas and motivations analyzed through discussion of movies (thesis). São Paulo: University of São Paulo Medical School; 2002. Available from: http://www.teses.usp.br/teses/disponiveis/5/5144/tde-31082009-085309/pt-br.php

[76] Blasco PG, Moreto G, Roncoletta AFT, Levites MR, Janaudis MA. Using movie clips to foster learners´ reflection: Improving Education in the Affective Domain. Family Medicine. 2006;**38**(2):94-96

[77] Available from: https://sobramfa.com.br/eng/articles/movies-in-medicaleducation/

Chapter 4

Role of Mentors in Undergraduate and Postgraduate Training

Anant Khot

Abstract

A career in academic medicine may take years to develop, as the skills it requires are often not taught at an early stage. Having a committed mentor is always a privilege and valuable to the students in medicine. Given the wide variety of mentoring relationships, they are broadly classified as formal and informal according to the way in which the relationship is formed. Mentoring relationships usually evolve in stages to ensure competencies are met before the mentees progress to the next part of their mentoring process. "Mentoring up" is a concept that empowers mentees to be active participants in their mentoring relationships. Also, the mentoring needs vary depending on the stage of professional development. Mentors have 7 roles to perform in this relationship. Despite the advantages, the mentoring process faces the challenges like unrealistic expectations from the mentees, lack of training and time constraint among the clinician educators, and so on. The challenges can be overcome by building structured mentorship programs, by organizing the faculty development programs, use of virtual platforms to facilitate the meeting and providing the academic recognition/financial incentives to the mentors providing the exemplary service.

Keywords: mentoring, medical education, respect, communication, technology, social media

1. Introduction

Mentorship is being defined as "a dynamic, reciprocal relationship in a work environment between an advanced career incumbent (mentor) and a beginner (protégé), aimed at the development of both" [1]. The first use of the term mentor was in the eighth century BC when Homer wrote his legend of the Trojan War. Odysseus, the King of Ithaca, left his infant son, Telemachus, and his wife, Penelope, under the care of his teacher, mentor. He was responsible not only for educating his son but also for helping to develop his character and for providing him with the knowledge with which he could build his wisdom and decisions [2]. Therefore, the word "mentor" came from mentor's name. In the present day, or a noun defined as: "An experienced and trusted adviser" [3]. As per the Standing Committee on Postgraduate Medical Education (SCOPME) in the United Kingdom, mentoring is a process whereby an experienced, highly regarded, empathic person, guides another individual in the development and helps in re-examining their ideas, learning, and personal and professional development [4].

A career in academic medicine may take years to develop, as the skills it requires are often not taught at an early stage [5]. Having a committed mentor is always a privilege and valuable to students in health care professional education [6]. Mutual trust, faith and respect while working towards a shared vision/goal is the main driving force of a mentoring relationship. According to the Vygotsky sociocultural theory, effective learning happens through interactive processes of discussion, negotiation and sharing [7]. Mentors not only promote mentees' academic development, performance, satisfaction, and success, but they also can help them cope with the conflicting demands of career development and private life [8]. In today's complex academic environments, a successful faculty career requires mentoring in multiple domains.

Mentoring relationships evolve in stages to ensure particular competencies are met before mentees progress to the next part of their mentoring process. There are four phases of mentorship:

1. **Phase I (preparatory phase)**: Here, mentees define their short-and long-term development objectives, evaluate their capabilities and understand their aspirations. With a goal in their mind, ideally, a mentee should select a mentor. But mostly, the mentor is allotted by the institution.

2. **Phase II (negotiating phase)**: Here, there is rapport building between the mentee and the mentor. At this stage, both the mentee and the mentor are uncertain about the future, but their attitude is usually upbeat. The mentor must explore the value base of the mentee and their goals in life to make this relation effective.

3. **Phase III (enabling growth/contracting phase)**: A formal structure is given to discuss the expected outcomes of this relationship. They will also define areas to be left out of such discussions. The most important part is building mutual trust and ensuring confidentiality. Mentee-mentor duo may also develop a checklist to document their progress and to get reassurance whether they are moving on the desired path for mutual benefit or not.

4. **Phase IV (coming to closure)**: The mentor-mentee duo assesses the value of partnership, identify areas of growth and learning and celebrate the achievement of learning outcomes [4].

2. Types of mentorships

Formal and informal.

Informal mentoring refers to the self-selection of mentors and mentees, particularly noting that the mentee typically initiates it.

Formal mentoring is a relationship in which a designated mentor and mentee are assigned to one another as part of an organizationally supported program [9].

3. Form of mentorship

a. **Dyadic mentoring**: A traditional mentoring model with a one-to-one relationship between mentor and mentee has influenced mentorship progress. It is relatively disadvantageous to some women because it emphasizes the challenge, competition and independence and highlights technical and informational conversation over psychosocial issues [10].

b. **Multiple mentoring**: Here, the mentee is mentored by several mentors simultaneously, noting that each mentor facilitates the development of a particular area. It provides an opportunity to have mentors who are in line with values and behaviors typically associated with females but also behaviors typically associated with males—equalizing or hierarchical relationships, collaboration and independence, encouragement and challenge.

c. **Mutual mentoring** is a specific type of multiple mentoring in which mentoring partnerships can be developed with a variety of individuals, including peers, near-peers, senior faculty, administrators, students and librarians [11].

d. **Apprenticeship**: It is when the mentee observes and emulates the skills of the mentor. In the apprenticeship model, the student initially becomes familiar with common medical problems, legitimately participates peripherally, performs under supervision and finally perform independently.

e. **Team mentoring**: Standardizes the concept of several mentors into a formal committee, just as in multiple mentoring.

4. Mentoring models

- **Classic model**: Formal approach, well planned with a specific setting, one-on-one mentoring and a more experienced mentor and less experienced mentee from the same field.

- **Shadowing**: Not a proper form of mentoring; it is based on the observation of skilled professionals.

- **Trans model**: Mentor works outside of the mentee's area of focus: for example, clinical research paired with a basic scientist. Fosters multidisciplinary and multi-departmental collaborations.

- **Networking model**: Less intense than traditional styles; less dependence on an individual mentor. It offers a broader range of perspectives.

- **Reverse mentoring**: Both the parties act in the capacity of mentor and mentee. The process recognizes that there are skills gaps and opportunities to learn on both sides of a mentoring relationship. Flipping the traditional format on its head can be very beneficial for both parties. It brings different employee generations closer together.

- **Group mentoring**: This style of mentoring involves one mentor working with several mentees in a group. Suitable in organizations with a lack of senior leaders. Delivery is either virtual or face to face and possess the advantage of rotating between mentors.

- **Spot (situational) mentoring**: It is a more casual approach, specific and focused. Seek out a senior leader as mentor and have one-off mentoring 'spot' meetings.

- **Peer mentoring**: It is collaborative and mutually beneficial as the relationship is formed among the mentors' peers or colleagues. Here mentees are inclined towards sharing their difficulties and questions with peers who are at an equal or similar level of knowledge and seniority [12].

- **Speed mentoring**: It allows groups of mentors and mentees to meet for a focused period with no expectation for ongoing mentoring follow-up [13].

- **Virtual mentoring**: It refers to digital platforms that facilitate communication between a mentee and a mentor, including emails, social media, short message service (SMS), app-mediated connections and computer platforms.

- It carries a few potential risks, which include miscommunication, slower development of the mentoring relationship, trust and confidence [14].

5. Changes in the culture of mentoring

Apprenticeship approach	Reflective-explorative approach
Instruction/instructor	Coaching/facilitator/partner
Hierarchy	Collaboration/mutual partnership
Individualistic focus ("I and my class")/ teaching development	Systemic focus ("I and my school")/school development
A classical form of mentoring (mentor-mentee)	Variety of forms (peer/team/e-mentoring, etc.)
Mentoring before or after student-teaching sessions/classes	Mentoring during student-teaching sessions/classes (co-planning/co-teaching)
Face-to-face mentoring	Professional learning communities
Modeling (learning by role model)	Dialogical learning

"Mentoring up" is a concept that empowers mentees to be active participants in their mentoring relationships by shifting the emphasis from the mentors' responsibilities in the mentor-mentee relationship to equal emphasis on the mentees' contributions.

Mentoring is usually accomplished through its sub role functions of "teaching, socializing, providing opportunity, sponsoring, coaching, guiding, protecting, advising and counselling, encouraging, inspiring, challenging, role modelling, supporting, and befriending" [15, 16].

6. 7 Roles of mentor

Teacher: Qualified doctors act as mentors by facilitating clinical skills sessions, bedside teaching and simulation. Mentoring can increase confidence and self-perceived preparedness for starting an independent practice as a doctor and reduce the performance gap. Also, positive mentoring can have a significant influence on speciality choices. The mentor knows well that education is not just the imparting of facts. Instead, the ultimate goal of education is to form character and attributes relevant to medicine.

Sponsor: Mentor introduces the fellow to a new social world.

Advisor: Mentor supplies the missing experience—as they have been there and successfully doing that. The fellow (mentee) does not need someone to pave the road but needs help in becoming a better navigator. The mentor helps the fellow to craft their solution—to become self-reliant.

Agent: The mentor removes obstacles, but only after the fellow has made a convincing attempt, and the mentor is careful to avoid spoon-feeding.

Role model: Values are best transmitted through deeds, not words—a how, not a what and role models are so important in medicine so that they are emulated by the mentees/students.

Coach: A professional coach motivates the players to win. The primary aim is to nurture a development-supporting professional self-understanding, looking at mentees as unique individuals and mentor as a coach raises the bar and sets high standards.

Confidante: A person with whom one shares a secret or private matter, trusting them not to repeat it to others. The mentor earns the fellow's trust through constancy, reliability, integrity and congruity [17].

7. Styles of mentoring

'Letting go' style: Mentor gets into the conversation by giving time to let things develop.

'Active listening' style: Mentor gets into the conversation by asking questions when things are unclear.

'Advisory' style: The mentor gets into the conversation by giving suggestions for good problem-solving.

'Prescribing' style: The mentor takes responsibility for solving the mentee's problems.

'Cooperative' style: Getting into the conversation by striving for a joint vision [18].

A truly great mentor has the dexterity to switch between the different styles when appropriate [19].

8. Role of mentee

The driver of relationship: He identifies the skills, knowledge and/or goals they want to achieve and communicates them to their mentor.

Development planner: Mentee works with his/her mentor on deficiencies and seeks resources for learning by identifying people and information.

Contributor: He looks for opportunities to give back to their mentor.

Life-long learner: The standards of the Liaison Committee on Medical Education (LCME) require the educational program must include instructional opportunities for active learning and independent study to foster the skills necessary for lifelong learning. By enrolling in the mentoring program, the mentee will gain the traits of life-long learner [20].

9. Mentoring needs at different stages of professional development

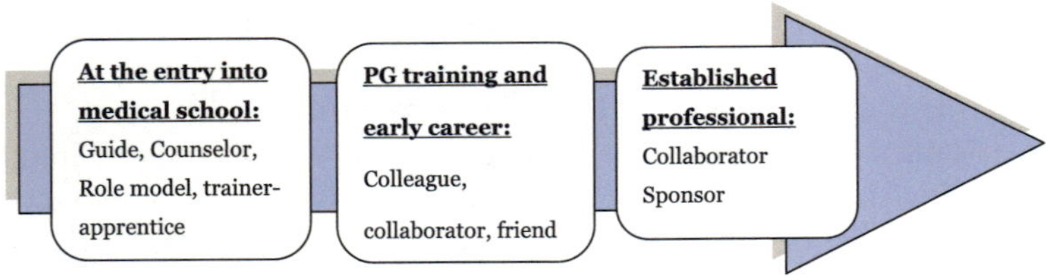

10. Do's and don'ts for mentees

Sl. no.	Do's	Dont's
1	Listen actively	Criticize or argue
2	Take initiative	Be passive
3	Openly and honestly share thoughts with the mentor	Have a hidden agenda
4	Be open to feedback and self-assess	Place blame on others
5	Respect your mentor's time	Ask for advice at the last minute
6	Show your gratitude	Compete with the mentor
7	Follow through on tasks	Overcommit
8	Have a positive attitude and enthusiasm	Stay in the relationship, out of obligation
9	Be respectful and polite	Burn bridges
10	Take risks	Stay in the comfort zone
11	Actively seek out different perspectives	Have a closed mind

Technology tools for mentoring: Advances in technology have provided many different tools that can be used in mentoring programs to improve connection and communication. From mobile technologies like Apps to video conferencing, scheduling of the meetings and mentoring software [21, 22].

Some examples of virtual mentoring platforms: Zoom, Skype, Trello, Slack, Blue Jeans, Twitter, Facebook, WeChat, WhatsApp, QQ, LINE, KAKAO talk, etc. [23].

The link for the above virtual platforms is given in the following table:

Sl. no.	Platform	Weblink
1	Zoom	https://zoom.us/
2	Microsoft teams	https://www.microsoft.com/en-in/microsoft-teams/download-app
3	Skype	https://www.skype.com/en/
4	Whatsapp	https://www.whatsapp.com/
5	Trello	https://trello.com/en
6	Slack	https://slack.com/intl/en-in/apps
7	Bluejeans	https://www.bluejeans.com/
8	Twitter	https://twitter.com/?lang=en

Sl. no.	Platform	Weblink
9	Facebook	https://www.facebook.com/
10	Wechat	https://www.wechat.com/
11	Google meet	https://apps.google.com/intl/en/meet/
12	Google classroom	https://edu.google.com/intl/ALL_in/products/classroom/
13	Tencent QQ	https://qq.en.uptodown.com/android
14	LINE	https://line.me/en/
15	Kakaotalk	https://www.kakaocorp.com/page/service/service/KakaoTalk?lang=en
16	GotoWebinar	https://www.goto.com/webinar
17	Gotomeeting	https://www.goto.com/meeting
18	Webex	https://www.webex.com/

11. Key elements to consider when choosing a mentor

Attraction: The mentee must be attracted to their mentor, so that they will emulate them.

Affect: The mentor should be positive, supportive and encouraging, displaying respect for the mentee.

Action: The mentor must be willing to invest time and energy into the mentee through guidance, teaching and counseling.

12. Desirable qualities/competencies required in a mentor

- Subject expertise: Recognized expertise in the field goes a long way in gaining the mentees respect and confidence
- Enthusiasm for sharing that expertise
- Approachable and pleasant personality
- Encouraging and open to new ideas
- Able to give constructive feedback
- Reflective listening and empathy
- Altruism
- Compassionate and genuine
- Person with interpersonal skills and networking abilities [24–26]

13. Models of mentoring

I. **The GROW model**: This coaching model designed by Sir John Whitmore. This coaching model can be used to structure mentoring conversations. The acronym “GROW“stands for

- **G**-Goal setting for the session as well as for the short and long term
- **R**-Reality checking to explore the current situation
- **O**-Options and alternative strategies, or course of actions
- **W**-What is to be done, when and by whom [27]

II. **Five-factor mentoring model**: It is meant for specific subject mentoring and includes the following:

- **Factor 1: Personal attributes** that are fundamental to the mentoring process includes the mentor need to be, (a) supportive, (b) attentive, (c) comfortable with talking about specific primary teaching practices, (d) instil positive attitudes and confidence in their mentees for teaching primary subjects, (e) assist the mentee to reflect more positively
- **Factor 2: System requirements**, which focus on aims for teaching the specific primary curriculum and school policies related to specific primary subject areas
- **Factor 3: Pedagogical knowledge**
- **Factor 4: Modeling**
- **Factor 5: Feedback** [28]

14. Benefits of mentorship program to the mentor

- Personal and professional development
- Development of communication and teaching skills
- Opportunity to build leadership skills
- Personal satisfaction
- Assistance on projects by the mentees
- Increased recognition
- Renewed interest in personal career, potential financial reward, and career advancement
- Giving back to the community
- Gaining insights and the different perspectives from future members of the profession

15. Benefits of mentoring for the mentee

- Provides assistance in defining the career goals, strategies and outcomes
- Develops a meaningful professional relationship with the mentor

- Increases professional network and connections
- Gains first-hand knowledge of workplace expectations
- Builds self-advocacy skills and confidence to be successful
- Access to potential internships and job opportunities [3]

16. Benefits to the institution

- Enhanced strategic planning based on the feedback
- Retention and recruitment of students and trainees
- Improved communication and organizational culture
- Widening access to medicine—forging links with under-represented communities to enable upward social mobility
- Accelerated training
- Professional development of employees
- Increased work performance and cost effectiveness

17. Factors influencing mentoring

- Goal and scope
- Mentor's behavior, skills and knowledge
- Mentoring structure/design/activities
- Commitment, gender and emotional intelligence
- Proactive personality, questioning and listening skills
- Reflection and 360° evaluation process
- Organizational closeness between both parties

18. Challenges to mentoring

- Unrealistic expectations from the mentees
- The administrative or infrastructural issues may remain unresolved at times and can have a negative effect on the relationship or might reduce the interest among both parties
- Time constraints and lack of training among the clinician-educators
- Unfair manipulation on the part of the mentor/mentee

- Exploitation by the mentor for personal gain and mentor may feel the mentee as his competitor.
- Incompatibility in personality/goals with mentee(s)
- Lack of incentives for successful mentorship
- Pressure to establish practice and excel academically, especially to the junior faculty
- Perceived (or real) competition
- Conflicts of interest, poor communication, lack of commitment
- Limited mentors with proven track record, especially work-life for women and URiM [29]

19. Strategies to overcome challenges

- **Orientation-cum-training programme for mentors**: In India, the University Grants Commission (UGC) has planned the orientation/induction programme of prescribed duration either MOOCs or online/offline/blended mode as approved by the concerned authority/body governing the higher education [30]
- To make the mentoring system efficient and transparent, a digital platform like the SWAYAM will help keep the database of mentees and their progress, a database of mentors, uploading learning resource material, assignments, etc.
- A peer-led structured academic mentoring program designed to provide educational assistance for new students
- **Comprehensive mentoring programs**: These are multi-faceted mentoring programs that offer academic, social and professional opportunities to traditionally underserved students
- Explained the reliability of the measurement tool used in determining outcomes and defined/assessed all operational definitions [31]
- **Collaborative problem solving**: The mentors to assist their mentees in identifying the root cause of the problem, thereby helping the peers to advance problem-solving skills [32]
- Seek feedback and strive for high-quality mentorship
- Build structured mentorship programs, provide funds and leadership presence, and celebrate mentor/mentee accomplishments
- Critically examine the value placed on high-quality mentorship in promotion and tenure policies
- Create structured virtual communities for mentorship
- Recognize exemplary mentorship with awards

20. Conclusions

Mentorship plays a critical role in the training and career development of physicians and scientists. It is increasingly recognized as a bidirectional process, benefiting both mentors and mentees. Despite the evidence of success, the current mentoring programs are facing real-time challenges like lack of formal training on mentoring and time constraint among the clinician-educators.

Some of the challenges can be overcome by organizing regular FDPs on mentoring and use of technology/virtual platforms to conduct meetings. Developing a culture of mentorship requires a strong commitment by leaders at all levels. The organization must frame the strategies for an effective mentorship program with regular feedback and evaluation. Also, the committed mentors need recognition and incentives from the organization.

Acknowledgements

I thank the management of the BLDE (Deemed to be University) for providing the opportunity to be the part of central core committee for the mentor ward system run by the institution.

Conflict of interest

The authors declare no conflict of interest.

Acronyms and abbreviations

MOOCs	massive open online courses
URiM	underrepresented students in medicine
UGC	the University Grants Commission
FDP	faculty development program
SCOPME	the Standing Committee on Postgraduate Medical Education

Author details

Anant Khot
Department of Pharmacology, AIIMS, Nagpur, India

*Address all correspondence to: anantkhot04@gmail.com

References

[1] Awasthi S. Mentoring in medical education: A neglected essentiality. Manipal Journal of Medical Sciences. 2017;**2**(1):5-7. Available from: https://ejournal.manipal.edu/mjms/docs/Vol2/MJMS Inside Pages/3-Editorial 3.pdf

[2] Irby BJ, Abdelrahman N, Lara-Alecio R, et al. Epistemological beginnings of mentoring. In: Irby BJ, Boswell JN, Searby LJ, et al., editors. The Wiley International Handbook of Mentoring, Paradigms, Practices, Programs, and Possibilities. 1st ed. USA: Wiley; 2020. pp. 19-28

[3] Nimmons D, Giny S, Rosenthal J. Medical student mentoring programs: Current insights. Advances in Medical Education and Practice. 2019;**10**:113-123

[4] Modi JN, Singh T. Mentoring in medical colleges: Bringing out the best in people. International Journal of User-Driven Healthcare. 2013;**3**(3): 106-115

[5] Leandro L, Joshi N, Zucker B. Mentoring undergraduates in academic medicine. Medical Teacher. 2018; **40**(10):1080-1081

[6] Swe KMM, Bhardwaj A. Mentoring undergraduate students: Perception of medical and dental faculties on undergraduate mentoring program. Journal of Education, Society and Behavioural Science. 2020;**33**(2):55-61

[7] Loosveld LM, Van Gerven PWM, Vanassche E, Driessen EW. Mentors' beliefs about their roles in health care education: A qualitative study of mentors' personal interpretative framework. Academic Medicine. 2020; **95**(10):1600-1606

[8] Straus S, Chatur F, Taylor M. Issues in the mentor-mentee relationship in academic medicine: A qualitative study. Academic Medicine. 2009;**84**(1):135-139

[9] Structures M. What forms does mentorship take. In: Winston AB, Dahlberg ML, editors. The Science of Effective Mentorship in STEMM. Washington, DC: The National Academies Press; 2019. pp. 75-102. DOI: 10.17226/25568

[10] Henry-Noel N, Bishop M, Gwede CK, Petkova E, Szumacher E. Mentorship in medicine and other health professions. Journal of Cancer Education. 2019;**34**:629-637. DOI: 10.1007/s13187-018-1360-6

[11] Blanco MA, Qualters DM. Mutual mentoring: Effect on faculty career achievements and experiences. Medical Teacher. 2020;**42**(7):799-805

[12] Burgess A, Diggele C, Mellis C. Mentorship in the health professions: A review. The Clinical Teacher. 2018; **15**:197-202

[13] Aylor M, Cruz M, Narayan A, et al. Optimizing your mentoring relationship: A toolkit for mentors and mentees. MedEdPORTAL. 2016; **12**:10459

[14] Straus SE, Johnson MO, Marquez C, Feldman MD. Characteristics of successful and failed mentoring relationships: A qualitative study across two academic health centers. Academic Medicine. 2013;**88**(1):82-89. DOI: 10.1097/ACM.0b013e31827647a0

[15] Brandau J, Studencnik P, Kopp-Sixt S. Dimensions and levels of mentoring: Empirical findings of the first German inventory and implications for future practice. Global Education Review. 2017;**4**(4):5-19

[16] Hayes EF. Approaches to mentoring: How to mentor and be mentored. Journal of the American Association of Nurse Practitioners. 2005;**17**(11): 442-445

[17] Tobin MJ. Mentoring: Seven roles and some specifics. American Journal of Respiratory and Critical Care Medicine. 2004;**170**:114-117

[18] Available from: https://www.google.com/search?q=Tool+%3A+Mentoring+styles+Goals+%3A+Conditions+%3A+Material&oq=too&aqs=chrome.0.69i59j46i433i512j0i20i263i512j69i57j46i

[19] Lin J, Reddy RM. Teaching, mentorship, and coaching in surgical education. Thoracic Surgery Clinics of North America. 2019;**29**(3):311-320. DOI: 10.1016/j.thorsurg.2019.03.008

[20] Available from: https://www.hsph.harvard.edu/

[21] Moores LK, Holley AB, Collen JF. Working with a mentor: Effective strategies during fellowship and early career. Chest. 2018;**153**(4):799-804. DOI: 10.1016/j.chest.2018.02.016

[22] Available from: https://www.togetherplatform.com/blog/mentoring-tools

[23] McReynolds MR, Termini CM, Hinton AO Jr, Taylor BL, Vue Z, Huang SC, et al. The art of virtual mentoring in the twenty-first century for STEM majors and beyond. Nature Biotechnology. 2020;**38**:1477-1484

[24] Cho CS, Ramanan RA, Feldman MD. Defining the ideal qualities of mentorship: A qualitative analysis of the characteristics of outstanding mentors. The American Journal of Medicine. 2011;**124**(5):453-458

[25] Holmes DR, Warnes CA, O'Gara PT, Nishimura RA. Effective attributes of mentoring in the current era. Circulation. 2018;**138**:455-457. DOI: 10.1161/CIRCULATIONAHA.118.034340

[26] Popescu-Mitroi MM, Mazilescu CA. Students-teacher perspectives on the qualities of mentor-teachers. Procedia - Social and Behavioral Sciences. 2013;**116**:3559-3563

[27] Cambridge International Examinations. Cambridge Professional Development Qualifications: A Guide for Mentors. 2015

[28] Hudson P. Specific mentoring: a theory and model for developing primary science teaching practices. European Journal of Teacher Education. 2004;**27**(2):139-146. DOI: 10.1080/0261976042000223015

[29] Ahmadmehrabi S, Farlow JL, Wamkpah NS, Esianor BI, Brenner MJ, Valdez TA, et al. New age mentoring and disruptive innovation—Navigating the uncharted with vision, purpose, and equity. JAMA Otolaryngology. Head & Neck Surgery. 2021;**147**(4):389-394. DOI: 10.1001/jamaoto.2020.5448

[30] University Grant Commission, Bahadur Shah Marg. Guidelines Mentor-Mentee Relation Vis-a Vis Life Long Learning. 2021

[31] Banu S, Juma FZ, Abas T. Mentoring in higher education. Advances in Medical Education and Practice. 2016;7:523-525

[32] George RS, Roy A, Lakshmi T. Mentor mentee strategy in academic success—A review. Indian Journal of Forensic Medicine and Toxicology. 2020;**14**:4746-4752

Chapter 5

How to Support Student Academic Success

Priyadarshini Dattathreya

Abstract

21st-century medical education is focused on healthcare equity by creating opportunities for students who are from underrepresented minority groups and non-traditional backgrounds to pursue medicine. Institutions that have spearheaded this movement have found a wide variation in the baseline knowledge, skills, and attitudes of their incoming medical students. Ensuring that these students meaningfully transition into and progress through medical school without negatively impacting their performance or wellness is a challenge that needs to be strategically addressed. This chapter will outline the challenges associated with the transition of matriculating medical students, the importance of a curriculum that promotes equity, the role of a developmental learning environment in supporting student academic success, and guidelines to use coaching to enhance student engagement.

Keywords: academic support, academic coaching, self-determination, student engagement, equity

1. Introduction

21st century medical education is responding to a global call to action against health disparities among racial and ethnic minorities [1]. This movement has highlighted the importance of increasing diversity and representation in the healthcare workforce. Consequently, it has also accentuated the historical underrepresentation of minority groups in medicine. In response, healthcare institutions have made concerted efforts to understand the factors influencing underrepresentation and explore strategies to overcome barriers to healthcare equity [2].

This chapter will outline how this movement has transformed the medical student profile and impacted how we envision student support and the learning environment. The value of providing flexibility and autonomy in the curriculum with opportunities for self-assessment in ensuring meaningful transition and progression of all students will also be emphasized.

2. Background

In 1990, the American Association of Medical Colleges (AAMC) initiated Project 3000 by 2000 which involved launching a national campaign to increase the annual matriculation number of underrepresented minority medical students from 1,485 to 3,000 by the year 2000. The goal of this project was to increase diversity

 IntechOpen

in healthcare in the US and create a culturally competent healthcare workforce that reflects the country's diverse population [3]. The AAMC also proposed a list of core competencies for students prior to entering medical school. This competency framework was intended to inform the medical school admissions processes and to deemphasize the importance of cognitive measures during admissions [4]. Similarly in 2009, the UK Government appointed a task force called the Panel on Fair Access to the Professions. The panel found that the individuals from non-privileged backgrounds had reduced access to various professions including healthcare [5]. This led to a program called Widening Access (WA). Similar to AAMC project, WA also encouraged increasing the fairness of the admissions process and providing more opportunities to students from lower socio-economic backgrounds entering medical school [6]. As a result of these projects, medical schools have witnessed a shift from knowledge-based admissions to holistic review of student applicants. Institutions have changed their admission policies to provide equal emphasis on skills and lived experiences. Measures such as situational judgment tests, multiple mini-interviews, and psychometric tests have been introduced to the admissions process to assess said competencies [7, 8].

These measures have widened the applicant pool which would otherwise have been limited due to grade-based admissions process. This resulted in a slight increase in students from underrepresented minority groups (URM) [9]. This has also opened up more opportunities for students who are non-science majors, have a lapse in education since graduation, or are of a higher age [10]. As more institutions embrace this movement towards widening access, predictably the medical student cohort will no longer be homogenous but would rather be comprise of unique individuals with diverse knowledge, skills, and abilities. As a result, institutions will have to make concerted efforts to support the appropriate progression of their students throughout the continuum of their medical education.

3. Supporting transition of matriculating medical students

While great strides have been made to widen access, attrition of URM and their underrepresentation in medical workforce continues to be a challenge [11]. For example, in the UK, ethnic minority medical students as a group on average were found to perform worse when compared to their white colleagues during medical school and training [12]. Similarly, URM students were more likely than non-URM students to experience graduation delays and failure [13]. In addition to the stress associated with adjusting to the rigor of medical school, URM students were more likely to view themselves as "fraud" and doubt their abilities to succeed [14]. This phenomenon has found to be secondary to systemic problems associated with factors such as low socio-economic status or quality of undergraduate studies etc. [15].

Institutions have strived to address these challenges and support meaningful transitions of their medical students. There has been an rise in innovative pipeline programs to increase the academic preparedness of URM students [16]. Academic enrichment programs on science and pre-med courses, and academic support programs have also been introduced to meet the diverse needs of matriculating students and support their transition into medical school [17]. Mentoring programs have been established to provide social support vital to professional identity formation of URM students [18, 19]. Several institutions have introduced pre-matriculation courses to increase student awareness on academic preparedness for medical school. These programs supported student transition by introducing knowledge and skills required for medical school, integrating students into the learning environment and/or helping them immerse into the community [17]. Some institutions have used these courses to proactively identify students who could potentially be at risk of academic difficulties during medical school [20]. Some have been designed to introduce the students to the rigors of the medical school curriculum. The goal of these programs were to "normalize the playing field" for students with diverse levels of pre-med knowledge and skills [21].

There were also several post matriculation remediation programs that were introduced to identify and support struggling medical students. These programs provided academic and emotional support, the outcomes of which were predominantly context dependent [22]. Due to the varying levels of success of these proactive and reactive approaches to supporting student success, institutions have grappled with the challenging question – how to support student academic success?

According to self-determination theory, student engagement in their own academic success is closely related to three basic psychological needs – autonomy, competence, and relatedness. Students who feel autonomous, competent and have a sense of belonging are typically more intrinsically motivated to maximize their potential [23]. The three psychological needs can be hindered by external pressures such as exceptionally challenging learning tasks, negative and disparaging feedback, judgments, threats, and punishments [24]. A learning environment that fails to address the three basic psychological needs of students could impact students' internal motivation and engagement in lifelong learning.

Therefore, the learning environment that is inherent to the traditional curriculum and its ability to support the progression of diverse group of students has come under scrutiny.

4. Shifting focus from equality to equity

Traditional US medical students have an average age of 24 and enroll in a medical program directly after completing college level pre-medical courses in science and math [25]. Similarly, in the UK, traditional medical students have an average age of 18–19 and have completed their schooling with necessary prerequisites [26]. With the move towards widening access and subsequent admission of non-traditional medical students, researchers have challenged the effectiveness of traditional curriculum to meet the diverse needs of 21st century student cohort [27]. The time-based curriculum assumes that all matriculating medical students have a homogenous level of knowledge, skills, and experiences, and therefore are able to progress through the continuum with a consistent pace. However, with the reforms in the admissions process and the reduced emphasis on standardized exam scores, the assumption of a "level playing field" seems to be no longer valid [28]. There is a greater need to shift from the one-size-fits-all approach of the traditional curriculum to individualization of learning experiences for medical students [29]. Recognition of these needs has led to the popularity of competency-based medical education (CBME).

CBME shifts the focus from knowledge-based standardized exams to holistic development of knowledge, skills and behaviors required to be a competent physician. The core elements of CBME include time variability, focus on outcomes, entrustability and professional identity formation [30]. Although CBME is time and resource intensive, several institutions have recognized the value of using core Entrustable Professional Activities (EPAs) and competency-based milestones in developing competent physicians while also honoring the existing multifariousness of medical student cohorts. In addition to providing tailored learning experiences, the greatest value of CBME lies within the opportunities for individualized formative feedback and real-time remediation for students [31].

Although CBME is a giant step towards equitable medical education, the challenges to its implementation lie in its trivia. Curriculum experts have stressed that there is no universal approach to CBME [32]. Institutions must set competency standards based on their unique contexts and implement their curriculum using several iterative cycles of planning and evaluation. Successful implementation of CBME lies in the ability to track assessment data of individual medical students in order to be able to assess their entrustability and progression. CBME researchers have promoted the use of learning analytics to integrate assessment data from multiple sources and provide visual representations of student progress [33]. Use of artificial intelligence in tracking student progress could be invaluable in providing individualized support to a 21st century medical student.

Therefore, a competency-based curriculum could support students' need for autonomy and competence and promote their progression and success.

5. Exploring student academic success factors

The ability to predict academic performance of medical students has been a significant topic of discourse among medical educators. Historically, academic achievements of students prior to medical school such as Medical College Admissions Test (MCAT) and Grade Point Averages (GPA) have been found to predictive of their academic performance and progression [34]. Similarly, the UK Clinical Aptitude Test (UKCAT) has also been found to be a predictor of student academic success [35]. These factors have been used as screening criteria for admissions or for identifying the need for additional academic support. With the introduction of non-cognitive measures in the admissions criteria, institutions began to explore traits or skills associated with motivation, attitude, and mindset as predictors of student academic success. There have been debates around the individual and/or collective roles of factors such as grit, perseverance, self-efficacy, and self-regulation in determining academic success [36]. Researchers have also explored the prospects of using these factors to identify students at-risk of experiencing academic difficulties in medical school [37].

Grit is defined as "perseverance and passion for long-term goals". Consistency of perseverance and effort has been positively related to academic performance and success [38]. This concept was further elaborated by the notion of academic psychological capital (PsyCap) and its impact on academic achievements. In addition to grit, the core constructs of PsyCap include positive psychological resources such as hope, efficacy, resilience, and optimism. All these factors have been shown to impact a student's response to challenges and adversity in pursuit of successful academic outcomes [39].

Metacognition or "thinking about thinking" has been another factor commonly researched as a predictor of high performance. Metacognition involves students' knowledge about cognitive strategies and their regulation of these strategies before, during and after learning events [40]. Researchers have attempted to compare metacognitive skills between high and low performing students to identify patterns that determine success [41]. Furthermore, the influence of self-regulation on learning has also been explored. Self-regulated learning builds on the concept of metacognition and also considers the influence of social and motivational factors on learning [42]. Self-regulated learning is generally described as a cyclical process, often triggered by the formulating of goals and the subsequent employment of strategies to achieve, and monitor advancement towards those goals, followed by engagement in reflection and the formulation of new learning goals. Among medical students a positive correlation has been identified between self-regulated learning and academic achievement [43]. Additionally, academic self-efficacy which is defined as learner's judgments about their ability to successfully attain educational goals has also been associated with academic performance [44]. Researchers have found associations between academic self-efficacy of students and their ability to self-regulate [45].

Essentially, the above non-cognitive factors have been found to have some degree of relationship with academic performance and success. Medical schools have used self-reported psychometric inventories to assess these factors in students. Some examples of self-reported inventories include Learning and Study Strategies Inventory (LASSI), Motivated Strategies for Learning Questionnaire (MSLQ), Academic Self-Efficacy Scale (AES) etc. [44, 46]. The psychometric data from the inventories have been combined with qualitative data from reflective journals, group discussions and interviews to assess these factors [47]. This data has been typically used to identify students who may be potentially at-risk of poor academic performance either to inform the admissions process or to direct remediation efforts.

However, the utilization of these factors as predictors of success among medical students, could impede the progress towards widening access. The reason for this argument is twofold. Firstly, self-efficacy is impacted by prior knowledge, experiences, and social support systems [48]. A diverse group of medical students with diverse levels of prior knowledge and experiences may not have uniform levels of self-efficacy. Secondly, literature has highlighted the domain-specificity of self-regulation and self-efficacy. Academic self-efficacy levels among students can vary depending on the context. It is found to be directly related to their "need for cognition", i.e., their inclination to enjoy tasks involving higher mental activity [49]. Besides motivation, persistence and effort, academic self-efficacy is also impacted by knowledge and regulation of metacognitive strategies [50]. The ability of students to regulate their own learning is dependent upon the specificity and complexity of the task [51]. Task-specific metacognitive strategies can be developed over time with practice and feedback. Therefore, the challenges to student development and progress could also be secondary to the learning environment including teaching and assessment practices [52]. Furthermore, reactive remediation approaches that are based on identification of "at-risk" students could have a negative impact on students' self-efficacy [53]. A learning environment that scaffolds the development of metacognition and self-regulation into the curriculum is vital to student success.

Therefore, shifting the focus from predicting outcomes to supporting student development might be beneficial in promoting student autonomy and sense of belonging.

6. Supporting student development through coaching

The factors associated with academic success of students can be complex and often unique to individual student context. Institutions have attempted to put several measures in place to support academic and psychosocial needs of students. Some examples include mentoring and assigning learning communities, special programs in study skills, academic advising by learning specialists, counseling support etc. There is also growing evidence that coaching practices can foster self-regulation and self-efficacy among medical students [54].

Academic coaching typically uses a different approach from the two common types of academic support namely advising, and mentoring. The most important difference is in the role of a coach when compared to that of an advisor or mentor. Mentors and advisors are typically subject matter experts and offer expert advice, insights, and directions to students in response to specific questions [55]. A coach on the other hand is not required to have subject matter expertise, but rather be equipped with coaching skills specifically questioning and challenging [56].

Several models of coaching have been highlighted in literature (**Table 1**) [57–59]. However, the fundamental principles to questioning skills in coaching are that of appreciative inquiry (AI) [60]. AI is a strength-based approach to change and development. At the core of AI are the assumptions that individuals are capable of imagining, and creating a desired future through questioning and dialog if change is focused on building on their strengths [61].

Institutions have introduced formal academic coaching to their students to support the development of lifelong learning skills [55]. However, student can also benefit from coaching conversations outside of a formal coaching setting. The following coaching guidelines can be used by clinicians when providing feedback in clinical settings or by mentors and advisors while working with students on an individual basis.

1. Collaboration: Academic coaching can promote accountability when the conversations are collaborative. In a coaching relationship, it is vital to create a space that is devoid of any form of power dynamics or hierarchy to build trust and collaboration [62].

2. Empowerment: Preventive academic coaching shifts the focus from learner remediation to learner empowerment. Coaching conversations when started earlier in a medical student's journey will assist them in proactively identifying threats or concerns that might lead to poor academic performance [63].

3. Student-centric: Academic coaching is a student-centered approach. The coaching conversations are typically based on the consideration that when students are aware of their own strengths and weaknesses, they are more likely to take accountability for their progress [64].

Coaching models	Stages
ACHIEVE	Assess current situation Creative brainstorming of alternative to current situation Hone goals Initiate options Evaluative options Valid action program design Encourage momentum.
GROW	Goal Current reality Options Wrap up
PRACTICE	Problem identification Realistic, relevant goals developed Alternative solutions generated Consideration of consequences Target most feasible solution(s) Implementation of chosen solution(s) Evaluation

Table 1.
Example of coaching models.

4. Reflection: Academic coaching takes a non-directive approach to help students set goals and reflect on their progress [65]. Therefore, asking open-ended reflective questions increases students' self-awareness.

5. Goal orientation: Academic coaching is typically a goal-oriented approach that is aimed at producing immediate adjustments that align students' learning to their long-term goals. Effective coaching conversations help individual students articulate their long-term and short-term goals, create action plans, and identify self-monitoring strategies [55].

Academic coaching is a powerful formative approach to provide individualized support to students. Effective and longitudinal coaching when introduced as a part of the curriculum, empowers students to maximize their own potential. Introducing regular non-directive coaching conversations as a part of the student's learning journey could support their autonomy, competence, and relatedness.

7. Summary

In summary, the 21st century medical student is less likely to conform to the norms of a typical medical student that institutions have observed in the past. Supporting the academic success of a 21st century medical student will require a paradigm shift in how we envision the curriculum, learning environment and support services. A one size fits all approach with a reactive response to remediation may not cater to the unique needs of a diverse student group.

Solutions might include curriculums that are competency-based, individualized, and time-flexible. Additionally, scaffolding self-regulated learning strategies into regular teaching can enhance student learning and retention. Formative assessments and feedback help student monitor their performance and progression. Feedback should compare their performance to a standard which can be set using competency-based curriculum. Additionally, creating a learning environment that provides longitudinal coaching support increases student self-awareness and empowerment.

8. Conclusions

Meaningful transition and progression of a diverse group of medical students is more about helping students set progressive goals for themselves rather than ensuring that everyone progresses at the same pace. If the ultimate goal of 21st century medical education is to provide an equitable learning environment, particular attention must be paid to increasing students' autonomy, competence, and relatedness.

Acknowledgements

I would like to acknowledge all our experienced academic coaches at the Academy for Teaching and Learning who inspired this chapter.

Conflict of interest

The author declares no conflict of interest.

Author details

Priyadarshini Dattathreya
Ross University School of Medicine, Bridgetown, Barbados

*Address all correspondence to: pdattathreya@rossu.edu

References

[1] Braveman P. What are health disparities and health equity? We need to be clear. Public Health Reports. 2014;129(1_suppl2):5-8.

[2] Williams JS, Walker RJ, Egede LE. Achieving equity in an evolving healthcare system: Opportunities and challenges. Am J Med Sci. 2016;351(1):33-43.

[3] Nickens HW, Ready TP, Petersdorf RG. Project 3000 by 2000 – Racial and ethnic diversity in US medical schools. Mass Medical Soc; 1994.

[4] Pierre JM, Mahr F, Carter A, Madaan V. Underrepresented in medicine recruitment: Rationale, challenges, and strategies for increasing diversity in psychiatry residency programs. Academic Psychiatry. 2017;41(2):226-232.

[5] Milburn A. Unleashing Aspiration: The Final Report of the Panel on Fair Access to the Professions. London: Cabinet Office. 2009.

[6] Nicholson S, Cleland JA. "It's making contacts": Notions of social capital and implications for widening access to medical education. Advances in Health Sciences Education. 2017;22(2):477-490.

[7] Webster ES, Paton LW, Crampton PES, Tiffin PA. Situational judgement test validity for selection: A systematic review and meta-analysis. Medical Education. 2020;54(10): 888-902.

[8] Powis D, Munro D, Bore M, Eley D. Why is it so hard to consider personal qualities when selecting medical students? Med Teach. 2020;42(4): 366-371.

[9] Smedley BD, Evans CH, Colburn L, Stith AY, Association of Academic Health Centers, Association of American Medical Colleges, et al. The Right Thing to Do, the Smart Thing to Do: Enhancing Diversity in the Health Professions – Summary of the Symposium on Diversity in Health Professions in Honor of Herbert W. Nickens, M. D. Washington, D.C.: National Academies Press; 2001 2001 Sep 29. 428 p.

[10] James D, Ferguson E, Powis D, Symonds I, Yates J. Graduate entry to medicine: Widening academic and socio-demographic access. Medical Education. 2008;42(3):294-300.

[11] Lett LA, Orji WU, Sebro R. Declining racial and ethnic representation in clinical academic medicine: A longitudinal study of 16 US medical specialties. PLOS ONE. 2018;13(11):e0207274.

[12] Stegers-Jager KM, Steyerberg EW, Cohen-Schotanus J, Themmen AP. Ethnic disparities in undergraduate pre-clinical and clinical performance. Med Educ. 2012;46(6):575-585.

[13] Orom H, Semalulu T, Underwood W, Iii Md MS. The social and learning environments experienced by underrepresented minority medical students: A narrative review. Acad Med. 2013;88(11):1765-1777.

[14] Mullangi S, Jagsi R. Imposter syndrome. JAMA. 2019;322(5):403.

[15] Woolf K. Differential attainment in medical education and training. BMJ. 2020;368:m339.

[16] Shields PH. A survey and analysis of student academic support programs in medical schools focus: Underrepresented minority students. Journal of the National Medical Association. 1994;86(5):373-377.

[17] Heck AJ, Gibbons L, Ketter SJ, Furlano A, Prest L. A survey of the design of pre-matriculation courses at US medical schools. Medical Science Educator. 2017;27(2):229-236.

[18] Elks ML, Herbert-Carter J, Smith M, Klement B, Knight BB, Anachebe NF. Shifting the curve: Fostering academic success in a diverse student body. Acad Med. 2018;93(1):66-70.

[19] Merchant JL, Omary MB. Underrepresentation of underrepresented minorities in academic medicine: The need to enhance the pipeline and the pipe. Gastroenterology. 2010;138(1):19-26.e3.

[20] Bennion LD, Torre D, Durning SJ, Mears D, Schreiber-Gregory D, Servey JT, et al. Early identification of struggling learners: Using prematriculation and early academic performance data. Perspectives on Medical Education. 2019;8(5):298-304.

[21] Williams MT. Pre-matriculation program at the University of South Florida College of Medicine. Academic Medicine: Journal of the Association of American Medical Colleges. 1999;74(4): 397-399.

[22] Stegers-Jager KM, Cohen-Schotanus J, Themmen APN. The Four-Tier Continuum of Academic and Behavioral Support (4T-CABS) model: An integrated model for medical student success. Acad Med. 2017;92(11): 1525-1530.

[23] Niemiec CP, Ryan RM. Autonomy, competence, and relatedness in the classroom: Applying self-determination theory to educational practice. Theory and Research in Education. 2009;7(2):133-144.

[24] Ten Cate TJ, Kusurkar RA, Williams GC. How self-determination theory can assist our understanding of the teaching and learning processes in medical education. AMEE guide No. 59. Med Teach. 2011;33(12):961-973.

[25] Mitchell KJ. Traditional predictors of performance in medical school. Academic Medicine. 1990.

[26] Mathers J, Sitch A, Marsh JL, Parry J. Widening access to medical education for under-represented socioeconomic groups: Population based cross sectional analysis of UK data, 2002-6. BMJ. 2011;342(feb22 1):d918-d.

[27] Tedesco JC, Opertti R, Amadio M. The curriculum debate: Why it is important today. Prospects. 2014;44(4): 527-546.

[28] Hodges BD. A tea-steeping or i-Doc model for medical education? Acad Med. 2010;85(9 Suppl):S34-S44.

[29] Ten Cate O, Gruppen LD, Kogan JR, Lingard LA, Teunissen PW. Time-variable training in medicine: Theoretical considerations. Acad Med. 2018;93(3S Competency-Based, Time-Variable Education in the Health Professions):S6-S11.

[30] Lucey CR, Thibault GE, Ten Cate O. Competency-Based, Time-variable education in the health professions: Crossroads. Acad Med. 2018;93(3S Competency-Based, Time-Variable Education in the Health Professions): S1-S5.

[31] Konopasek L, Norcini J, Krupat E. Focusing on the formative: Building an assessment system aimed at student growth and development. Academic Medicine. 2016;91(11):1492-1497.

[32] Dagnone JD, Chan M-K, Meschino D, Bandiera G, Den Rooyen C, Matlow A, et al. Living in a world of change: Bridging the gap from competency-based medical education theory to practice in Canada. Academic Medicine. 2020;95(11):1643-1646.

[33] Thoma B, Ellaway RH, Chan TM. From Utopia through dystopia: Charting a course for learning analytics in competency-based medical education. Academic Medicine. 2021;96(7S):S89-S95.

[34] Patterson F, Knight A, Dowell J, Nicholson S, Cousans F, Cleland J. How effective are selection methods in medical education? A systematic review. Medical Education. 2016;50(1):36-60.

[35] Tiffin PA, Mwandigha LM, Paton LW, Hesselgreaves H, McLachlan JC, Finn GM, et al. Predictive validity of the UKCAT for medical school undergraduate performance: A national prospective cohort study. BMC Medicine. 2016;14(1).

[36] Ferguson E, James D, Madeley L. Factors associated with success in medical school: Systematic review of the literature. BMJ. 2002;324(7343):952-957.

[37] Cariaga-Lo LD, Enarson CE, Crandall SJ, Zaccaro DJ, Richards BF. Cognitive and noncognitive predictors of academic difficulty and attrition. Academic Medicine. 1997;72(10): S69-S71.

[38] Duckworth AL, Peterson C, Matthews MD, Kelly DR. Grit: Perseverance and passion for long-term goals. Journal of Personality and Social Psychology. 2007;92(6):1087.

[39] Luthans KW, Luthans BC, Chaffin TD. Refining grit in academic performance: The mediational role of psychological capital. Journal of Management Education. 2019;43(1): 35-61.

[40] Ozturk N. Assessing metacognition: Theory and practices. International Journal of Assessment Tools in Education. 2017;4(2):134-148.

[41] Dattathreya P, Shillingford S. Identifying the ineffective study strategies of first year medical school students. Medical Science Educator. 2017;27(2):295-307.

[42] Bransen D, Govaerts MJB. How to conceptualise self-regulated learning: Implications for measurement. Med Educ. 2020.

[43] Cho KK, Marjadi B, Langendyk V, Hu W. The self-regulated learning of medical students in the clinical environment – A scoping review. BMC Med Educ. 2017;17(1):112.

[44] Elias SM, Macdonald S. Using past performance, proxy efficacy, and academic self-efficacy to predict college performance. Journal of Applied Social Psychology. 2007;37(11):2518-2531.

[45] Honicke T, Broadbent J. The influence of academic self-efficacy on academic performance: A systematic review. Educational Research Review. 2016;17:63-84.

[46] González-Torres MC, Torrano F. Methods and instruments for measuring self-regulated learning. Handbook of instructional resources and their applications in the classroom. 2008:201-219.

[47] Cazan A-M. Teaching self regulated learning strategies for psychology students. Procedia – Social and Behavioral Sciences. 2013;78:743-747.

[48] Pajares F, Schunk D. The development of academic self-efficacy. Development of achievement motivation United States. 2001;7:1-27.

[49] Elias SM, Loomis RJ. Utilizing need for cognition and perceived self-efficacy to predict academic performance. Journal of Applied Social Psychology. 2002;32(8):1687-1702.

[50] Linnenbrink EA, Pintrich PR. The role of self-efficacy beliefs in student engagement and learning in the

classroom. Reading and Writing Quarterly. 2003;19(2):119-137.

[51] Poitras EG, Lajoie SP. A domain-specific account of self-regulated learning: The cognitive and metacognitive activities involved in learning through historical inquiry. Metacognition and Learning. 2013;8(3):213-234.

[52] Steinert Y. The "problem" learner: Whose problem is it? AMEE Guide No. 76. Med Teach. 2013;35(4):e1035-e1045.

[53] Chou CL, Kalet A, Costa MJ, Cleland J, Winston K. Guidelines: The dos, don'ts and don't knows of remediation in medical education. Perspectives on Medical Education. 2019;8(6):322-338.

[54] Barato JB, Rodríguez Moneo M. Can coaching contribute to the development of self-regulation? Similarities and differences between these two processes. Coaching: An International Journal of Theory, Research and Practice. 2021:1-14.

[55] Deiorio NM, Carney PA, Kahl LE, Bonura EM, Juve AM. Coaching: A new model for academic and career achievement. Med Educ Online. 2016;21:33480.

[56] Wolff M, Morgan H, Jackson J, Skye E, Hammoud M, Ross PT. Academic coaching: Insights from the medical student's perspective. Med Teach. 2020;42(2):172-177.

[57] Palmer S. Revisiting the P in the PRACTICE coaching model. The Coaching Psychologist. 2011;7(2): 156-158.

[58] Grant AM. Is it time to REGROW the GROW model? Issues related to teaching coaching session structures. The Coaching Psychologist. 2011;7(2): 118-126.

[59] Dembkowski S, Eldridge F. Achieving tangible results: The development of a coaching model. The Philosophy and Practice of Coaching: Insights and Issues for a New Era. 2012:195-215.

[60] Sandars J, Murdoch-Eaton D. Appreciative inquiry in medical education. Med Teach. 2017;39(2): 123-127.

[61] Gordon S. Appreciative inquiry coaching. International Coaching Psychology Review. 2008;3(1):17-29.

[62] Wolff M, Stojan J, Buckler S, Cranford J, Whitman L, Gruppen L, et al. Coaching to improve self-directed learning. Clin Teach. 2020;17(4): 408-412.

[63] Lovell B. What do we know about coaching in medical education? A literature review. Med Educ. 2018;52(4): 376-390.

[64] Spence GB, Oades LG. Coaching with self-determination theory in mind: Using theory to advance evidence-based coaching practice. 2011.

[65] Ives Y. What is 'coaching'? An exploration of conflicting paradigms. International Journal of Evidence Based Coaching and Mentoring. 2008;6(2).

Chapter 6

Clinical Curriculum Revolution to Integrity and "Attunity"

Samhaa Abd Elmoneim

Abstract

Reviewing the history of clinical educational curricula reveals enormous change and progress through successive antiquity up-to the current 21th century. Surely, there are stable fundamental criteria which are pillars in designing any curriculum; however there are torrential inevitable reforms which are important in filling the changeable gaps and fulfilling the ecological and temporal aspects. Over the last 20th century, numerous new paradigms for curricula reforms were constructed to adapt ebullient millennium needs, interactive pedagogical approaches and psychological/sociological learning theories. These reforms fostered clinical practice, integrating core competencies and reflection on designing, and achieving clinical curricula depending on outcome-based models such as clinical competences milestones. On the other hand, systematic approach of Kern's framework adopts curriculum development through six consecutive interlinked and intersected steps which are refined to eight steps later. Moreover, taking contextual factors into account during curricula planning was evolved in other models such as PRISMS model. Despite all these pearly efforts, there are still caveats about inclusive gaps negligence between education process and overall health system. 3P-6Cs toolkit is deemed a recent novel paradigm that enrolls this role of health systems in clinical training during curricula design.

Keywords: medical education, curriculum reforms, 21th century, history, curriculum, criteria, types, clinical training, Kern's framework, PRISMS, 3P-6Cs

1. Introduction

1.1 Overview

Medical education process has faced many challenges which have to be considered and have not to be omitted in the current 21th century by clinical educators and administrators. Pandemic covid-19 has invaded the earth and has made forcibly its own characteristic troublesome era [1]. Technology has disseminated and has profoundly integrated in the whole life; social, educational, political, societal, and professional/clinical life with its positive and negative impacts [2, 3]. Moreover, there are other deeply forked challenges into medical education practice, likewise the challenge of practicing clinical education being a secondary mission by many clinicians after their primary clinical profession, the challenge of commercialization of many health institutions, the challenge of narcissism overwhelming phenomenon in clinical skills education regardless ethics regard, the challenge of marketing which has been exploded and has devitalized emotional intelligence, ethical values and humane morals in medical field communication and the challenge of multitude of variable curricula types, thoughts, models, and aspects that have to be merged to achieve overarching holistic safe and successful medical practice [4, 5]. Continuous change of the medical education process, which has depended and has reflected mainly on curricula reforms, has become indispensable to meet stakeholders and societies' needs.

Indeed, explicit (formal) aligned to implicit (informal) curricula are the flux and estuary of medical education and clinical training that link between educational and administrative aspects [6]. Explicit curriculum is considered the organized systematic plan model that most institutions follow in clinical training [6]. However, implicit curriculum is always extracted and is never separated from practicing the explicit one despite practicing it unconsciously and unsystematically in most times in real world. So, achieving an ideal curriculum is prospective complex aspiration within the upcoming medical education renaissance that has been evolved to encompass many aspects not only knowledge.

Curriculum design, being a sophisticated structure, should be planned considering multitude of factors, not related to content only but also to stakeholders (medical trainees, trainers, patients, administrators, and other healthcare workers) and institutional, environmental and local and global societies' needs [7]. Hence, planning an ideal curriculum, which is suited all these factors, is somehow fallacious and antiquated and this requires pragmatic changes to execute individual, local and global benefits from it. This is closely related to the standpoint in the written articles about general learning issues by the writer, May Zyiada within the first half of 20th century. She advocated, at that time, that "not all learning rules and projects that show success in west mean achieving the same success in east, however coping up what are updated is mandatory to apply what is suited with each community". Accordingly, there is no ideal universal curriculum for every place or every time, because of many social, societal, cultural, political, economic, intellectual, emotional and psychological contexts that have to be considered [7, 8]. So, the impact of considering these detailed variables in tandem in each curriculum is reflected positively on medical education and health not only locally but also globally.

Despite the associated logic caveats on standardization a universal curriculum, outlining a contextual framework connecting the most fundamental elements can empower broad and profound success through constructing it in an organized coherent manner [9, 10]. Moreover, each curriculum should be supplied by metacognitive thinking about soft system approaches which interconnect all these elements and associated factors together in a coherent comprehensive emerging plan [11, 12]. These recent upcoming approaches are expected to tower curricula designs up to higher levels of thinking theoretically and achievement pragmatically through integrating health system care with clinical knowledge and skills.

In this chapter we will retrieve curriculum etymology origin and its historical story. We will touch on crucial curriculum criteria regardless the place of its execution. We will elucidate the importance of curricula designs in educational process. We will demonstrate diverse curricula types and frameworks, particularly Kern's foundational six steps framework and PRISMS strategy. Emerging metacognition within the already used curricula designs is the recent trajectory in clinical education to interconnect all elements of curricula and surrounding factorial circumstances to be attuned, so we will read this out under the term 3P-6Cs toolkit. Hoping this chapter will be a catalyst to invest ecology in constructing more effective and efficient curricula ideas in this widely opened era that only accepts everlasting adventurous progress. Finally, you will face some footnotes through reading this chapter which are little bit away from medical writing rules. However these are not so far from the aim of this chapter which is to interlink medical to societal, psychological, administrative or even literary aspects. These footnotes help to approximate the meaning of integrating ecological life into medical practice.

1.2 Etymology and history

1.2.1 Etymology

"Curriculum" with its Latin root means race. It is derived from "currere" word which means to run or to proceed or "curricle" which means chariot. "Curriculum vitae" is also a mutual term which shares the same meaning of progressive continuity, hence; this meaning reflects that it is a continuous evolving not-stationary not stagnant process, so it needs endless assessment and improvement to maintain and metastasize its virtues and to overcome its shortcomings [13].

Footnote: *Do not be stagnant in this turbulent race, think about curriculum reform.*

1.2.2 History

Earliest ancient centuries, Before Common Era (BCE), testified the outset of medicine by Egyptian and Babylonian priests in ancient Egypt and Iraq. Evolving of medical knowledge and development of medical education started and transferred by Hippocrates during Greece culture then by Galen which was eminent during Roman Empire [14, 15]. Islamic civilization had a potent influence on medical education especially after its invasion to Europe. Revolution was transmitted from Arabian to European areas between the ninth to fourteenth centuries. Razi and Ibn Sina, excelled at this time, in diagnosis, management and in medical education [14, 16, 17]. Then, in Europe, 19th century came to prove, classify, develop and apply the educational theories in a frame of systematized educational practice [14, 15]. With the beginning of 20th century, Flexner exploded his report for medical education reform to be applied in all US areas and all medical institutions without distinction or segregation [18]. In 1949, Tyler started structuring curriculum in a four-staged organized framework. Then Harden 10 question adjusted in depth and breadth more details about content of each of Tyler's 4 stages considering the relation between curriculum elements and stakeholders, institution support and community conditions to be more reflective on practice [8, 19]. Later, Kern developed the six steps framework which has been become the popular systematized framework in medical education till our current days [8, 20].

The current open 21th century mandates continuous life-long learning in medical education. This requires contemplation of history' events to confront the present facilities and challenges and to adapt the everlasting changing future without missing the fundamental rules, without omission of basic knowledge and theories monograph and without neglecting the variables of stakeholders needs.

Footnote: *Be firm in roots (by applying what is sturdy from curriculum history), flexible in twigs (by continuous required reforms).*

1.3 Importance

The educational process is complex and is loaded by many elements which need to be determined, organized and linked together. These elements include defining goals and objectives, content intelligibility, targeting general and learners' needs, detection of educational strategies, implementation and assessing of the whole educational process [9]. Inter-link between all these elements in a clear organized plan is what ended by a curriculum design [8]. Repercussions are obviously attained in educational process if there is no clear specific organized plan. The role of curriculum plan is to organize *what to be learned (content of program, learners will do), who will receive this (learners, stakeholders), how to learn this (strategies, methods, and implementation), why this important to be learned (goals, objectives and assessment), when (timetable, environment and resources)* and *where the learning process (environment, resources)* are carried out in a conceptual framework. Moreover there are many factors and forces that should be considered during achieving this sophisticated process [21]. These factors entail social, societal, political, commercial (which is obvious in private institutions), academic and health service aspects [8]. Consideration of all these factors, during curriculum mapping, is important to reveal curriculum translation into practice and to reflect the practice impact on curriculum development as well [8, 21, 22]. Recently in addition to these factors consideration in curricula planning, system based thinking and regulation are overarched to fill gaps in health care system [23].

Footnote: *Practicing education, using elements without knitting each of them in comprehensive organized steps, resembles breaking up of one bead from a continuous necklace beads. Other elements (or beads) will be easily lost.*

So, connect all elements (beads) to construct useful curriculum (necklace).

2. Curriculum classification

2.1 Criteria

There are many curricula classification and types, each determines the way of preparation and delivery of the education process. Each curriculum -to be effective- requires fulfilling specific criteria of different aspects [24]. Although there is an evolving renaissance in medical education and curricula designing, there is still no evidence that the new curricula are more effective than the iterative old ones [25]. On the other hand, following fundamental criteria (in **Figure 1**) for curriculum planning and achievement guarantees -to greater extent- a realistic, not only a theoretic, curriculum which is attuned with contexts. These criteria include the relevance of curriculum to health service and learners' needs, filling gaps to reach outcomes, flexibility with surrounding changes, relatedness to practice, organized timetabled plans and continuous assessment and remediation at each curriculum stage in addition to final assessment as well [24].

Footnote: *Each body –to be healthy- requires basic balanced mixtures of different sorts of diet, each soul –to be sober- requires acquiring perceptions from different*

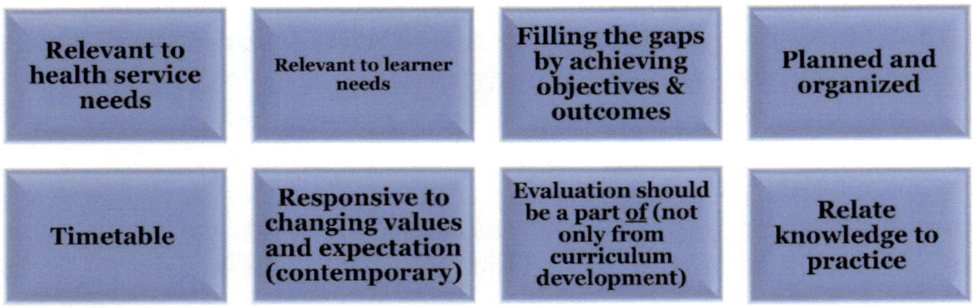

Figure 1.
Fundamental criteria.

cultures. Likewise, each curriculum -to be effective- requires matching specific criteria of different aspects.

So, make your curriculum effective by considering its fundamental criteria.

2.2 Curriculum models

There is continuous mounting in classification of various curriculum types and in development of different frameworks. The most of these curricula variants are derived from the following two models; prescriptive and descriptive [26].

2.2.1 Prescriptive model

It is the origin of outcome based curricula which is commonly used in the present medical education. It depends on objectives and goals (intent) rather than other affecting factors on the process (context). Objectives are determined using behavioral verbs. Tyler four staged curriculum, in 1949, is the initial example of this objective model which fosters the intended clinical competencies, knowledge, skills and/or attitude outcome [7, 26, 27].

2.2.2 Descriptive model

It depends robustly on internal and external contextual factors analysis of curriculum situation in addition to the intent which is the target of the prescriptive model. This model describes and analyses the context of different interlinked elements (including intent, content, teaching strategies and assessment) of curriculum design regardless the definite ordered manner of these elements [7, 26, 27].

Table 1 outlines the differences between perspective and descriptive models.

2.3 Curriculum types

Under and post-graduate medical education can be delivered depending on different curricula types or categories. Each curriculum type has its pros and cons; there is no ideal or perfect curriculum one hundred percent. Some medical schools or institutes use single standalone curriculum, whereas integrating two or more of these types are more consistent with contemporary milieu and expanding medical health system and education needs [4, 10, 26].

Common curricula types are listed and described briefly in **Figure 2**.

Prescriptive	Descriptive
Rely on intent (outcome)	Rely on context (means)
Concerned with objectives and outcome rather than content and process	Concerned with internal and external factors affecting content and process
Translate curriculum to practice (obligatory)	Reflect practice into curriculum (reflective)
What will be done	How this will be done
Core Competencies	PRISMS models

Table 1.
Perspective and descriptive curricula models differences.

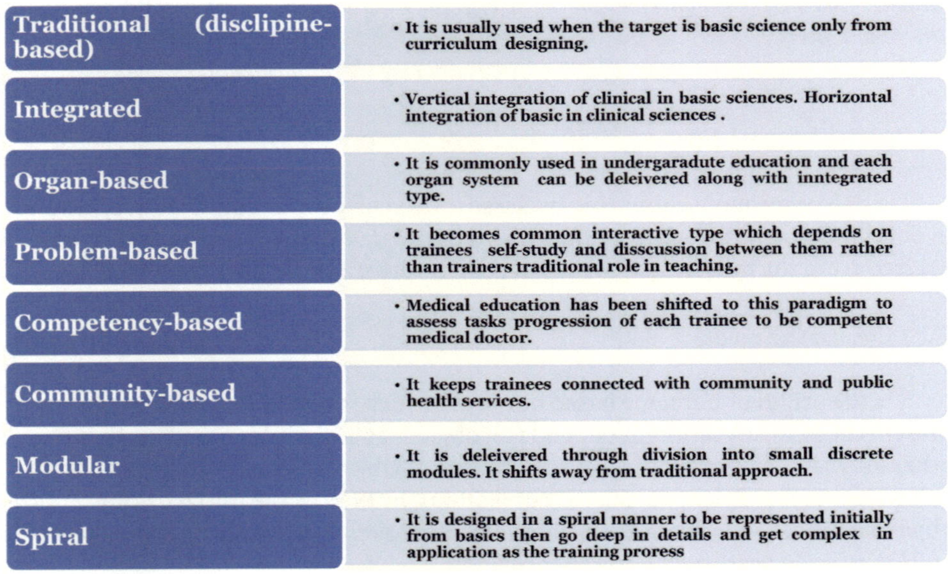

Figure 2.
Curriculum types.

3. Modern curriculum frameworks

Flexner started and reported in the last century that clinical education has to be reformed to transmit practice into curricula and the reverse. He stated that it is important to standardize any reform on all health care service and medical educational institutions regardless the socioeconomic status [18]. Evolving leap has been occurred in medical educational curricula designing to cope patient care, clinician competency and local/global health service [28]. However, in each design there is still a gap which can be filled and remediated by coherence and interrelation between other elements included in the design [4]. Indeed, keening in the details of only one or two aspects prohibits clear viewing the whole process. It is the conception, regarding clinical curricula reforms, that is appeared in the current 21th century to construct overarching curricula [4]. This reminds me by Indian quote "Sometimes you just need to distance yourself to see things more clearly".

Diverse curricula frameworks have been arisen in modern era of medical education [29]. These curricula have endeavored to flourish professional practice which is composed of knowledge, skills and attitude based on adult learning theories and active teaching methods and are oriented by ecological and communities' circumstances [30, 31]. We will elucidate in the first subsection 3.1, Kern's six steps and outline PRISMS models being a recent and advanced framework in clinical education. Then, in the following subsection 3.2, we will invite you to create your conceptive curriculum thoughts in a way that integrates health systems within clinical training. This invitation will be through the catalyst which will be demonstrable in the novel creative 3P-6C toolkit [11].

3.1 Modern frameworks examples

3.1.1 Kern's six steps framework

Kern declared that, systematic approach helps profoundly in reaching the objectives. This systematic approach of curriculum design and development is formed of six steps in a sequence manner. However working on one step and looking at other step/s at the same time can promote the whole process by intersection between the targeted all steps [20, 29]. Six steps are usually started by **problem identification and general need assessment** [20] step while you are sitting back and contemplating on the whole situation. This helps in picking up *the start of the knot* (problem) based on health care problem, quality of clinical training, clinical outcome, and incongruent clinical practice with health care system and your community' needs. In this first step, it is important to identify who are affected by this problem (patients, learner, trainers, and administrators) and to reveal the current and the ideal approach to treat this problem [20, 32].

From the first step, identifying **target need assessment** being the second step is the cue and clue to construct goals and objectives in the third step. This step aims at assessing needs of two bases of education process; learners/stakeholders and learning environment. Learners' needs are detected by discovering their experiences, expectation, actual competencies and their learning style. Regarding learning environment, identifying availability of the required resources is inevitable to proceed in curriculum process, in addition to manifest barriers and enablers. Various methods for assessing needs can be achieved, for instance, by formal interviews, observation, informal discussion, audits and/ or questionnaires [20, 32, 33]. Without **goals and objectives**, content are not clearly structured, training methods and strategies cannot be chosen properly and assessment is got unfair. Goals aim at putting broad non measurable lofty vision of curriculum [20, 33]. Objectives target outcomes and have to be specific, measurable, attainable, realistic and timetable regarding cognitive, psychomotor and/or affective domains [34]. Levels of objective selection according to Bloom taxonomy are determined by the desired outcomes and needs assessment [35].

The fourth step; **educational strategies** pertain content with its resources and events, and plan to use multiple interactive teaching methods which are suitable to connect objectives with outcome depending on brain storming and metacognition [20, 29]. Going from the designed plan to achieving it is what is occurred in the fifth step; **implementation** wherein it checks resources for obtaining financial, administrative, material and political support in addition to addressing barriers to solve them. Piloting curriculum before executing it with friendly audience can be helpful to predict its success and to provide a chance for improvement and remediation [20, 32]. Last but not least, assessment is the sixth step where the curriculum is ended and is started by for development. **Assessment** is performed to assess learners and program using different summative and formative methods through the whole program. Learners' assessment depends on correlation between objectives and what they actually perform. On the other hand, program is assessed regarding the quantity and quality of every achieved step. All assessed data have to be collected and analyzed to be used for further **maintenance** (the seventh step) and **dissemination** (the eighth step) in other institutions locally and globally, in the case that this curriculum proves its success [20, 32].

Six steps kern's framework with the main elements of each step are outlined in **Figure 3**.

3.1.2 PRISMS model

By the start of 21th century, **PRISMS** model asserted on the importance of clinical practice reflection on clinical training program, integrating modern active teaching methods and modern technology in an evidence-based symbiotic learning, considering needs of learners, patients and health services. **PRISMS** acronym refers to the six elements of this model; wherein **P** refers to Product-based which means that learning focus on clinical practice rather isolated knowledge only and that assessment focus on doing rather knowing. **R** refers that learning has to be Relevant to learners,

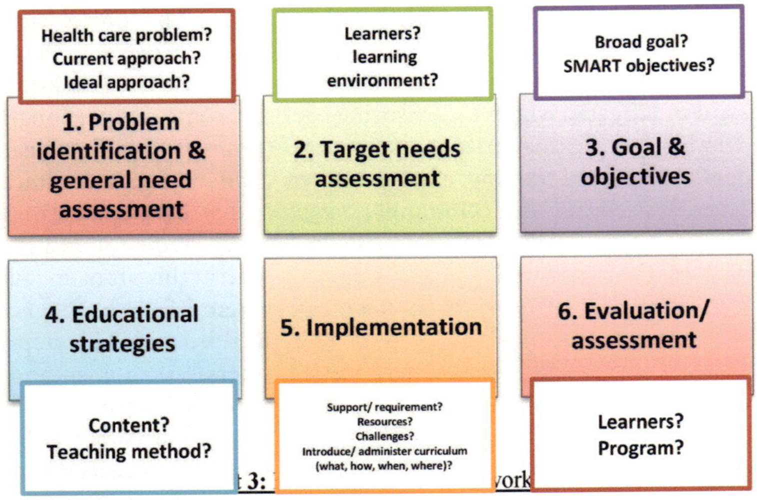

Figure 3.
Kern's six steps framework.

communities and updating evidence based knowledge, skills and behavior. **I** refers to inter-professional collaboration in learning process and teamwork role between clinical, academic research and administrative members. **S** refers to **S**horter courses duration of learning combined with **S**maller groups of learners to ensure interactive teaching and conform the millennium needs. **M** refers to **M**ultisite learning to expand learning from larger academic hospitals to involve rural areas and smaller hospitals and units using information technology. Lastly, **S** refers to **S**ymbiotic actions of the above five items to be incorporated with each other. Prideaux resembled PRISMS model by prism which encloses and radiates the light elements! [29, 36].

3.2 Upcoming system thinking curricula (3P-6Cs)

Awakening of consciousness and metacognition help in continuous probing and picking up gaps in previous plans to go through higher stages and to profound details to fill these gaps efficiently and effectively. This inducts what is continuously desired in medical curricula reforms in 21th century of coping with patients and learners needs, to overcome learning environment challenges and recently to integrate health system into clinical education process [37]. Curricula which are called system thinking curricula aim at filling gaps of health system to be attuned within clinical curricula. Thus, curricular designers, trainers and learners (clinician) are able to broaden their conception to regard health system needs parallel to the desired progressive life-long knowledge, skills and attitude outcomes [38], so the upcoming learning process tends to bind *ecology* with *clinic-ology*.

3P-6Cs Systems Thinking Toolkit is deemed a paradigm of soft thinking reforms that connects the all fragmented elements together in a comprehensive curriculum that is used in clinical training and practice to express how these elements work together [39]. 3P-6Cs systems thinking toolkit is assumed to be able to resist any affection by unpredicted environmental change. The acronym 3P refers to cohere between the main three aspect; **Personal** (learner or clinician learning), **Program** (curriculum outcome and assessment) and **Practice** (system and teamwork) [11].

So learners' **Personal** aspect reflects what they know, how they learn and assure their learning by assessment (**3C**: **C**ontent, **C**ognition and **C**onfirmation). **Program** aspect targets **6Cs** as the study reported; the first **3Cs** targets training outcomes, relation to contextual environment and what are the teaching methods and strategies (**3C**: **C**ommand, **C**ontextualization and **C**oordination) and the other **3Cs** targets the summative/formative assessment of each learner, connects different competencies and activities and relates all these to program evaluation (**3C**: **C**ollection, **C**ollation and **C**onnection). Finally, to close this connected circuit, **Practice** aspect calibrates learners outcome in relation to circumstances and program goals/objectives, assesses the role of teamwork/communication and confirms the existence of long-life learning through (**3C**: **C**alibration, **C**ollaboration and **C**ontinuous development) [11]. Although there is no enough evidence in real world that 3P-6C toolkit is more practical, but it is a great chance to assess this new perception in practice and to create new ones.

Footnote: *Designed clinical curricula are truncate without coherence of clinical knowledge with ecological, ethical, emotional, intellectual, social, societal contexts. Unleash your thoughts and apply new overarching reforms to foster attuned health system in clinical curricula.*

4. Conclusion

Clinical education no longer persuades by copying and imitation, hence creative overarching smart thoughts have been the ways for comprehensive improvement. Expressing and applying these thoughts in planned designs and realistic manner is an art which requires overview and in depth look in past, present and future clinical curricula. So, you, being curriculum designer or clinical educator, start now and unleash your thoughtful imagination and cultivate new thorough curricular design which emerges health system in clinical training curricula based on your practical experience and evidence based medical education research.

Conflict of interest

There is no conflict of interest.

Notes/thanks/other declarations

I would like to note that **Table 1**, **Figures 1–3** and footnotes are my work, and are not quoted or paraphrased from other references. The purpose of these footnotes is to get you overwhelmed that clinical education is not separated from daily life and other fields. They act like metaphors to make the meanings more obvious by interlinking medical to societal, psychological, administrative and even literary aspects which are not separated from daily practice.

I dedicate this work to my father's soul, my mother, my inspiring brother and my darling family.

Special thanks to the sincere multi-talented members of the team; (Training Of Teachers for medical education) at Princess Fatimah Academy at Egypt.

Appendices and nomenclature

PRISMS	Product based, Relevance to learners, Inter-professional collaboration, Shorter courses Smaller Groups, Multisite, Symbiosis.
3P-6Cs	(Personal, Program, Practice, Command, Contextualization and Coordination, Collection, Collation and Connection).

Author details

Samhaa Abd Elmoneim
Zagazig Ophthalmology Hospital, Ministry of Health, Zagazig, Egypt

*Address all correspondence to: dr.samhaa@yahoo.com

References

[1] Alsoufi, A., Alsuyihili, A., Msherghi, A., Elhadi, A., Atiyah, H., Ashini, A., ... & Elhadi, M. (2020). Impact of the COVID-19 pandemic on medical education: Medical students' knowledge, attitudes, and practices regarding electronic learning. PloS one, 15(11), e0242905.

[2] Han, E. R., Yeo, S., Kim, M. J., Lee, Y. H., Park, K. H., & Roh, H. (2019). Medical education trends for future physicians in the era of advanced technology and artificial intelligence: an integrative review. BMC medical education, 19(1), 1-15.

[3] Fallavollita, P. (2017). Innovative Technologies for Medical Education. Human Anatomy: Reviews and Medical Advances, 22-36.

[4] Buja, L. M. (2019). Medical education today: all that glitters is not gold. BMC medical education, 19(1), 1-11.

[5] Podzimek, M. (2019). Problems of narcissism in education: the culture of narcissism as a dangerous global phenomenon for the future. Problems of education in the 21st century, 77(4), 489.

[6] Herr, K. D., George, E., Agarwal, V., McKnight, C. D., Jiang, L., Jawahar, A., ... & Ganeshan, D. (2020). Aligning the Implicit Curriculum with the Explicit Curriculum in Radiology. Academic radiology, 27(9), 1268-1273.

[7] Koens, F., Mann, K. V., Custers, E. J., & Ten Cate, O. T. (2005). Analysing the concept of context in medical education. Medical education, 39(12), 1243-1249.

[8] Obadeji, A. (2019). Health professions education in the 21st century: A contextual curriculum framework for analysis and development. J Contemp Med Edu, 9(1), 34-40.

[9] General Medical Council. (2017). Excellence by design: standards for postgraduate curricula.

[10] Walsh, K. (Ed.). (2013). Oxford textbook of medical education. Oxford University Press.

[11] Khanna, P., Roberts, C., & Lane, A. S. (2021). Designing health professional education curricula using systems thinking perspectives. BMC Medical Education, 21(1), 1-8.

[12] Cooper, R. A., & Tauber, A. I. (2007). Values and ethics: A collection of curricular reforms for a new generation of physicians. Academic Medicine, 82(4), 321-323.

[13] Prideaux, D. (2003). Curriculum design. Bmj, 326(7383), 268-270.

[14] Fulton, J. F. (1953). History of medical education. British medical journal, 2(4834), 457.

[15] Yavuz, R., & TONTUŞ, H. (2014). Examinations and curriculum in medical education and learning-assessment relations. Journal of Experimental and Clinical Medicine, 31(1), 1-5.

[16] Leiser, G. (1983). Medical education in Islamic lands from the seventh to the fourteenth century. Journal of the History of Medicine and Allied Sciences, 38(1), 48-75.

[17] AL BINALI, H. A. H., ERDEMIR, A. D., KAADAN, A. N., Oncel, O., Aksoy, S., Al-Ghazal, S. K., ... & DOGAN, H. (2004). JOURNAL OF THE INTERNATIONAL SOCIETY FOR THE HISTORY OF ISLAMIC MEDICINE (JISHIM). JISHIM.

[18] Barzansky, B. (2010). Abraham Flexner and the era of medical education reform. Academic Medicine, 85(9), S19-S25.

[19] Stone, M. K. (1985). Ralph W. Tyler's principles of curriculum, instruction and evaluation: past influences and present effects.

[20] Thomas, P. A., Kern, D. E., Hughes, M. T., & Chen, B. Y. (Eds.). (2016). Curriculum development for medical education: a six-step approach. JHU Press\

[21] World Health Organization. (2009). WHO patient safety curriculum guide for medical schools.

[22] Plack, P. T., Margaret, M., & Scott, R. (2019). Systems thinking in the healthcare professions: A guide for educators and clinicians.

[23] Gonzalo, J. D., Haidet, P., Papp, K. K., Wolpaw, D. R., Moser, E., Wittenstein, R. D., & Wolpaw, T. (2017). Educating for the 21st-century health care system: an interdependent framework of basic, clinical, and systems sciences. Academic Medicine, 92(1), 35-39.

[24] English, J. (1990). Criteria for Comprehensive Health Education Curricula.

[25] Norman, G. (2017). The birth and death of curricula.

[26] Arja, S. (2017). Undergraduate Medical Education and Curricula. Immunother Res, 1(1), 3.

[27] Prideaux, D. (2003). ABC of learning and teaching in medicine. BMJ, 326(1), 268-270.

[28] Ten Cate, O. (2017). Competency-based postgraduate medical education: past, present and future. GMS journal for medical education, 34(5).

[29] Li-Sauerwine, S., & King, A. (2018). Curriculum development: Foundations and modern advances in graduate medical education. In Contemporary Topics in Graduate Medical Education. IntechOpen.

[30] Abela, J. C. (2009). Adult learning theories and medical education: a review.

[31] McCoy, L., Pettit, R. K., Kellar, C., & Morgan, C. (2018). Tracking active learning in the medical school curriculum: a learning-centered approach. Journal of medical education and curricular development, 5, 2382120518765135.

[32] Sweet, L. R., & Palazzi, D. L. (2015). Application of Kern's six-step approach to curriculum development by global health residents. Education for Health, 28(2), 138.

[33] Robertson, A. C., Fowler, L. C., Niconchuk, J., Kreger, M., Rickerson, E., Sadovnikoff, N., ... & Urman, R. D. (2019). Application of Kern's 6-Step Approach in the Development of a Novel Anesthesiology Curriculum for Perioperative Code Status and Goals of Care Discussions. The journal of education in perioperative medicine: JEPM, 21(1).

[34] Orgill, B. D., & Nolin, J. (2020). Learning Taxonomies in Medical Simulation.

[35] Adams, N. E. (2015). Bloom's taxonomy of cognitive learning objectives. Journal of the Medical Library Association: JMLA, 103(3), 152.

[36] Bligh, J., Prideaux, D., & Parsell, G. (2001). PRISMS: new educational strategies for medical education. Medical Education, 35(6), 520-521.

[37] Fernandez, C. M. (2012). Literature Review: Trends in 21st Century Medical Education. Touro College Lander Center for Educational Research, 1-4.

[38] Cabrera D, Colosi L, Lobdell C. Systems thinking. Eval Program Plann. 2008; 31(3):299-310.

[39] Pourdehnad, J., Wexler, E. R., & Wilson, D. V. (2011). Integrating systems thinking and design thinking. The Systems Thinker, 22(9), 2-6.

Chapter 7

Students Guided Learning for Medical Students - Novel Teaching for the 21st Century

Lior Naamati-Schneider and Adaya Meirovich

Abstract

The changing demands of the Western organizational and academic world are having a great impact on the medical profession. Adapting medical students' learning to as-yet-unknown future needs requires changes in learning objectives, methods, and assessment and the development of new skills. Students frequently express initial opposition to paradigms that require them to take responsibility for their learning process and invest greater effort. They may be uncooperative, and this may impede their training and the adoption of such changes in other courses. This qualitative study examines changes in attitudes toward student-centered learning among 120 medical students who experienced student-guided learning (SGL), a novel method emphasizing the student's primary role and self-expression, in a 3-unit course titled Patient–Therapist Relationship. The data were gathered from reflective journals the students kept during the course. The application of SGL methods resulted in changes in students' attitudes toward adopting new teaching methodologies. Their initial opposition was expressed in low motivation, lack of cooperation, negative attitudes toward assignments, and lack of motivation toward adopting changes. At the end of the course there was an improvement in students' openness to change, and they showed a greater desire and higher motivation to adopt new paradigms and innovative methodologies.

Keywords: Student-Guided learning (SGL), student centered learning (SCL), Life Long Learner, Innovative teaching methods, medical education

1. Introduction

The outbreak of the COVID-19 pandemic in December 2019 heightened the need of education systems worldwide to adapt rapidly to a changing situation and to the demands of the Western business and academic world. Even before that, the relevance of the teaching methods and content in academe was becoming increasingly crucial. To adapt learning to future needs that are changing and largely unknown today, we must change its goals, methods, and assessment [1, 2].

Academic institutions are more than transmitters of knowledge to students: They are also agents of cultural change. As such, they must consistently ensure that students develop new skills [3]. Adapting to the labor market requires 21st-century skills, such as problem solving in real time, synthesizing existing knowledge with changing situations, integrating material studied and applying it as part of a team, acquiring managerial abilities, and engaging in self-regulation [2]. Changes in teaching methods, combined with training in learning skills and construction of a learning toolbox, will enable students to remain relevant in the work force and become lifelong learners [4–6].

The outbreak of the COVID-19 pandemic created an opportunity for quickly introducing such changes by taking advantage of a variety of constraints, such as digital platforms and synchronous and asynchronous distance learning. This chapter describes an intervention program in the undergraduate course titled Patient–Therapist Relationship, taught in the Department of Management of Service Organizations, Health Track. The intervention changed the teaching and learning in the course from traditional frontal teaching to active student-centered learning. This chapter describes the effect of the intervention on students' perceptions, as revealed in reflective journals kept during the course, and students' willingness to adopt innovative teaching methodologies in the wake of this experience.

2. Theoretical background

The dominant conceptual approach today [7] is that most learning should be active so as to enhance the student's abilities and adapt them to the period and its demands [8]. This approach challenges both teachers and students because of the total change in the setting of learning goals and the perception of the learning process. The change requires a shift from teacher-centered pedagogical approaches to approaches in which the students and the development of their learning abilities are at the center. This shift constitutes an important element in adapting academic teaching to 21st-century needs and ensuring that the student becomes a lifelong learner [9].

Student-centered teaching methodologies have existed for years to various extents in educational institutions, but most teachers view them with suspicion and prefer to cling to traditional methodologies [10]. Resistance to student-centered methodologies exists at three levels: teachers, students, and the teaching environment. Many faculty members fear losing their power as the sole authority in learning and knowledge [11]. They also find it difficult to adapt curricula and courses to more innovative methods [12]. Students are deterred by the intensive work deriving from the requirement that they invest resources and time and take personal responsibility for the course of their studies [13]. In addition to this resistance to change on the part of faculty and students, often the academic learning environment does not make it easy to implement the necessary changes. Among these obstacles are budget constraints, a large number of students in a course, fear of students' objections to the many course requirements, research pressure, and other academic demands. All these create strong competition for the teacher's time and abilities [14]. These sources of resistance constitute an obstacle to implementing broad changes in academe, where the extent to which changes are adopted varies from one discipline to another.

3. The needs of the 21st century in medical education

The requirements of medical systems worldwide have changed in recent years along with global changes in the needs and demands of the general labor market [2]. The localized organizational changes that health organizations are undergoing as part of becoming patient-centered affect the character of the medical staff, medical management, and paramedical professions and training [15]. These changes require health-related higher education to adapt accordingly. This adaptation includes broadening students' set of abilities and skills and making them lifelong learners [16]. The set of abilities required in medical education includes coping with dilemmas, solving complex problems, teamwork capability, self-regulation, medical literacy, individual and managerial flexibility, and the ability to cope effectively daily with the challenges of a new and constantly changing world, under conditions of pressure and ever-expanding knowledge [17, 18].

The changes in the labor market's requirements and the consequent need to change teaching methods have moved the center of gravity in the class from the teacher to the student. This change is the basis for the change in approach in learning strategies. Student-guided learning (SGL) refers to a methodology that combines several teaching methodologies, such as problem- or project-based learning (PBL), cooperative learning, and creating a toolbox of skills. In using SGL, the student is guided by the teacher from the very beginning through the stages that include choosing a topic for the course and the learning materials, setting goals, students' acceptance of responsibility for the process of learning, and presentation of the product of learning. This methodology requires the teacher's constant supervision and oversight while leading the student on a long, active journey to the goals defined in the course [1].

Methodologically, SGL includes a combination of project-based learning [19] and models of learning collaboration. This combination enables the students to achieve a shared goal [20]. Achieving the goal requires positive interdependence among the students, in which each individual is responsible for his or her own learning and for the contribution to the group [21]. This learning emphasizes the process of learning and is characterized by active learning. The teacher is not the sole source of knowledge, and the learning is led by the students' choices, with direction from the teacher.

In SGL, the teacher sets the learning goals and broad topics that constitute the values and learning framework of the course. The study topics problem and cases to be written by students and will be presented within these boundaries. The teacher guides the student throughout the process [22].

This methodology has nine stages that constitute points for guidance and interface between teacher and student: describing an individual's experience, turning the experience into an event or dilemma, making the student an expert in the selected area/building a knowledge base, learning collaboratively, discussing and decision-making as a group, carrying out a summary project, presenting the project by the group, and evaluating the project by peers. This semester-long process is accompanied by maintenance of a reflective journal that describes the process of individual and group learning [1].

4. The current study and its methodology

This qualitative study used a case study of the implementation of an intervention program in the course titled Patient–Therapist Relationship. The case study, through observations and data gathering, makes it possible to draw conclusions regarding human activity [23]. The data gathered describe patterns and attitudes that enable understanding of broader phenomena. Analysis of the data gathered in categories at two time points makes it possible to form generalizations and deductions on the basis of quotations from the data [24, 25].

4.1 Participants

The participants were 120 students in a three-credit course titled Patient–Therapist Relationship. The students are second-year undergraduates in the department of Management of Service Organizations, with a subspecialty in health.

The course content pertains to the patient–therapist relationship in health contexts and how it is meaningful in healing and support.

The data in this chapter were gathered in four courses over two academic years. The courses were taught simultaneously by both authors. The data were gathered at two time points: the beginning of the course, before the students had any experience of the teaching method, and the end. The students were told that the materials would be analyzed anonymously and that they were free to refuse to allow the use of the materials for research purposes.

4.2 The intervention program

The SGL methodology—a combination of problem-based learning (PBL) and collaborative-learning methodologies—is at the heart of the intervention program. This intervention program focuses on a dilemma in the profession, based on the personal experience of the student, with an emphasis on experiences related to patient–therapist relationships. The use of this personal basis make possible an immediate and personal connection to the course content combined with acquisition of knowledge and development of critical thinking in a PBL environment [19, 26]. The students, divided into groups, examine the experience/dilemma from three perspectives characteristic of the course: the clinician, the patient, and the organization. Each student is responsible for sharing with the group the data he or she has gathered at each stage of the program. In this way, the students become experts within the group on their knowledge area. Sharing with the group enables a broadening of the members' knowledge, collaborative learning, discussion, and group decision-making. The process makes the students experts in their area as they prepare to present the final project (including the intermediate stages) to the other students in the course. The final project presents by digital visual mean—for example, a digital poster or a digital thought map—the examination of the selected experience from three perspectives (therapist, patient, organization). The last stage of the program is the peer review, in which the students evaluate each other in accordance with guidelines set in advance [1]. Students are also asked to maintain a reflective journal and to record in it their individual learning process in each stage of the project, describing their experiences, feelings, attitudes, and challenges.

4.3 Data analysis

The students' reflective journals were collected and analyzed at two time points: the start of the course and its conclusion. The texts underwent thematic analysis, which leads to categorization of the text. The relations between the categories were examined and mapped, and the two time points were compared. In this process, information is constructed and interpreted [27, 28]. Categories were constructed by identifying main themes and consolidating them in main categories. The following is a description of the main categories and the change in the students' perceptions and attitudes regarding the innovative learning methodology.

5. Findings

The content analysis of the reflective journals revealed six main categories: active learning as opposed to passive learning, previous experience of active learning, feeling of capability, collaboration, a learning experience, and adopting innovative learning methodologies. The analysis of the findings is presented by category in relation to the two time points.

5.1 Active learning as opposed to passive learning

At the first time point, most of the students wrote that their previous experience was largely of passive learning. Thus, for example, they noted that the structure of the course was new to them and that they were used, generally, to other teaching methods:

> *I'm full of anxiety about the learning because it is much easier to learn in frontal learning. I prefer getting the material from the teacher and not having to search for some of the material.*

> *This is the first time that I personally am learning with this method. Usually the teacher gives us the material for the whole semester.*

> *I'm already used to learning differently, used to receiving the material, learning for an exam and then for a final exam, or doing homework on the material taught and then taking a final exam.*

> *My feelings about the manner of the course are complicated. They evoke various feelings because it's a new style and different from what we were used to until now.*

> *The method I jibe with the most is the traditional method of frontal teaching: learning on set days and hours in a classroom facing the lecturer with exercises and an exam—unlike independent learning in which there is no set time for study and therefore I tend to procrastinate until the last minute.*

At the first time point, the students pointed out their anxiety and fear regarding the innovative teaching method and the assignments and difficulties that lay ahead, in their view, from studying in this manner.

> *When we started the course I walked into the classroom with anxieties and fears. I'm a third-year student and I'm making up a course with second-year students whom I don't know. It's hard enough already ... definitely with this method of learning, with many assignments in a group.*

> *True, this is an opportunity for me to contend with the fear and face the commitment that the course requires, but I'm not certain I'll be able to express myself fully.*

> *I was anxious because in the exam we are required to regurgitate in writing material that we've learned throughout the semester, whereas a paper requires you to gather articles from various sources and sometimes even in other languages (something that in itself frightens me).*

In the examination of this category at the second time point, it seemed that most of the students related to the course as a positive experience. They revealed that, despite their initial concerns, they succeeded in coping well with the learning processes and the assignments.

> *In the beginning it seemed beyond my abilities and rather exhausting, but after we got the first assignment I discovered that it was actually a pleasant and interesting assignment. This teaching method made me remember an event and reconstruct the feelings I experience during it and thus gave me a different perspective on the event.*

In the beginning there was anxiety over this learning format which is not necessarily for an exam, "blind learning" just to answer questions automatically, but rather, really, a true process of learning with yourself, with other students in the class as a team, and actually causes the student to be more involved in the assignments in the course of the semester and also to be more involved socially and mutually with the group members.

The students also pointed out the difficulties; these included the level of difficulty involved in active learning, the level of involvement in the course, and the time commitment in such learning.

It's much easier to get the material from the lecturer.

It was hard for me to think on my own how I should find the material.

Undoubtedly this course requires a greater investment than do other courses that are taught frontally. We had to invest more time.

5.2 The experience of active learning

Already at the first time point, students with previous experience of this method noted that their prior positive experience was a mediating factor that eased their learning.

From my past experience, when I wrote a paper it helped me to understand the material better. And like this project, it helps me because every student can say what helps them learn, more or less, and also the students have an opinion about which method is good for studying.

I already had experience with a course in which you had to work independently, so I was less scared.

5.3 Adopting innovative teaching methodologies

Adapting to innovative learning methodologies often sparks antagonism and concerns, as was evident in the reflective journals and was presented above. The students wrote that they were used to relying on learning by receiving material from the lecturer. This learning process was seen as easier, in comparison to the process of active learning. This worldview is presented in the analysis of the students' reflections at the first time point:

There's tremendous pressure of papers during the semester. Therefore I prefer not to be part of a large project but simply to write an exam.

It's preferable to write one exam, and that's it. I have no desire to work like this.

It scares me to deviate from the usual drill of an exam and to write a paper instead. True, the lecturer explained in class that the paper would be submitted in a process that she supervised, but still there is the concern that I will make a mistake and will not do things properly because I'm not used to writing papers. I think it takes more time than studying for an exam, because there's always something that [needs to be] changed or improved.

At the second time point, toward the end of the semester, because of the positive experience the students had in the course, one can see a change in their attitudes and their willingness to adopt innovative methodologies. Thus, for example:

We've come a long way, but I have the desire to learn more.

I feel that I want to learn like this in other courses.

I really loved how the course was taught. The assignments we have had thus far give us an opportunity to express ourselves and are not too burdensome.

Nevertheless, students still note difficulties and challenges, which they ascribe to this method and which will make it difficult, in their view, to adopt innovative methods in the future.

The planned teaching method is interesting and breaks up the routine, and in my view it will be nice and will lead to a deeper understanding of the material. In my view, when it is fun to learn, the material is absorbed better. But on the other hand, getting used each time to a different learning method can be confusing and take up a lot of time.

5.4 The learning experience

This category appeared in the analysis of the reflections at the second time point, in which the students wrote their views of the learning experience in the course in comparison to courses with frontal teaching.

The method of study is a breath of fresh air in comparison to the lessons that are frontal only and tend to be boring. In the lesson there is lively discussion by everyone, with personal experiences that contribute to the learning atmosphere.

I am very satisfied that there is a course like this in which the teaching method is different from the usual. It allows you to formulate opinions, feelings, and various reflections.

For example, this exercise enables me to speak freely, think, and be creative. I feel free and confident that I can speak and also recommend and suggest new ideas.

The course is different and I interpret this as refreshing and as a different way of learning that has thought behind it. On the one hand, it really enabled us, the students, to contend with assignments that require thought and to be active partners in the lesson and the entire course, and not just to mark our attendance. I see this as something very positive, especially since it's a very important lesson for the profession we chose and which we'll probably work in in the future.

5.5 A sense of capability

The beginning of the course was accompanied by fears, concerns, and even hesitation regarding the capability of completing the course and meeting its goals. "I asked not to have to present." "I really didn't think I would succeed."

Such feelings were not evident in the analysis of the reflections at the second time point.

Although I didn't think that I would want to present, I enjoyed it and wasn't even concerned about presenting before the president of the college.

I surprised myself while presenting the project.

I think that the time has come to work this way, to prepare both an individual paper and a group paper and to present what we prepared, and to be exposed directly to the responses and questions of the audience, lecturers, students.

5.6 Teamwork/collaborative learning

The analysis of the reflective journals at the first time point showed that the students related also to the category of collaborative learning and to teamwork, and noted diverse attitudes toward them.

I like to work in a group because there is support from the team members and exposure to a range of different ideas. Also, if there is something I didn't understand in a certain way, there are other people who can interpret it.

I see the work in groups as something slightly threatening: Beyond the grade that is given for it, it requires interaction and contending with other people. I'm a person for whom it is easy to express myself when I am not in a group. Perhaps I am different from many others and my coping is different in this respect, but I'm a little hesitant about it.

At the second time point, too, the students addressed this category, indicating the problems and challenges in relation to it, on the basis of their experience. Their opinions regarding this category were varied. Some wrote that they prefer working on their own, whereas others wrote that the experience of learning in groups was positive for them.

For me the work in groups was less convenient because to this day I have proved to myself that I work better on my own. I rely only on my own work ... I felt that most of the work anyway fell on my shoulders so that the work didn't take less time, it took even longer than usual.

It's hard for me to coordinate a time that is convenient and suits everyone to sit and discuss the assignment. And in the end, even when you succeed in setting a time with everyone a lot of time is wasted on chitchat—unlike my own work in which I work according to a timetable that is convenient for me.

Learning in groups helps a lot in understanding the material because each one explains the material in a way that everyone can understand.

6. Discussion

The analysis of the students' reflective journals at two time points, the beginning and end of the course, showed a change in attitudes. At the start of the process, their attitudes toward adopting innovative methodologies of teaching were based on perceptions and attitudes formed in response to their acquaintance with traditional teaching methods. At this stage, the students' worldview was determined, inter alia, by the teaching methods customary in the process of socialization, starting with the preschool, through elementary school, high school, and academe. These attitudes shaped their perception of teaching methods and contributed to their resistance and concerns regarding the adoption of other teaching methods.

During the course, while using SGL methodology, and at the end, the students displayed a change in attitudes, perceptions, and experiences in relation to adopting active teaching methodologies and the process of individual learning. Also, students who had studied in the past with this method, or who had prior experience with various methods of active learning, showed from the start less resistance and greater willingness to cooperate with this teaching method.

Support for the findings can be found in earlier studies on the student-centered class, according to which students reveal behaviors characteristic of the stages of mourning and trauma at being forced to take responsibility and a degree of independence in learning as an alternative to the use of traditional learning methodologies [29].

The students' responses are subjective. Some went through all the stages smoothly, whereas others remained a longer time in a specific stage, or in several of them. Passage through the various stages of the program is essential and constitutes a substantial part in the student's growth and turning into a lifelong learner [30, 31]. Therefore, the aim is to lower the level of resistance, on the one hand, and to ease the process of independent learning, on the other. Students should be allowed this type of learning as part of a structured, guided framework [23].

The students' attitudes toward collaborative learning also changed. In the beginning of the course many students wrote that because of the difficulties and challenges in the process, they rely primarily on themselves and prefer to carry out the assignments and learning processes on their own. At the end of the experience, the students wrote that the collaborative learning contributed to their feeling of vitality, their openness, and their ability to learn from others. As the learning process continued, the students were exposed through a collaborative learning framework to a variety of opinions of group members. This process exposed the complexity of the dilemma and the understanding that it might have various interpretations and various solutions [32].

7. Conclusions

This study examined the change that took place in the attitudes of students following an intervention program that changed the teaching framework in a course from frontal learning to SGL methodology, which combines PBL with collaborative learning [1]. The study demonstrated how attitudes can be changed and resistance and concerns can be reduced with regard to adopting innovative teaching methodologies, while creating a positive collaborative experience of active learning.

The use of SGL methodology, which enables individual learning as described in this chapter, offers a learning framework that is structured but sufficiently broad, combined with leadership and clear guidance by the lecturer. Choosing the dilemma relevant to the course content on the basis of students' experiences (personal stories) enables them to connect individually to the topic studied and to maximize their learning abilities. These experiences contribute to changing the perceptions and obstacles to adopting innovative teaching methodologies like this one. In addition, they expose the students to a positive experience of learning and to a sense of capability. All these lead to the removal of students' resistance and to their willingness and desire to adopt innovative active-learning methodologies.

It is very important to adapt learning and teaching methods to the changing needs of the labor market and the academic world. Adopting these methodologies, in which the emphasis in learning moves to the student and the lecturer's role becomes more of a support and guide, encountered students' resistance, negative attitudes, and low motivation to adopt them [12, 26, 31].

Widespread adoption of such methodologies in academe, and in medical education in particular, is a step toward making academe more relevant than ever and training graduates suited to a changing market. Adopting methodologies of active learning such as SGL from the earliest stages of professional training may increase the potential for change and transform students into lifelong learners, thus enabling graduates in the field of health to cope better with the future needs of the health system.

Author details

Lior Naamati-Schneider* and Adaya Meirovich
Department of Management of Service Organizations, Health Track, Hadassah Academic College, Jerusalem, Israel

*Address all correspondence to: liorna@hac.ac.il

References

[1] Schneider LN, Meirovich A. Student Guided Learning: From teaching to E-learning. Revista Romaneasca pentru Educatie Multidimensionala. 2020;12(1Sup2):115-121. DOI: https://doi.org/10.18662/rrem/12.1sup2/254

[2] Alt, D, Naamati-Schneider L. Health management students' self-regulation and digital concept mapping in online learning environments. BMC Medical Education. 2021; 21:10. https://doi.org/10.1186/s12909-021-02542-w

[3] Bruffee KA. Collaborative Learning: Higher Education, Interdependence, and the Authority of Knowledge. 2nd ed. Baltimore, Md.: Johns Hopkins University Press; 1999. 344 p.

[4] Friedman T. The World Is Flat: A Brief History of the Twenty-first Century. New York: Farrar, Straus and Giroux; 2007. 660 p.

[5] Vaira M. Globalization and higher education organizational change: A framework for analysis. Higher Education. 2004;48:483-510. DOI:10.1023/B:HIGH.0000046711.31908.e5

[6] McArthur JW, Sachs J. Needed: A new generation of problem solvers. Chronicle of Higher Education. 2009;55:1-4. Available from https://www.chronicle.com/article/needed-a-new-generation-of-problem-solvers/

[7] McWilliam E. (2017). Today's children, tomorrow's creatives: Living, learning and earning in the conceptual age. In: Choo, S, Sawch D, Villanueva A, Vinz R, editors. Educating for the 21st Century. Singapore: Springer. p. 7-23.

[8] Harris N, Bacon CEW. Developing cognitive skills through active learning: A systematic review of health care professions. Athletic Training Education Journal. 2019;14:135-148. https://doi.org/10.4085/1402135http://doi.org/10.4085/1402135

[9] Donahue–Di Conti V. Experiential education in a knowledge-based economy: Is it time to reexamine the liberal arts? Journal of General Education. 2004;53:167-183. DOI: 10.1353/jge.2005.0003

[10] Johnson A, Kimball R, Melendez B, Myers L, Rhea K, Travis B. Breaking with tradition: Preparing faculty to teach in a student-centered or problem-solving environment. Primus. 2009;19:146-160. https://doi.org/10.1080/10511970802409164

[11] Estes CA. Promoting student-centered learning in experiential education. Journal of Experiential Education. 2004;27:141-160. https://doi.org/10.1177/105382590402700203

[12] Breunig M. Turning experiential education and critical pedagogy theory into praxis. Journal of Experiential Education. 2005;28:106-122. https://doi.org/10.1177/105382590502800205

[13] Weimer M. Learner-centered Teaching: Five Key Changes to Practice. San Francisco: Jossey Bass; 2002. 258 p. Available from https://tlap.ksu.edu.sa/sites/tlap.ksu.edu.sa/files/attach/ref17.pdf

[14] White FA. Tenure and promotion 101: What you need to know. 2008. (ERIC Document Reproduction Service No. ED502681).

[15] Naamati-Schneider L. Strategic management as adaptation to changes in the ecosystems of public hospitals in Israel. Israel Journal of Health Policy Research. 2020;9:65. https://doi.org/10.1186/s13584-020-00424-y

[16] Reis S. The doctor in the digital age: competencies needed and a road map for their achievement [review].

Harefuah. 2019;158:648-53. Hebrew. PMID: 31576710

[17] Vaira M. Globalization and higher education organizational change: A framework for analysis. Higher Education. 2004;48:483-510. DOI:10.1023/B:HIGH. 0000046711.31908.e5

[18] Friedman T. The World Is Flat: A Brief History of the Twenty-first Century. New York: Farrar, Straus and Giroux; 2007. 660 p.

[19] Jalinus N, Nabawi RA, Mardin A. The seven steps of project based learning model to enhance productive competences of vocational students. In International Conference on Technology and Vocational Teachers (ICTVT 2017). 2017;251-256. https://doi.org/10.2991/ ictvt-17.2017.43

[20] Brody CM, Davidson N. Introduction. In: Brody CM, Davidson, N, editors: Professional Development for Cooperative Learning: Issues and Approaches. Ithaca, NY: State University of New York Press; 1998. ERIC Number: ED422319

[21] Slavin RE. Instruction based on cooperative learning. In: Mayer R, editor, Handbook of Research on Learning and Instruction. London: Taylor and Francis; 2010. p. 344-360.

[22] Utecht JR. (2003). Problem-based learning in the student-centered classroom. Research in Education Journals. Available from http://www. jeffutecht. com/docs/PBL. pdf

[23] Yin RK. Case Study Research Design and Methods (5th ed.). Thousand Oaks, CA: Sage; 2014. 282 p.

[24] Lincoln YS., Guba EG. Naturalistic Inquiry. Beverly Hills, CA: Sage;1985. 416 p.

[25] Strauss A, Corbin J. Grounded theory methodology: An overview. In: Denzin NK, Lincoln YS, editors. Handbook of Qualitative Research. Sage;1994. p. 273-285.

[26] Woods DR. Problem-based Learning: How to Gain the Most from PBL. Waterdown, Ontario: Woods Publishing; 1994. Distributed by McMaster University Bookstore.

[27] Shkedi A, editor. The Meaning behind the Words: Methodologies of Qualitative Research: Theory and Practice. Tel Aviv, Israel: Ramot—Tel Aviv University; 2011. Hebrew.

[28] Shleski S, Alpert B. Paths in Writing Qualitative Research: From Deconstruction of the Reality to Construction of the Text. Tel Aviv, Israel: Mofet Institute; 2007. Hebrew

[29] Utecht, JR. Problem-based learning in the student centered classroom. 2003. Retrieved from http://www.jeffutecht. com/docs/PBL. pdf

[30] Kloss, RJ. A nudge is best: Helping students through the Perry scheme of intellectual development. College Teaching. 1994;424:151-158. https://doi. org/10.1080/87567555.1994.9926847

[31] Hains BJ, Smith B. Student -centered course design: Empowering students to become self-directed learners. Journal of Experiential Education. 2012; 35:357-374. https://doi.org/10.1177/ 105382591203500206

[32] Kim HY, LaRusso MD, Hsin LB, Harbaugh AG, Selman RL, Snow CE. Social perspective-taking performance: Construct, measurement, and relations with academic performance and engagement. Journal of Applied Developmental Psychology. 2018; 57: 24-41. https://doi.org/10.1016/j. appdev.2018.05.005

Chapter 8

Congruence of Nurse Staffing and Activities with Patient Needs

Melita Peršolja

Abstract

This study aimed to discover the correlation between patient satisfaction with nursing care activities and staffing patterns. The research was conducted at the medical ward of a secondary care regional hospital in Slovenia over one month. Data was collected with regard to the following: (1) patients cared for daily and number of hours/patients day at the ward level, (2) patient needs (using a classification system), (3) nurse activities as observed at 10-minute intervals, and (4) the Patient Perception of Hospital Experience with Nursing tool. A total of 218 patients were involved, and their satisfaction with nursing care was found to be high. Patient satisfaction was negatively correlated with the number of patients cared for at the unit daily, but positively with the number of care hours per patient day, the proportion of registered nurses in the nursing team, the realized percentage of the registered nurse personnel requirements, and with some direct care activities. The correlation also revealed three process items (undivided attention, explanation, and things are done without asking) being the special strengths of nursing care activities. The results show that nurse-staffing and process patterns affect patient experience. It is thus recommended to increase the amount of nursing care offered by registered nurses, while nurses' competences can affect the process of care, and thus patient satisfaction.

Keywords: evidence-based healthcare management, nursing service hospital, patient satisfaction, quality of healthcare

1. Introduction

Patient satisfaction with hospital care has been defined as the degree of alignment between the care expected and actual care received, as perceived by patients [1]. Nurses have thus been recognized as the key factors influencing patient satisfaction because they are involved in almost every aspect of the healthcare process [2]. Although nursing care processes are integrated with other healthcare processes, when the quality of nursing care is poor, patients' satisfaction has been found to be low [3].

The use of a good structure increases the likelihood of good processes, and good processes increase the likelihood of good outcomes [4]. The best criteria with regard to reflecting the structure and process of nursing care and the related patient outcomes are the nursing-sensitive indicators [5]. The literature describes two general nursing-sensitive patient outcomes: adverse and positive. Some adverse patient outcomes that are potentially sensitive to nursing care are urinary tract infections, pneumonia, shock, upper gastrointestinal bleeding, longer hospital stays, failure to rescue, and 30-day mortality [6]. The main positive nursing-sensitive patient outcome is patient satisfaction with nursing care quality.

Structure in a healthcare context refers to the attributes of various material resources (facilities, equipment, money), human resources (supply of nursing staff, the skill level of staff, education of staff), and organizational factors (staff organization, methods of peer review, methods of reimbursement). In contrast, process denotes what is done in giving and receiving care. It includes patient activities in seeking care and receiving it, as well as practitioner activities in making the diagnosis and recommending or implementing treatment. An outcome denotes the effects of care on the health status of patients, including improvements in the patients' knowledge, and positive changes in their health status and behavior, as well as greater patient satisfaction with care [4].

According to the Donabedian model [7], some nursing care structural and process features are associated with the quality of care and thus capable of increasing patient satisfaction in hospitals. Regarding structure, the number of patients per nurse in a hospital [8–10], the nursing care hours per patient day [11], the proportion of registered nurses [8, 12], and the presence of registered or specialist nurses [13–15] all influence the quality of care as perceived by patients. Researchers have also associated nurse staffing with various patient, suggesting that a higher proportion of registered nurses could reduce preventable in-hospital deaths [8, 16–18], prevent falls [15], decrease the percentage of care left undone [19], and increase patient satisfaction [8–10]. Regarding the relevant processes, the total amount of direct patient care [20, 21], frequency of communication [22, 23], and organizational priorities with regard to the quality of care [8] have also been documented as affecting patients' satisfaction with nursing care.

However, the amount of nursing care and the mix of skills of the staff providing it are only proxy measures for what the nursing staff actually does daily at the bedside, and nursing activities can include both contact and no-contact time, as well as unproductive time [24]. In fact, according to published studies hospital nurses spend from 7.3% [25] to 54.2% [26] of their time on direct patient care, from 0% [27] to 59% [28] on indirect care, and from 14% to 17% on personal time [29]. Patient satisfaction is influenced by factors identified at the patient level [2, 30–33] along with nurses' kindness and competence with regard to performing technical procedures [34]. When items in the instrument represent patients' perceptions, there are no criteria against which criterion-related validity could be tested [3].

In Slovenia, a post transitional European country, the number of practicing nurses per 1 000 population is 8.8, and the ratio of nurses to physicians is 3.2 [35]. The problem is that when officially counting the number of nursing professionals, the nursing assistants (called health technicians) are included, and therefore the ratio between registered nurses and health technicians (which is currently 35:65) is in favor of the latter [36]. The Slovenian Chamber of Nursing and Midwifery prepared a proposal of human norms, where one of the four basic criteria was the calculation of staff needs resulting from patient classification system [37]. But although the percentage of categorized patients in hospitals is high, the collected data are not used for staff planning [38].

2. Aim

This study aimed to examine the connection between nurse staffing patterns, their process characteristics and the quality of care with regard to patient satisfaction with the nursing care received.

The specific objectives of this study were: [1] to identify the relevant nursing staff structural conditions (patient to nurse ratios, skill mix, and educational level); [2] to examine the nursing care activities performed by distinguishing those direct and indirect care activities; [3] to examine patients' actual nursing care needs; and [4] to measure patient outcomes (with a focus on satisfaction with the nursing care received).

It was assumed that higher nurse staffing and more direct care activities are associated with an increased likelihood of meeting patient needs, and that higher perceptions of fulfilled needs would be reflected in higher patient satisfaction with nursing care.

3. Methods

3.1 Study design

A cross-sectional study was conducted in a Slovenian secondary care regional hospital, in 2014.

3.2 Setting

The researched hospital had 24 specialty departments with approximately 400 beds. Approximately 350 nursing care personnel rendered the services (mostly nursing technicians (n = 224; 66.47%), with a third of them being registered nurses (n = 103; 30.57%) and ten of them (2.97%) being support staff. The hospital dealt with nearly 15,000 prospective payment system episodes in one year. The annual bed occupancy was approximately 80%. This research focused on a medical ward with three units, a 94-bed capacity and nearly five hundred (n = 498) hospitalized patients during the research month. The medical unit participated in this study based on the criteria identified by a hospital expert advisory panel. The unit was selected based on the feasibility of the research process and the availability of participants. The hospital was anonymized at the request of the management of the institution.

3.3 Participants

As the study target, two populations were identified: (a) nursing staff and (b) patients.

a. Nursing staff: All registered nurses and nursing technicians (hereafter called *nursing staff*) were eligible. All nursing staff participated as subject matter experts over a total of nine observational days in one month. Sample size (43 subjects) was calculated based on the confidence level (95%), confidence interval (5%), and the number of total nursing staff employed (45 individuals) in the medical department. Two subjects (the department head nurse and an unlicensed practitioner) were excluded from the study because of their specific tasks.

b. Patients: A sample size of 217 subjects was calculated (confidence level (95%), confidence interval (5%), with an expected patient population of around 500 individuals in a one-month observation period). Therefore, all patients who were (I) admitted to the ward for at least 24 hours, (II) staying in the medical ward during the study period, (III) capable of communicating, and (IV) willing to participate, were invited to take part in the study. Out of the total 484 patients admitted to the ward during the study period, 218 were eligible.

On the research day, the researcher personally contacted all hospitalized patients capable of communicating. The patients were informed that a *study on nursing care* was being conducted, and offered the name of the person responsible and their contact details when requested, and provided with details regarding what would happen to the information provided. If willing to cooperate, patients were offered a questionnaire to complete. When a patient was unable or unwilling to participate, one of their visitors was invited to complete the questionnaire instead.

3.4 Variables

3.4.1 Records

The daily census report, bed occupancy, and patient needs classification using the Slovenian patient classification system [39] were collected from the hospital every day. Data from nursing schedules and hospitalized patient numbers allowed the calculation of the number of patients per nursing staff (registered nurse, nursing technician), staff hours per patient day (registered nurse, nursing technician), and the proportion of graduate nursing staff hours. The principal investigator of the study collected data daily after the study approval and by contacting the chief nurse.

3.4.2 Observations

At the nursing staff level, we used the Maribor Primary Health Care Patient Classification System instrument to measure the nursing care activities performed [40]. This instrument measures the nursing care activities divided into four categories:

1. Care contact time (direct patient care) includes all hands-on care, one-to-one observation or support for patients, and direct communication with patients.

2. Indirect contact time (indirect patient care) includes patient documentation, professional discussions to plan patient care, discharge planning, communication with patients' relatives and friends, ordering investigations, and shift handovers.

3. Other nursing activities: other patient-focused activities (completing nursing audits, checking clinical equipment), staff-focused activities (student support, giving and receiving training sessions, personal development reviews, rounds), and ward-focused activities (ensuring environmental safety and cleanliness, ordering or unpacking stock).

4. Unproductive time: personal staff time (staff meals, breaks) and wasted time (waiting for equipment, waiting for colleagues, etc.).

For the aims of the study, we planned 16 hours of observations in the research days, including morning and afternoon shifts (from 06:00 to 22:00). Observations were performed in such a way that all working days of the week were included in a range of one month, randomly selected by the principal investigator of the study. Throughout the observations, activities were recorded at intervals of 10 minutes (allowing six observations per hour). Data collection was performed by 18 third-year pre-trained nursing students who previously had at least eight weeks of clinical practice at the ward.

3.4.3 Survey

At the patient level, the 15-Item Single-Factor Patient Perception of Hospital Experience with Nursing (PPHEN) [3] tool was used. The tool was developed in the English language, and was translated into Slovenian according to standard procedures for forward and backward translation [41]. The tool was piloted in a preliminary way in a group of 15 patients (not involved in this study) to test its comprehensibility and feasibility. The Cronbach's alpha for the PPHEN questionnaire in the Slovenian language was 0.905 (n = 15).

Patients' satisfaction was reported using a five-point Likert scale (1 = strongly disagree/not at all satisfied, 5 = strongly agree/completely satisfied). The responses to this were then turned into a patient satisfaction index including all the variables and ranging from 1 to 5, with higher scores indicating a higher degree of satisfaction with nursing care. Patients also answered some questions exploring demographic variables (e.g., age and gender) as well as data regarding whether the respondent was the patient or one of their relatives.

The questionnaires were distributed by nine third-year nursing students, who were not included in direct observations or in nursing care. On the research days, nursing activities were observed, and the patients included in the study (or their relatives) were invited to complete the questionnaire.

3.5 Ethics

Institutional review board approval was obtained from the Faculty of Health Sciences, University of Primorska, Slovenia, and from the hospital administration prior the start of the study. The study was conducted following the Code of Ethics for Nurses and Nurse Assistants, as well as the Declaration of Helsinki: Ethical Principles for Medical Research Involving Human Subjects [42]. Patient and nurse consent was obtained on-site.

3.6 Statistical methods

Reliability was reached in the data analysis, with the exclusion of three of the nine (i.e., 30%) previously selected observational days. These days were selected casually in advance before the data collection phase. Only the principal investigator was aware of which days were chosen. Therefore, a total of 7,732 (78.4%) out of 9,866 observed nursing activities were used in the final analysis. As a consequence, 149 (68.4%) out of the total of 218 gathered questionnaires were used.

Exploratory data analyses were performed to inspect the data and identify inconsistencies. IBM SPSS Statistics, version 21.0 (IBM Corp., Group NY, USA) was used for data analysis to consider the three levels of analyses, namely: the hospital unit, the individual nurse, and the patient. Preliminary data analyses were completed using descriptive and bivariate analysis techniques.

Quantitative data analysis was performed using descriptive methods: mean (M), standard deviation (SD), frequency (n), percentage (%), Pearson's correlation (r), and Spearman's correlation (R). Correlation strengths were set as follows: 0–0.09 not correlated, 0.1–0.3 weak, 0.31–0.6 medium, and 0.61–1 strong correlation [43]. The significance was set at $p < 0.05$.

4. Results

4.1 Nursing structure

Seven registered nurses worked regularly across the observed medical ward, aided by 36 nursing technicians. Therefore, a total of 43 individuals participated in this study, representing 95.6% of the nursing population.

In the 94 available beds there were, on average, 80 patients/day. The nursing teams consisted mostly of nursing technicians (64%), which delivered 61.3% of nursing care. Each member of nursing staff cared for an average of three patients/day, and every registered nurse was responsible for an average of 8.5 patients/day.

The mean number of nursing staff hours per patient day was 3.64 hours, of which 1.41 hours were provided by registered nurses. The average percentage of registered nurse hours was 38.74%, ranging from 38.05% to 39.9% of total nursing staff hours (**Table 1**).

4.2 Nursing care process

About 36.8% (n = 2,842) of all nursing staff activities involved direct contact with patients, and hands-on care represented 27.5% of all recorded nursing activities. One-to-one observation was identified 336 times (4.2%), direct communication with patients 294 times (3.8%), and support being given to patients 98 times (1.3%).

About 18.5% of all nursing activities were indirect patient care. A large number of these were represented by dealing with patient documentation, professional discussion to plan patients' care, discharge planning, and communication with patients' relatives and friends (n = 538, 6.9%). Shift handovers were identified 469 times (6.1%) and ordering investigations and preparing for medical/technical procedures performed independently by nursing staff were recorded 425 times (5.5%).

Other nursing activities were recorded 2,013 times (26%): patient-focused activities 1,470 times (19%), ward-focused activities 446 times (5.8%), and staff-focused activities 97 times (1.2%). Unproductive time represented 9.5% (n = 735) of all observed activities, including personal staff time (n = 729, 9.4%) and wasted time (n = 6, 0.1%). Information was missing with regard to staff activities for 9.2% of the observations (n = 710) (**Table 2**).

Independent Variable / Constant	**Total**	
	n	**%**
Total hospitalized patients[1] (average/day)	484 (80.67)	100
Category 1[2]	237	49.2
Category 2[2]	123	25.4
Category 3[2]	124	25.6
Total staff in unit[1] (average/day)	160 (26.67)	100
Total RNs[1]	57	35.63
Total NTs[1]	103	64.38
No. patients/nursing staff	3.03	—
No. patients/RN	8.49	—
No. patients/NT	4.7	—
Average nursing care hours/patient day	3.64	—
RN hours	1.41	38.74
NT hours	2.23	—

[1]*Summary for 6 research days, 2 day shifts.*
[2]*patients classified using the Slovenian patient classification system; RN = graduated (registered) nurse; NT = nursing technician; nursing staff = RN and NT; Average nursing care hours/patient day = (((total nursing care staff on duty, 6 research days, 2 shifts) x no. hours worked per day) x 1,5) /No. hospitalized patients.*

Table 1.
Independent variable characteristics.

Nursing care activities		% (n)
Direct patient care	Hands-on care	27.5 (2124)
	One-to-one observation	4.2 (326)
	Direct communication with patients	3.8 (294)
	Support to patients	1.3 (98)
	Sub-total direct patient care	*36.8 (2842)*
Indirect patient care	Patient documentation & professional discussion [a]	6.9 (538)
	Shift handovers	6.1 (469)
	Ordering investigations [b]	5.5 (425)
	Sub-total indirect patient care	*18.5 (1432)*
Other nursing activities	Other patient-focused activity	19 (1470)
	Ward-focused activity	5.8 (446)
	Staff-focused activity	1.2 (97)
	Sub-total other nursing activities	*26 (2013)*
Unproductive time	Personal staff time	9.4 (729)
	Wasted time	0.1 (6)
	Sub-total unproductive time	*9.5 (735)*
Missing data [c]		*9.2 (710)*
Total		100 (7732)

%, percent; n, number; [a] includes: patient documentation, professional discussion to plan patients' care, discharge planning, and communication with patient's relatives and friends; [b] includes individual medical–technical procedures done independently by nursing staff; [c] nursing activities that could not be observed, as the RN or the NA was not in the medical ward.

Table 2.
Proportions of nursing care activities.

4.3 Patient needs

Nurses documented and evaluated the needs of 378 patients. Another 106 (21.9%) patients were evaluated during the exploratory data analysis, based on the documented relations between categories within the unit. Unit A had the highest (27%) percentage of patients classified into category 2 – which meant that the patients were assigned by default and received supportive or partial assistance from nurses. In unit B, more than half (55%) of the hospitalized patients were assigned to category 1, which meant that they did not receive assistance with hygiene care, mobility, elimination, and feeding, they did not have infusion lines, and their vital signs were monitored less than six times every 24 hours. A few patients were assigned to the demanding category 3. In unit C, more than two fifths (42%) of patients were assigned to category 3, and these required complete assistance with regard to hygiene care, mobility, elimination, and feeding; the patients received tube care, or their vital signs were monitored more than six times every 24 hours.

The number of required staff was calculated by adjusting the factors from three to two shifts (from 24 to 16 hours) based on the patient needs classification system and the standards of staff requirements [39]. The index of the actual and required quantity of nursing staff showed that the medical ward deficit ranged from 22% to 43%, and none of the observed units had enough nursing staff.

Patient satisfaction variables	M	Sd	Nursing staff hours/patient day (r)			Frequency of nursing staff activities (R)	
			RN	NT	RN + NT	All activities	Direct activities
The nurses helped me feel at ease in the hospital.	4.65	0.62	0.184**	0.059**	0.169**	0.025	0.006
The nurses' actions made me feel cared for.	4.59	0.66	0.122**	0.083**	0.098**	0.031	0.001
I was sure that nurses would be there when I needed them.	4.52	0.75	0.067**	0.044*	0.053**	−0.013	0.060**
The nurses made me feel relaxed when treatments were being done.	4.51	0.67	0.143**	0.142**	0.143**	0.025	0.031
The nurses gave me their undivided attention while caring for me.	4.50	0.72	0.075**	0.038	0.052*	−0.044*	0.028
The nurses helped my outlook become more realistic.	4.49	0.70	0.131**	0.128**	0.130**	0.008	0.039
The nurses helped me better deal with the unknowns of this hospitalization.	4.47	0.72	0.008	0.014	0.012	0.011	0.036
The nurses' explanations helped put me at ease.	4.44	0.87	0.049*	0.018	0.030	−0.010	0.033
My requests were promptly attended to by the nursing staff.	4.42	0.78	0.113**	0.104**	0.108**	0.011	0.028
The nursing staff helped me manage the fears I had about my illness.	4.35	0.91	0.126**	0.104**	0.113**	0.022	0.011
I know that due to the nurses' efforts some problems were avoided.	4.30	0.81	0.009	0.012	0.011	0.006	0.016

Patient satisfaction variables	M	Sd	Nursing staff hours/patient day (r)			Frequency of nursing staff activities (R)	
			RN	NT	RN + NT	All activities	Direct activities
I feel that the nurses understood what this illness means to me.	4.29	0.89	0.088**	0.069**	0.077**	0.003	0.017
I was sure that the nurses alerted others to my needs and requests.	4.27	0.81	0.106**	0.078**	0.089**	0.027	−0.013
Little things were done for me without asking.	4.21	0.91	−0.025	−0.050*	−0.041*	−0.015	0.055*
The nurses thought ahead about what I needed.	4.18	0.93	0.218**	0.190**	0.202**	0.023	0.051*
Patient satisfaction index	*4.42*	*0.53*	*0.143***	*0.125***	*0.132***	*0.008*	*0.042*

*RN, graduated (registered) nurse; NT, nursing technician; Nursing staff, includes RN and NTs; r, Pearson's correlation coefficient; R, Spearman's correlation coefficient; Statistical significance set at.95: ** < .00; * < .050; Correlation strength: .0–.09 not correlated, .1–.3 weak, .31–.6 medium, .61–.1 strong correlation [43]; Patient satisfaction index, includes all 15 variables measuring patient satisfaction.*

Table 3.
Relations between the patient satisfaction, nursing staff hours and nursing care activities.

4.4 The patients' perception of nursing quality

The respondents were mostly women (n = 82, 56.9%), with an average age of 67.4 years (SD = 14.7). Fifteen (6.9%) questionnaires were filled in by relatives, 95 (43.6%) patients were helped by the researchers to fill in the form, and the remaining 110 (50.5%) questionnaires were filled in by the patients. The variable patient satisfaction was computed by aggregating all the items from the questionnaire.

The mean of the perceived nursing quality rating was 4.74 (*above good/high*) (SD = 0.49) and ranged from 3 (*good*) to 5 (*high*). The highest average score was for the item concerning the nurses' ability to help make the patients feel at ease, but the lowest average score was for the item concerning the nurses' prediction regarding what the patients needed.

Patient satisfaction with nursing care was associated with the respondents' status (patient or relative) ($r = 0.278$, $p < 0.000$), negatively correlated with the number of patients present daily at the unit level ($r = -0.172$; $p < 0.00$) and was predicted in nearly 10% ($R^2 = 0.098$) from the number of patients in 2nd to 4th category.

In contrast, the patient satisfaction index was positively correlated with the number of nursing care hours per patient day ($r = 0.118$; $p < 0.01$), significantly for both profiles. Registered nurses' and nursing technicians' hours per patient day, along with the index of registered nurses' needed (needed vs. real number of registered nurses) predicted 5% ($R^2 = 0.054$) of patient satisfaction with nursing care.

Moreover, *undivided attention* and *explanation* were positively correlated only with the volume of registered nurses' work hours. However, the item *things are done without asking* was negatively correlated with the working hours of nursing technicians. Patients' satisfaction with nursing care was not significantly correlated with the frequency of nursing staff activities in general, while significant correlations were found between the patients' satisfaction variables and the frequency of some direct patient care activities (**Table 3**).

If selected items from the questionnaire are added to the three presented nursing staff structural variables (registered nurses and nursing technicians' hours on patient day, the index of registered nurses' need) – namely *The nurse, helped my outlook become more realistic; Little things were done for me without asking; I was sure that nurses would be there when I needed them; I know that due to the nurses' efforts some problems were avoided; The nursing staff helped me manage the fears I had about my illness; The nurses made me feel relaxed when treatments were being done* – then together they could predict 96% ($R^2 = 0.961$; $\alpha = 0.747$) of the hospitalized patients' perception of the quality of nursing care.

5. Discussion

This study describes the correlation between patient perceptions of the quality of nursing care and nurse structure and process variables. Hospitalized patients' perceptions of nursing care quality was measured with a questionnaire, the nursing process was directly observed, and the data on nursing workforce and patient structure were obtained from routine hospital data. The results indicate a significant association between certain constants (actual and needed staffing levels, some nursing activities) and patient satisfaction.

In the researched medical ward the average number of patients per registered nurse was high, and only a third of the overall nursing hours were conducted by nurses with a bachelor's degree. Although, the number of staff did not deviate from that expected in European hospitals [44], the observed staffing levels could provoke rushed judgments about low quality of care. However, it should be noted that in the observed hospital the management calculates the number of registered nurses and nursing technicians together (as nursing staff), ignoring evidence on higher nurse staffing levels being reflected in better patient outcomes [8, 15, 18, 45, 46]. With the use of two profiles of nursing staff, the productivity levels, number of nurse working hours and nurse–patient ratios appear to be good. But this hospital is employing cheaper nursing technicians instead of registered nurses, and this low-cost approach ignores actual patients care needs, actual unit occupancy rates, and staff competences and, as a consequence, the graduate staff are overloaded.

This study showed also that patients were more satisfied when the proportion of baccalaureate nurses in the nursing workforce was higher. While these results support the findings of previous studies [10, 47, 48], there is limited evidence correlating hospital nurse staffing with patient satisfaction in the literature [8, 30, 49, 50]. This study also found that patient satisfaction is positively correlated with the number of registered nurse working hours, with the index of actual and required registered nurses, and with the number of registered nurse and nursing technician working hours per patient day. Research reports positive patient outcomes when staffing levels allow a maximum of six patients to one registered nurse on a medical ward [51]. Similarly, other research finds that more patients per nurse result in higher rate of care left undone [19].

Observations suggest that registered nurses need to engage in a great variety of tasks, and spend a great deal of time locating the information needed for individual patients. Health education, clinical references, consulting, and coaching were the least frequent activities in the registered nurses' working days. We were not able to observe a fifth of the registered nurses' activities, as these were done outside the medical ward. These activities could thus not be classified in the observations, but were described by the staff as nursing tasks on other medical units, meetings with management, quality teams, and so on. Moreover, the results show that the patients noticed the individual attention they received from registered nurses while they cared for them, and that their explanations helped them feel more at ease. Nurses are known to spend more time with patients than other health professionals, and that enables them to show the caring attitude which is sensitive to patients' reports of quality of nursing care [52]. Registered nurses have a wide range of nursing knowledge and good communication skills, are alert to changes in the patients' status and have the competencies needed to do all the activities that arise in nursing care. Nursing technicians have fewer competencies, and care for fewer patients than registered nurses – certain tastes are thus not delegated from registered nurses to technicians, but the vice versa. This could mean that patients would benefit if mixed staffing models, like the one observed in this study, would include more nurses with bachelor's degrees.

We used a hierarchical four-grade nursing care classification system to assess nursing care levels for patients at different acuity levels. This system identifies the staffing levels required to achieve appropriate nursing care, although unfortunately it is not used in practice yet. When we compared the actual nursing levels, the conventional patient-to-nurse ratio and the nurses needed on the basis of patients' classification, we found severe shortages. Individual patient requirements were not respected, as a 38% shortage of registered nurses was measured. Therefore, nursing staff requirements should be considered as a predictor of the quality of nursing services [53], and having enough nurses to meet patient needs could be reflected in higher patient satisfaction with nursing care [8, 54].

According to the findings of the current study, patient satisfaction was not correlated with the frequency of contact care activities performed by the entire nursing staff. Contrary to what is documented in studies in high-income countries [13, 21], where the time that nurses spend in direct care activities was found to be a determinant of patient satisfaction, our patients valued the number of hours worked by nurses. The proportion of direct patient care activities performed by all nursing staff was higher (36.8%) than that documented previously [29]. However, the majority of observed contacts included hands-on-care and were focused on the patient's physical needs (e.g. hygiene, food intake, mobility, medical/technical procedures), while a limited proportion of activities was devoted to regular patient observations, communication, or support. In contrast, some authors [55] have found that nurses spend most time communicating with patients and charting or reviewing information. The different findings could be the result of different research protocols, where communication is documented as an individual task, as in our study, instead of being a part of a multitasking activity.

The results of the correlations also revealed three process items (*undivided attention, explanation,* and *things are done without asking*) that are the special strengths of nursing care. Some authors [33, 56] have also stated that the most important factors that influence patient satisfaction are perceived nurse caring, nursing kindness, and the technical aspects of care, while others focus on individual patient characteristics [2, 30, 31].

In general, the patients in this study reported high satisfaction with the nursing care they received. Some previous research also reported a comparable average satisfaction index, ranging from 4.0 to 4.5 [3], but other studies also reported lower perception levels [48, 57]. It was found that the quality of bedside nursing care is also affected by the related hospital services such as the quality of beds, the quality and cleanliness of bed linens, the number of bathrooms available, and the quality of the bathrooms available, cleanliness of the toilets, and ventilation and lighting in the wards [52]. The high satisfaction perceived by our patients could therefore reflect good hospital services or, at contrary, a paternalistic perspective, where patients believe that healthcare workers are doing their best with the limited resources available [58], and therefore are less demanding.

6. Conclusion

This paper supports nursing management efforts for a higher proportion of registered nurses in the nursing staff structure, and an increased volume of overall nursing staff working hours. The results show that the more the needs of patients that are detected, the higher the satisfaction regarding nursing care. Managers could use the patient needs categorization system as in this study to facilitate decisions on staffing requirements and therefore predict patient satisfaction.

Patients do not only perceive the presence and value of registered nurses when they are at their bedsides. The competencies registered nurses acquire at the academic level can also affect the care given, and thereby the perceptions of patients, who feel higher levels of satisfaction. Overall, our findings suggest that the health system requires more highly skilled healthcare professionals.

Acknowledgements

Special thanks for article revision and professional consulting to Prof. Mirko Markič, Ph.D.; and Dragica Blatnik, the head nurse of Izola hospital for support in organizing the study; and to patients and nurses in the researched hospital units.

Conflict of interest

The author declares no conflict of interest.

Author details

Melita Peršolja
Faculty of Health Sciences, University of Primorska, Unit Nova Gorica, Delpinova, Nova Gorica, Slovenia

*Address all correspondence to: melita.persolja@fvz.upr.si

References

[1] Al-Qahtani M, Dahi A, Khalil S. Satisfaction with nursing care from the inpatients' perspective in Prince Salman Armed Forced Hospital Tabuk, Saudi Arabia. Middle East Journal of Family Medicine. 2015;13(2):13-17.

[2] Atallah MA, Hamdan-Mansour AM, Al-Sayed MM, Aboshaiqah AE. Patients' satisfaction with the quality of nursing care provided: the Saudi experience. Int J Nurs Pract. 2013;19(6):584-590.

[3] Dozier AM, Kitzman HJ, Ingersoll GL, Holmberg S, Schultz AW. Development of an instrument to measure patient perception of the quality of nursing care. Research in Nursing & Health. 2001;24(6):506-517.

[4] Donabedian A. Quality of care: problems of measurement. II. Some issues in evaluating the quality of nursing care. Am J Public Health Nations Health. 1969;59(10):1833-1836.

[5] Klaus SF, Dunton N, Gajewski B, Potter C. Reliability of the nursing care hour measure: A descriptive study. International Journal of Nursing Studies. 2013;50(7):924-932.

[6] Jones TL. Outcome Measurement in Nursing: Imperatives, Ideals, History, and Challenges. Online J Issues Nurs. 2016;21(2):1.

[7] Donabedian A. Evaluating the Quality of Medical Care. The Milbank Quarterly. 2005;83(4):691-729.

[8] Aiken LH, Sermeus W, Van den Heede K, Sloane DM, Busse R, McKee M, et al. Patient safety, satisfaction, and quality of hospital care: cross sectional surveys of nurses and patients in 12 countries in Europe and the United States. BMJ. 2012;344:e1717.

[9] Kraska RA, Weigand M, Geraedts M. Associations between hospital characteristics and patient satisfaction in Germany. Health Expect. 2016;20(4):593-600.

[10] Hockenberry JM, Becker ER. How Do Hospital Nurse Staffing Strategies Affect Patient Satisfaction? ILR Review. 2016;69(4):890-910.

[11] Kalisch BJ, Lee KH. Nurse staffing levels and teamwork: a cross-sectional study of patient care units in acute care hospitals. J Nurs Scholarsh. 2011;43(1):82-88.

[12] Palese A, Gonella S, Fontanive A, Guarnier A, Barelli P, Zambiasi P, et al. The degree of satisfaction of in-hospital medical patients with nursing care and predictors of dissatisfaction: findings from a secondary analysis. Scand J Caring Sci. 2017;31(4):768-778.

[13] Penque S, Kearney G. The effect of nursing presence on patient satisfaction. Nurs Manag. 2015;46(4):38-44.

[14] Kostovich CT, Dunya BA, Schmidt LA, Collins EG. A Rasch Rating Scale Analysis of the Presence of Nursing Scale-RN. J Appl Meas. 2016;17(4):476-488.

[15] Butler M, Collins R, Drennan J, Halligan P, O'Mathúna DP, Schultz TJ, et al. Hospital nurse staffing models and patient and staff-related outcomes. Cochrane Database of Systematic Reviews [Internet]. 2011; (7). Available from: http://onlinelibrary.wiley.com/doi/10.1002/14651858.CD007019.pub2/abstract.

[16] Needleman J, Buerhaus P, Pankratz VS, Leibson CL, Stevens SR, Harris M. Nurse staffing and inpatient hospital mortality. N Engl J Med. 2011;364(11):1037-1045.

[17] Aiken LH, Sloane DM, Bruyneel L, Van den Heede K, Griffiths P, Busse R,

et al. Nurse staffing and education and hospital mortality in nine European countries: a retrospective observational study. The Lancet. 2014;383(9931):1824-1830.

[18] Cho E, Sloane DM, Kim E-Y, Kim S, Choi M, Yoo IY, et al. Effects of nurse staffing, work environments, and education on patient mortality: An observational study. Intern J Nurs Stud. 2015;52(2):535-542.

[19] Ausserhofer D, Zander B, Busse R, Schubert M, De Geest S, Rafferty AM, et al. Prevalence, patterns and predictors of nursing care left undone in European hospitals: results from the multicountry cross-sectional RN4CAST study. BMJ Qual Saf. 2014;23(2):126-135.

[20] Negarandeh R, Hooshmand Bahabadi A, Aliheydari Mamaghani J. Impact of regular nursing rounds on patient satisfaction with nursing care. Asian Nurs Res (Korean Soc Nurs Sci). 2014;8(4):282-285.

[21] Staniszewska S, Ahmed L. Patient expectations and satisfaction with health care. Nurs Stand. 1998;12(18):34-8.

[22] Davidson R, Mills ME. Cancer patients' satisfaction with communication, information and quality of care in a UK region. European Journal of Cancer Care. 2005;14(1):83-90.

[23] Attree M. Patients' and relatives' experiences and perspectives of 'Good' and 'Not so Good' quality care. J Adv Nurs. 2001;33(4):456-466.

[24] England N. Safer staffing: a guide to care contact time. In: Cummings J, editor. Health Services, Social Work, Social Care and Social Services. Quarry House: NHS England, 2014.

[25] Sulmasy DP, Sood JR. Factors associated with the time nurses spend at the bedsides of seriously ill patients with poor prognoses. Medical Care. 2003;41(4):458-466.

[26] Hoffman FM. Setting nursing hours standards. Part 2. J Nurs Admin. 1986;16(2):17-9.

[27] Munyisia EN, Yu P, Hailey D. How nursing staff spend their time on activities in a nursing home: an observational study. J Adv Nurs. 2011;67(9):1908-1917.

[28] Dellefield ME, Harrington C, Kelly A. Observing how RNs use clinical time in a nursing home: a pilot study. Geriatric Nursing. 2012;33(4):256-263.

[29] McCloskey JC, Bulechek GM, Moorhead S, Daly J. Nurses' use and delegation of indirect care interventions. Nurs Econ. 1996;14(1):22-33.

[30] Laal M. Inpatient's Perspective on Nursing Care; Affecting Factors. Procedia - Social and Behavioral Sciences. 2013;84:243-247.

[31] Ham HS, Peck EH, Moon HS, Yeom HA. Predictors of patient satisfaction with tertiary hospitals in Korea. Nurs Res Pract. 2015;2015:749754.

[32] Berg GM, Spaeth D, Sook C, Burdsal C, Lippoldt D. Trauma patient perceptions of nursing care: relationships between ratings of interpersonal care, technical care, and global satisfaction. J Trauma Nurs. 2012;19(2):104-110.

[33] Papastavrou E, Andreou P, Tsangari H, Merkouris A. Linking patient satisfaction with nursing care: the case of care rationing - a correlational study. Bio Med Central Nursing. 2014;13:26.

[34] Al-Abri R, Al-Balushi A. Patient satisfaction survey as a tool towards quality improvement. Oman Med J. 2014;29(1):3-7.

[35] OECD. Health at a Glance 2019: OECD INDICATORS. Paris: OECD Publishing, 2019.

[36] Turk E, Habjanič A. Slovenia. In: Rafferty A, Busse R, Zander-Jentsch B, et al., editors. Strengthening health systems through nursing: Evidence from 14 European countries. Copenhagen: European Observatory on Health Systems and Policies, 2019.

[37] Starc A. Nursing professionalization elements in Slovenia. In: Štemberger Kolnik T, Majcen Dvoršak S, Klemenc D, editors. From evidence to Practice. Ljubljana: Nurses and Midwives Association of Slovenia, National Center for professional, career and personal development of nurses and midwives, 2012:83-87.

[38] EPCN. Blue Book of Standards and Norms in Nursing and Midwifery. Ljubljana: Nurses and Midwives Association of Slovenia, Trade Union of Workers in Health care of Slovenia, 2013.

[39] Klančnik-Gruden M, Bregar B, Peternelj A, Marinšek N, Zaletel M, Skela-Savič B. Slovenian Categorization of Complexity in Hospital Nursing: Handbook. Ljubljana: Slovenian Chamber of Nursing and Midwifery, 2011.

[40] Zorec M, De Miranda OR, Filej B, Van den Hout AC. Razvoj metodologije merjenja kolicine dela v zdravstveni negi v mednarodnem projektu = Development of methodology to measure quantity of the work in nursing care in an international project. Slov Nurs Rev. 2001(35):181-184.

[41] WHO. Process of translation and adaptation of instruments. 2013. Available from: http://www.who.int/substance_abuse/research_tools/translation/en/.

[42] WMA. World Medical Association Declaration of Helsinki, ethical principles for medical research involving human subjects. Jama. 2013;10(22):2191-2194.

[43] Field A. Discovering statistics using SPSS. London: SAGE Publications Ltd., 2009.

[44] Sermeus W, Aiken LH, Van den Heede K, Rafferty AM, Griffiths P, Moreno-Casbas MT, et al. Nurse forecasting in Europe (RN4CAST): Rationale, design and methodology. BMC Nursing. 2011;10(1):1-9.

[45] Andersen MH, Lonning K, Bjornelv GM, Fagerstrom L. Nursing intensity and costs of nurse staffing demonstrated by the RAFAELA system: liver vs. kidney transplant recipients. J Nurs Manag. 2016;24(6):798-805.

[46] Griffiths P, Ball J, Drennan J, Dall'Ora C, Jones J, Maruotti A, et al. Nurse staffing and patient outcomes: Strengths and limitations of the evidence to inform policy and practice. A review and discussion paper based on evidence reviewed for the National Institute for Health and Care Excellence Safe Staffing guideline development. Int J Nurs Stud. 2016;63:213-225.

[47] You LM, Aiken LH, Sloane DM, Liu K, He GP, Hu Y, et al. Hospital nursing, care quality, and patient satisfaction: cross-sectional surveys of nurses and patients in hospitals in China and Europe. Int J Nurs Stud. 2013;50(2):154-61.

[48] Clark PA, Leddy K Fau - Drain M, Drain M Fau - Kaldenberg D, Kaldenberg D. State nursing shortages and patient satisfaction: more RNs--better patient experiences. J Nurs Care Qual. 2007;22(2):119-127.

[49] Martsolf GR, Gibson TB, Benevent R, Jiang JH, Stocks C, Ehrlich ED, et al. An Examination of Hospital Nurse Staffing and Patient Experience with Care: Differences between Cross-Sectional and Longitudinal Estimates. Health Services Research. 2016;51(6):2221-2241.

[50] Ball J, Griffiths P, Hope J. Evidence on the effect of nurse staffing levels on patient outcomes. Nursing Times. 2017;113(1):48-49.

[51] Shekelle PG. Nurse-patient ratios as a patient safety strategy: a systematic review. Ann Intern Med. 2013;158 (5 Pt 2):404-409.

[52] Al-Hussami M, Al-Momani M, Hammad S, Maharmeh M, Darawad M. Patients' perception of the quality of nursing care and related hospital services. Health and Primary Care. 2017;1(2):1-6.

[53] Peršolja M, Markič M, Blatnik D, Palese A. Patient satisfaction with nursing care delivered in medical units in post-transitional country: a correlational study. Acta Medit Medic. 2018;6:2045.

[54] Aiken LH, Sloane DM, Ball J, Bruyneel L, Rafferty AM, Griffiths P. Patient satisfaction with hospital care and nurses in England: an observational study. BMJ open. 2018;8(1):e019189.

[55] Yen P-Y, Kellye M, Lopetegui M, Saha A, Loversidge J, Chipps EM, et al. Nurses' Time Allocation and Multitasking of Nursing Activities: A Time Motion Study. AMIA Annual Symposium proceedings AMIA Symposium. 2018;2018:1137-1146.

[56] Berg GM, Ekengren F, Lee FA, Acuna D, Burdsal C. Patient satisfaction with surgeons in a trauma population: testing a structural equation model using perceptions of interpersonal and technical care. J Trauma Acute Care Surg. 2012;72(5):1316-1322.

[57] Jha AK, Orav EJ, Zheng J, Epstein AM. Patients' perception of hospital care in the United States. N Engl J Med. 2008;359.

[58] Albreht T, Pribakovic Brinovec R, Josar D, Poldrugovac M, Kostnapfel T, Zaletel M, et al. Slovenia: Health System Review. Health Systems in Transition. 2016;18(3):1-207.

Chapter 9

Item Analysis: Concept and Application

Assad Ali Rezigalla

Abstract

In the field of medical education, Item analysis is a statistical analysis of student's responses on exam items and the relationship between them. It provides constructive feedback about items quality, increases the effectiveness of the exam, and supports exam validity and reliability. The decision of adding or removing an item should depends mainly on the result of the item analysis. The feedback of item analysis can support modification of instruction methods. This chapter provides a comprehensive review of item analysis (psychometric analysis) and also can be used as methodological guidance to perform an informative analysis. The chapter discusses item analysis under the following headings, importance of item analysis, factors affecting item analysis, parameters of item analysis and application. The parameters of item analysis includes the indices of the internal consistency, difficulty, discrimination, and distractor analysis.

Keywords: item analysis, difficulty index, reliability, discrimination index, KR20

1. Introduction

"Assessment is a central component of the teaching and learning" process. It is defined as "the systematic collection and analysis of information to improve student learning" [1]. Test (exam) is a part of student assessment and should be "An objective and standardized measure of a sample of behavior" [2]. Item analysis is a post-examination evaluation and can provide information about the quality of tests.

Item analysis is a statistical analysis of the student's responses on a test. Collection and summarization of students' responses can provide quantitative objective information that is useful in deciding the quality of the test items and increasing the assessment's efficiency [3, 4]. Also, Item analysis "investigates the performance of items considered individually either in relation to some external criterion or the remaining items on the test" [5].

2. Importance of psychometric analysis

Any educational test should measure students' achievement in content material. Also, it leads to an overall assessment of students' development to decide their academic status [6, 7].

The importance of item analysis is determined by the objective of the assessment [8]. In summative assessment, the assessment results should be reliable and valid because incorrect decisions about the academic status will lead to negative consequences [9]. While for the formative evaluation where the target is students learning, the item analysis has no much importance in giving feedback about items construction to test composers.

In literature, many reasons were reported for the conduction of item analysis, including examining if the item is functioning as intended, did it assess the required concepts (content)?, did it discriminate between those who master the content material and those who were not? was it within the acceptable level of difficulty?, whether the distracters are functioning or not? [10, 11].

3. Factors affecting item analysis

Many factors can affect item analysis and hence its interpretation [8]. Difficulty and discrimination indices were constantly changing per administration and influenced by the ability and number of the examinee, the number of items, and the quality of instructions [8, 12].

Whatever the exam or test blueprinting (item selection) method, exam items remain a sample of the needed content material. The number of items (item sampling) carries excellent importance because one cannot ask about all contents. With a too-small number of items, the results may not be enough to reflect true student ability [8]. Technical item flaws are divided into two major types, test wiseness, and irrelevant difficulty. Test wiseness flaws can result in more easy items. Faults related to irrelevant difficulty can result in more challenging items unrelated to the content under assessment. It was reported that item analysis of exam with 200 examinees is stable, and with fewer than 100 examinees should be interpreted with caution (item difficulty or item discrimination index). While Downing and Yudkowsky described that even for a small number of the examinee (e.g., 30) still, the item analysis can provide a piece of a helpful information to improve item [13, 14].

4. Parameters of item analysis

The item or psychometric analysis parameters include difficulty index, reliability, discrimination index, distractor efficiency [2]. The descriptive statistics of the exam are important and can provide helpful generalized information [2]. The descriptive statistics include scores frequency, the mean, the mode, the median, and the standard deviation.

5. Cronbach's alpha (Index of reliability)

Cronbach's alpha (KR20) is widely accepted and used estimate of test reliability (the internal consistency) and reported to be superior to the split-half estimate [15, 16]. Although validity and reliability are closely associated, the reliability of an assessment does not depend on its validity [16, 17]. Coefficient alpha is known to be equal to Kr-20 if the item has a single answer, such as in the case of type A MCQs or binary [18–21].

Coefficient alpha reflects the degree to which item response scores correlate with total test scores [15]. It also describes the degree to which items in the exam measure the same concept or construct [22]. Therefore, it is connected to the inter-relatedness and dimensionality of the items within the exam [16, 20]. Cronbach's alpha is affected by exam time, the number and inter-relation of the items (dimensionality) and easy or hard, poorly written or confusing items, Variations in examinee responses, curriculum content not reflected in the test, Testing conditions, and Errors in recording or scoring [22–24]. The value of alpha is decreased in the exam with fewer items and increased if items assessing the same concept (unidimensionality of the exam) [16]. Other factors were reported to impact alpha value, such as item difficulty, number of the examinee, and student performance in the exam time. It was argued that very high alpha values could indicate lengthy exams, parallel items, or a narrow coverage of the content material [22].

The alpha value of the exam can be increased by increasing the number of items with a high p-value (difficulty index). It was reported that items with moderate difficulty could maximize alpha value and while those with zero difficulties or 100 can minimize it [15]. In the same way, deletion of faulty items can increase alpha value. It should be considered that repetition of items in the same exam or using items assessing the same concept can increase alpha value.

6. Interpretation of Cronbach's alpha

The interpretation of reliability is the correlation of the test with itself. When the estimate of reliability increases, the portion of a test score related to the error will decrease. Wise interpretation of alpha needs an understanding of the interrelatedness of items and whether the items measure a single latent trait or construct. Exam or test with different content materials such as integrated courses, for example, in the musculoskeletal system course, although is dominated by anatomy it contains other subjects of basic medical and clinical sciences that have different contains. Therefore, interpretation of such a course exam needs deep looks beyond the alpha figure. It was reported that KR20 of 0.7 is acceptable to short test (less than 50 items) and KR20 of 0.8 for an extended test (more than 50 item-test) [25]. Moreover, it was documented that a multidimensional exam does not have a lower (**Table 1**) alpha value than a unidimensional one [30].

A low alpha value can be due to a smaller number of items, reduced interrelatedness between items, or heterogeneous constructs [22]. A high value of alpha can suggest exam reliability, and some items are non-functional as they are testing the same content but in a different guise or repeated ones [16, 22]. Also, a high value indicates items with high interrelatedness, indicating a limited coverage of the content materials [22].

7. Improving Cronbach's alpha

Adding new items with an acceptable difficulty index, high discrimination power and distractor efficiency can increase the test reliability [22, 31, 32]. In addition, deletion of faulty items or those with low or very high p-value can improve Cronbach's alpha. Items with poor correlation or are not related should be revised or discarded from the exam.

8. Distractor analysis

Commonly are formed of a stem with or without leading question and five or four alternatives (type A MCQs). Among item's alternatives, only one is the key answer and others are called distractors [4]. Distractors should carry or convey a miss concept about the key answer and appear plausible. The distractors should appear similar to the key answer in terms of the used words, grammatical form,

Author	Interpretation of Cronbach's alpha (KR20)
Robinson, Shaver et al. [26]	≥0.80 Exemplary
	0.70–0.79 Extensive
	0.60–0.69 Moderate
	<0.60 Minimal
Cicchetti [27]	<0.70 Unacceptable
	0.70–0.80 Fair
	0.80–0.90 Good
	< 0.90 Excellent
Axelson and Kreiter [28]	>0.90 is needed for very high stakes tests (e.g., licensure, certification exams)
	0.80–0.89 is acceptable for moderate stakes tests (e.g., end-of-year summative exams in medical school, end-of-course exams)
	0.70–0.79 would be acceptable for lower stakes assessments (e.g., formative or summative classroom-type assessments created and administered by local faculty
	<0.70 might be useful as one component of an overall composite score.
Obon and Rey [12]	>0.90 Excellent reliability
	0.80–0.90 Very good for a classroom test
	0.70–0.80 good for a classroom test
	0.60–0.70 Somewhat low (The test needs to be supplemented by other measure)
	0.50–0.60 Suggests need for revision of test (unless it is quite short, ten or fewer Items).
	0.50 < Questionable reliability.
Hassan and Hod [29]	> 0.7 is excellent
	0.6–0.7 is acceptable
	−0.5-0.6 is poor
	< 0.5 is unacceptable
	< 0.30 is unreliable

Table 1.
Reference values and interpretation of Cronbach's alpha (KR20).

style, and length [19]. Distractor efficiency (DE) is the ability of incorrect answers to distract the students [12].

A functional distractor (FD) the distractor that is selected by 5% or more of the examinee [4, 33]. At the same time, those chosen by less than 5% of the examinee are considered non-functional (NFD) [4]. In comparison, other authors reported 1% of the examinee as the demarcation of functional distractors [34, 35]. Commonly items are categorized based on the numbers of NFDs in the item (**Table 2**) [12, 26, 36, 37].

The occurrence of NFD makes the item easier and reduces its discrimination power, while FD distractors are making it more difficult [36, 38]. It was reported that non-functional distractors are negatively correlating with reliability [38]. The presence of non-functional distractors can be related to two main causes. First is the training and construction ability of the item writer or composer. Second, the miss-match between the target content and the possible number of a distractor created. Thus, training and more effort in item writing and construction can decrease NFDs [36]. Other causes were related to NFDs, including the low cognitive level of the item, irrelevant or limited number of plausible distractors, or presence of logic cues [39]. Another possibility of NFDs is mastering the content material of the item, and students can identify the distractor as the wrong one. If no other cause (s) for NFDs, they should be removed or changed with a more plausible option because it has no contribution to the measurement of the test [12]. If a distractor is selected more frequently than the key answer by a higher-scoring examinee, this may indicate poor constructions or a misleading question or miss or double-keyed [12, 40]. In this, concerning the use of three options is more practical than four, does not affect reliability, and does not affect the discrimination index significantly [26, 35–37].

Furthermore, it was reported that there is no psychometric reason that all items in the exam should have the same number of distractors [26, 41]. The required number of options in an item should be considered according to the content material from which plausible distractors can be developed [33, 40, 42].

Reducing the number of options/distractors will result in other important benefits such as reducing the answering time of the test and safe time can be used to cover more content material, reduce the burden on item composers, and have items with more acceptable parameters [43, 44].

Puthiaparampil et al. reported a non-high significant negative and positive correlation between the number of functional distractors and difficulty and discrimination indices, respectively [34]. While a significant positive correlation was reported between the DIF and the number of NFDs [45].

Many authors concluded that no predictable relationship between DE and difficulty index and discrimination index [26, 31, 40, 46, 47]. In addition Licona-Chávez et al. did not find a parallel performance between DE and other parameters of item analysis including Cronbach alpha [46]. In contrast, some authors claimed that low DE decreases the difficulty index [47, 48].

9. Improving distractor analysis

Restoring the optimal DE of the item can be achieved by identifying flaws related to the NFDs and correcting them or removing the NFDs from the item [39].

Number of NFD	Percentage	Interpritation
3	0	Poor
2	33.3	Moderate
1	66.6	Good
0	100	Excellent

Table 2.
Classification of items according to thee number of the nonfunctional distractors (NFD).

10. Difficulty index

The item difficulty (easiness, facility index, P-value) is the percentage of students who answered an item correctly [6, 40]. The difficulty index ranges from 0 to 100, whereas the higher the values indicate, the easier the question and the

Number of options	The ideal (optimal) difficulty level	
	[46, 47]	[24]
2	—	0.75
3	0.77	0.67
4	0.74	0.63
5	0.70	0.60

Table 3.
The ideal (optimal) difficulty level (for tests with 100 items).

low value represents the difficulty of hard items. The ideal (optimal) difficulty levels for type A MCQs is varying according to the number of the options (**Table 3**) [49, 50]. The range of items difficulty can be categorized into difficult, moderate, and easy. Easy and difficult items were reported to have very little discrimination power [48]. Item difficulty is related to the item and the examinee that took the test in the given time [24]. Thus, reusing of the item depending on its difficulty index should be controlled. Some authors found that difficulty indices of items assessing high cognitive levels in Bloom's taxonomy such as evaluation, explanation, analysis, and synthesis are lower than those assessing remembering, understanding, and applying [51, 52].

During item or exam construction, the constructor should aim for acceptably level of difficulty [6]. Sugianto reported that items within the exam could be distributed according to difficulty to moderate level (40%), easy and challenging levels (20%), and easier and more challenging levels (10%) [6]. Other authors reported that most items should be of moderate difficulty or 5% should be in the difficult range [50, 53]. Some authors found that difficulty indices of items assessing high cognitive levels in Bloom's taxonomy such as evaluation, explanation, analysis, and synthesis are lower than those assessing remembering, understanding, and applying [51, 52]. Regarding the general arrangement of test or examination, easy items start first then are followed by difficult ones. At the same time, in the case of diagnostic assessment, the sequence of the learning material is more important [6, 7].

Easy and difficult items affect the item's ability to discriminate between students and show low discrimination power. Some reports described a negative correlation between exam reliability and difficult and easy items [38]. Oermann et al. reported that educationalists must be careful in deleting items with poor DIF because the number of items has more effect on test validity [54]. It is recommended that difficult items should be reviewed for the possible technical and content causes [50]. Possible causes of low difficulty index include uncovered (taught) content material, challenging items, missed key or no correct answer among the item options [55]. Easy items (high P-value) can be due to technical causes, or the concerned learning objective (s) were achieved or revisited in coverage that is more superficial [55].

11. Interpretation of difficulty index

In literature including medical education, many ranges of difficulty indices were reported (**Table 4**).

Author	Difficulty index	Interpretation
Uddin et al. [50]	>80%	Easy
	30–80%	Moderate
	<30%	Difficult
Kaur, Singla et al. [56]	>80	Easy
	40–80	Moderate
	<39	Difficult
Sugianto [6]	90	Easy
	50	Moderate
	10	Difficult
Date, Borkar et al. [37] and Kumar, Jaipurkar et al. [36]	<30	Too difficult
	>70%	Too easy
	50–60%	Excellent/ideal
	30–70%	Good/acceptable/average
Obon and Rey [12]	> 0.76	Easy (Revise or Discard)
	0.26–0.75	Right difficult (Retain)
	0–0.25	Difficult (Revise or Discard)
Bhat and Prasad [57]	>70%	Easy
	30–70%	Good
	<30%	Difficult

Table 4.
Reference values and interpretation of difficulty index (p-value).

12. Discrimination index (Power)

Item discrimination (DI) is the ability of an item to discriminate between higher achiever (good) students and low ones. It was defined as "stated that item discrimination is a statistic that indicates the degree to which an item separates the students who performed well from those who did poorly on the test as a whole" [6]. The discrimination power of an item is calculated by categorizing the examinee into upper 27% and lower 27% according to their total test score. The difference between the upper and lower group is divided by the number of the examinee in the upper group or the larger group or by half of the total number of the examinee or even by the total number [4, 6, 58, 59]. Obon and Rey [12] calculated the discrimination index as the difference of difficulty index between the upper and lower groups [12]. In literature, both 25 and 27% were reported as possible percentages of examinee categorization [60, 61]. The 27% is commonly used to maximize differences in normal distributions and increase the number of examinees in each category. The discrimination index range from 1.0 to −1.0. The positive discrimination index indicates that high achievers answer the item correctly more than those in the lower ones, which is desirable. The negative discrimination index reflects that lower achiever examinees answer the item more correctly, while zero discrimination indicates equal numbers of students in the upper and lower groups [36, 37]. Negative discrimination is thought to be due to item flaws or inefficient distractors, miss keys, ambiguous wording, gray areas of opinion, and areas of controversy [12, 62]. Nevid and McClelland [52] reported that items assessing evaluation and explanation domains could discriminate between high and low performers, while Kim et al. [51] comments that items assessing remembering and understanding levels have low discrimination power [52, 54].

It was reported that discrimination indices are positively associated with difficulty index and distractor efficiency [39, 63]. The discrimination power of the item is reduced by the increased number of non-functional distractors [36].

A test with poor discriminating power will not provide a reliable interpretation of the examinee's actual ability [6, 64]. In addition, discrimination power will not indicate item validity, and deletion of items with poor discrimination power negatively impacts validity due to a decrease in the item number [65].

13. Discrimination coefficients

Discrimination coefficients can evaluate item discrimination. The discrimination coefficients include point biserial correlation, biserial correlation, and phi coefficient. Although point biserial correlation is used interchangeably with the discrimination index, discrimination coefficients are considered superior to the discrimination index [24]. The superiority came from the fact that discrimination coefficients are calculated using all examinees' responses in the item rather than only 54% of the examinees such as in the discrimination index.

The difference between Point-biserial correlation (rBP) and discrimination indexes is that rBP is the correlation between an item in the exam and the overall student score [2, 66]. In cases of highly discriminating items, the examinees who responded to the item correctly also did well on the test. In general, the examinees who responded to the item incorrectly also tended to perform poorly on the overall test. It was suggested that point biserial can express the predictive validity better than Biserial correlation coefficients [61, 67].

14. Interpretation of discrimination index

Discrimination power of items more than 0.15 was reported as evidence of item validity [50, 53]. While any item with less than 0.15 or negative should be reviewed [50] (**Table 5**).

When interpreting the discrimination power of an item to decide about, especial consideration should be related to its difficulty. Items with a high difficulty index (most of the examinee answer it right) and those with low difficulty index (most of the examinee answer it wrong) commonly have low discrimination power [35, 63]. In both cases, such items will not discriminate examines as the majority are on one side. Thus items with a moderate difficulty index are more likely to have good discrimination power.

The common causes of poor discrimination power of item include technical or writing flaws, untaught or not well covered content material, ambiguous wording, gray areas of opinion and controversy, and wrong keys [12, 50, 62, 66].

In general, the statistical data obtained from item analysis can help item constructors and exam composers to detect defective items. The decision to revise an item or distractors must be based on the difficulty index, discrimination index, and distractor efficiency. Revision of items can lead to modification in the teaching method or the content material [68].

Author	Discrimination power	Interpretation
Elfaki, Bahamdan et al. [53]	≥0.35	Excellent
	0.25–0.34	Good
	0.21–0.24	Acceptable
	≤ 0.20	Poor
Obon and Rey [12]	≥ 0.50	Very Good Item (Definitely Retain)
	0.40–0.49	Good Item (Very Usable)
	0.30–0.39	Fair Quality (Usable Item)
	0.20–0.29	Potentially Poor Item (Consider Revising)
	≤ 0.20	Potentially Very Poor (Possibly Revise Substantially or Discard)
Bhat and Prasad [57]	> 0.35	Excellent
	0.2–0.35	Good
	< 0.2	Poor
Sugianto [6]	>0.40	Very good
	0.30–0.39	Reasonably good possibly need to improvement
	0.20–0.29	Marginal item usually needing and being to improvement
	<0.19	Poor item rejected or improved by revision
Aljehani, Pullishery et al. [66] and Sharma [4]	≥ 0.40	Very discriminating, very good item(Keep)
	0.30–0.39	Discriminating item, good item (Keep)
	0.20–0.29	Moderately discriminating, fair item (Keep)
	< 0.20	Not discriminating item, marginal item (Revise/Discard)
	Negative	Worst/ defective item (Definitely Discard)
Ramzan, Imran et al. [63]	> 0.30	Excellent discrimination
	0.20–0.29	Good discrimination
	0–0.19	Poor discrimination
	00	Defective
Uddin et al. [50]	≥ 0.35	Excellent
	0.25–0.34	Good
	0.21–0.24	Acceptable
	< 0.20	Poor

Table 5.
Reference values and interpretation of discrimination index (power).

15. Item analysis application

Figure 1:
In this Example 1.
The number of examinees was 21.
The number of test items (Total possible) is 40.

Exam Item Analysis Report				Exams Graded: 21				
Instructor:	0	Total Possible:	40	Average:	30.3 (75.83%)			
Exam Name	0	Highest Score:	38(95%)	Median:	30(75%)			
Exam Date:	0	Lowest Score:	14(35%)	KR20:	0.8238477			
Correct responses are shown in bold and italics					Pt. Biserial	Disc. Index	Correct	Pct. Incorrect
Q1	***A (18, 85.71%)***	B (0, 0.00%)	C (0, 0.00%)	D (3, 14.29%)	0.58	0.6	18, 85.7%	14.3%
Q2	A (0, 0.00%)	B (0, 0.00%)	C (0, 0.00%)	***D (21, 100.00%***	0	0	21, 100.0%	0.0%
Q3	A (1, 4.76%)	***B (20, 95.24%)***	C (0, 0.00%)	D (0, 0.00%)	0.1	0.2	20, 95.2%	4.8%
Q4	A (4, 19.05%)	***B (15, 71.43%)***	C (0, 0.00%)	D (2, 9.52%)	-0.02	0	15, 71.4%	28.6%
Q5	A (0, 0.00%)	***B (15, 71.43%)***	C (3, 14.29%)	D (3, 14.29%)	0.29	0.25	15, 71.4%	28.6%
Q6	A (2, 9.52%)	B (2, 9.52%)	C (3, 14.29%)	***D (14, 66.67%)***	0.43	0.6	14, 66.7%	33.3%
Q7	A (8, 38.10%)	B (4, 19.05%)	***C (6, 28.57%)***	D (3, 14.29%)	0.39	0.67	6, 28.6%	71.4%
Q8	A (0, 0.00%)	***B (16, 76.19%)***	C (4, 19.05%)	D (1, 4.76%)	0.04	-0.33	16, 76.2%	23.8%
Q9	A (0, 0.00%)	B (1, 4.76%)	***C (20, 95.24%***	D (0, 0.00%)	0.06	0	20, 95.2%	4.8%
Q10	***A (19, 90.48%)***	B (1, 4.76%)	C (0, 0.00%)	D (1, 4.76%)	0.27	0.2	19, 90.5%	9.5%

Figure 1.
Standard item analysis of mid-course examination. The total number of items is 40, and the total number of the examinee is 21. The KR20 is 0.82. Pt.Biserial: Point biserial correlation, Disc Index: discrimination index, Correct: number and percentage of the correct answer (difficulty index), Pct. Incorrect: percentage of an incorrect answer.

The highest and lowest scores were 38 and 14 respectively.

The class average (mean) (30.3) is more than the class median (30) which represents a positively skewed distribution of examinee scores. Despite this, examinee scores may show normal ball-shape distribution. If the median is larger than the average (mean), the examinee scores will be negatively skewed distribution. Average equals median, the examinees' scores are symmetrically (zero skewed) and normally distributed with ball-shaped.

The KR20 (Cronbach's alpha) is 0.82 which is an acceptable value for most of the authors. Such value of internal consistency of exam allows deciding pass/fail. Lower values put the exam in questionable status.

- Item 1: the difficulty index is 85.7% (easy). Although it has high discrimination power (DE = 0.6, Pbiserial = 0.58), two distractors are non-functional (B, C).

  Comment: the item needs reediting. Distractors B and C need to be revised or changed by more plausible ones before being re-used.

- Item 2: the difficulty index is 100% (easy). It has low discrimination power (DE = 00, Pbiserial = 00), all distractors are non-functional.

  Comment: the item needs major revision or rewriting. This item is absolutely easy with no difficulty or discrimination index. Such items should be removed from the question bank and removal from the exam is considered valid.

- Item 6: the difficulty index is 66.7% (moderate). It has high discrimination power (DE = 0.6, Pbiserial = 0.43) and all the distractors are functional.

  Comment: The item has acceptable indices. Such items can be saved in the question bank for further use. The distractors need to be updated to have more efficiency.

- Item 7: the difficulty index is 28.6% (difficult). Although it has high discrimination power (DE = 0.67, Pbiserial = 0.39), all the distractors are functional.

Comment: The item has acceptable indices. Such items can be saved in the question bank for further use. The distractors need to be updated to have more efficiency.

- Item 8: the difficulty index is 76.2% (moderate). This item has a negative discrimination index (−0.33) and poor Pbiserial (0.04). Only one distractor is functional (C). The negative discrimination index is caused by the increased number of students in the lower account (27%) than those in the upper account (27%).

  Comment: although the item has a moderate difficulty index, but is poorly discriminating. Such an item needs major revision.

Exam Item Analysis Report					Exams Graded: 25			
Instructor:	0	Total Possibl	40	Average:	24.6(61.40%)			
Exam Name:	0	Highest Scor	33(82.5%)	Median:	25(62.50%)			
Exam Date:	0	Lowest Score	13(32.5%)	KR20	0.7409171			
	Correct responses are shown in bold and italics				Pt. Biserial	Disc. Index	Correct	Pct. Incorrect
Q1	A (1, 4.00%)	B (4, 16.00%)	C (1, 4.00%)	***D (19, 76.00%)***	0.39	0.5	19, 76.0%	24.0%
Q4	A (0, 0.00%)	B (2, 8.00%)	C (1, 4.00%)	***D (22, 88.00%)***	0.36	0.5	22, 88.0%	12.0%
Q5	A (2, 8.00%)	***B (22, 88.00%)***	C (0, 0.00%)	D (1, 4.00%)	0.2	0.33	22, 88.0%	12.0%
Q8	***A (1, 4.00%)***	B (18, 72.00%)	C (1, 4.00%)	D (5, 20.00%)	-0.06	-0.17	1, 4.0%	96.0%
Q9	A (11, 44.00%)	B (7, 28.00%)	***C (5, 20.00%)***	D (2, 8.00%)	0.09	0.17	5, 20.0%	80.0%
Q10	***A (3, 12.00%)***	B (6, 24.00%)	C (10, 40.00%)	D (6, 24.00%)	0.32	0.17	3, 12.0%	88.0%
Q11	***A (11, 44.00%)***	B (1, 4.00%)	C (3, 12.00%)	D (10, 40.00%)	0.01	0	11, 44.0%	56.0%
Q12	A (5, 20.00%)	B (1, 4.00%)	***C (13, 52.00%)***	D (6, 24.00%)	0.19	0.33	13, 52.0%	48.0%

Figure 2.
Standard item analysis of Mid-course examination. The total number of items is 40, and the total number of examinee is 25. The KR20 is 0.74. Pt.Biserial: Point biserial correlation, Disc Index: discrimination index, Correct: number and percentage of the correct answer (difficulty index), Pct. Incorrect: percentage of an incorrect answer.

Figure 2:
In this Example 2.
The number of examinees was 25.
The number of test items is 40.
The highest and lowest scores were 33 and 13 respectively.

The class average (mean) (24.6) is more than the class median (25), distribution of examinee scores is skewed to the left. Despite this, examinee scores may show normal ball shape distribution.

The KR20 (Cronbach's alpha) is 0.74 which is an acceptable value for most of the authors. Such a value of internal consistency is suitable for class tests.

- Item 8: the difficulty index is 4.0% (difficult). It has negative discrimination power (DE = -0.17, Pbiserial = −0.06), one distractors is non-functional (C).

  Comment: the correct answer is (A) while most of the examinees chose (B). According to distractor analysis, this item is miss-keyed rather than an implausible distractor.

- Item 9: the difficulty index is 20% (difficult). It has low discrimination power (DE = 0.17, Pbiserial = 0.09), all distractors are functional.

  Comment: distractor analysis show option number (A) and (B) are more selected by examinees. This can be due to implausible. The presence of implausible can affect the item difficulty index. Distractors in this item should be revised or changed with plausible ones.

- Item 11: the difficulty index is 44.0% (moderate). It has low discrimination power (DE = 0.0, Pbiserial = 0.01) and only one the distractors is non-functional.

  Comment: The item has an acceptable difficulty index. Distractor (D) is more selected by upper examinee such as the key answer. Such a situation can favor missed key or implausible distractors. The distractors need to be updated to have more efficiency.

Author details

Assad Ali Rezigalla
Department of Basic Medical Sciences (Unit of Anatomy), College of Medicine, University of Bisha, Saudi Arabia

*Address all correspondence to: assadkafe@yahoo.com

References

[1] Stassen, M.L., K. Doherty, and M. Poe, *Program-based review and assessment: Tools and techniques for program improvement*. 2004: Office of Academic Planning & Assessment, University of Massachusetts Amherst.

[2] Tavakol, M. and R. Dennick, *Post-examination analysis of objective tests.* Med Teach, 2011. **33**(6): p. 447-58.

[3] Benson, J., *A comparison of three types of item analysis in test development using classical and latent trait methods*, in *GRADUATE COUNCIL OF THE UNIVERSITY OF FLORIDA*. 1978, UNIVERSITY OF FLORIDA: FLORIDA, USA. p. 134.

[4] Sharma, L.R., *Analysis of difficulty index, discrimination index and distractor efficiency of multiple choice questions of speech sounds of english.* International Research Journal of MMC, 2021. **2**(1): p. 15-28.

[5] Thompson, B. and J.E. Levitov, *Using microcomputers to score and evaluate items.* Collegiate Microcomputer archive, 1985. **3**.

[6] Sugianto, A., *Item analysis of english summative test: Efl teacher-made test.* Indonesian EFL Research, 2020. **1**(1): p. 35-54.

[7] Kumar, H. and S.K. Rout, *Major tools and techniques in educational evaluation*, in *Measurement and evaluation in education*. 2016, Vikas Publishing House Pvt. Ltd.: India. p. 256.

[8] Case, S.M. and D.B. Swanson, *Constructing written test questions for the basic and clinical sciences*. 3 ed. 1998, United States of America: National Board of Medical Examiners Philadelphia, PA. 129.

[9] Kruyen, P.M., *Using short tests and questionnaires for making decisions about individuals: When is short too short?* 2012, Netherlands Ridderprint BV, Ridderkerk.

[10] Akinboboye, J.T. and M.A. Ayanwale, *Bloom taxonomy usage and psychometric analysis of classroom teacher made test.* AFRICAN MULTIDISCIPLINARY JOURNAL OF DEVELOPMENT, 2021. **10**(1): p. 10-21.

[11] Brookhart, S.M. and A.J. Nitko, *Education assessment of students*. New jearsey: Merrill prentice hall. 2018, New Jersey: Pearson; 8th edition.

[12] Obon, A.M. and K.A.M. Rey, Analysis of multiple-choice questions (mcqs): Item and test statistics from the 2nd year nursing qualifying exam in a university in cavite, philippines. Abstract Proceedings International Scholars Conference, 2019. 7(1): p. 499-511.

[13] Downing, S. and R. Yudkowsky, *Assessment in health professions education*. 2009, New York and London: Routledge and Taylor & Francis

[14] Silao, C.V.O. and R.G. Luciano, *Development of an automated test item analysis system with optical mark recognition (omr)* International Journal of Electrical Engineering and Technology (IJEET), 2021. **12**(1): p. 67-79.

[15] Reinhardt, B.M., *Factors affecting coefficient alpha: A mini monte carlo study*, in *The Annual Meeting of the Southwest Educational Research Association (January 26, 1991)*. 1991, University of Texas: San Antonio, Texas, USA. p. 31.

[16] Tavakol, M. and R. Dennick, *Making sense of cronbach's alpha.* International journal of medical education, 2011. **2**: p. 53-55.

[17] Graham, J.M., *Congeneric and (essentially) tau-equivalent estimates of*

score reliability: What they are and how to use them. Educational and Psychological Measurement, 2006. **66**(6): p. 930-944.

[18] Rezigalla, A.A., A.M.E. Eleragi, and M. Ishag, *Comparison between students' perception toward an examination and item analysis, reliability and validity of the examination.* Sudan Journal of Medical Sciences, 2020. **15**(2): p. 114-123.

[19] Considine, J., M. Botti, and S. Thomas, *Design, format, validity and reliability of multiple choice questions for use in nursing research and education.* Collegian, 2005. **12**(1): p. 19-24.

[20] Cortina, J.M., *What is coefficient alpha? An examination of theory and applications.* Journal of applied psychology, 1993. **78**(1): p. 98.

[21] McNeish, D., *Thanks coefficient alpha, we'll take it from here.* Psychol Methods, 2018. **23**(3): p. 412-433.

[22] Panayides, P., *Coefficient alpha: Interpret with caution.* Europe's Journal of Psychology, 2013. **9**(4): p. 687-696.

[23] Al-Osail, A.M., et al., *Is cronbach's alpha sufficient for assessing the reliability of the osce for an internal medicine course?* BMC research notes, 2015. **8**(1): p. 1-6.

[24] McCowan, R.J. and S.C. McCowan, *Item analysis for criterion-referenced tests*. 1999, New York: Center for Development of Human Services.

[25] Salkind, N.J., *Encyclopedia of research design*. Vol. 1. 2010: sage.

[26] Robinson, J.P., P.R. Shaver, and L.S. Wrightsman, Scale selection and evaluation, in Measures of political attitudes, J.P. Robinson, P.R. Shaver, and L.S. Wrightsman, Editors. 1999, Academic Press: USA. p. 509.

[27] Cicchetti, D.V., Guidelines, criteria, and rules of thumb for evaluating normed and standardized assessment instruments in psychology. Psychological assessment, 1994. 6(4): p. 284.

[28] Axelson, R.D. and C.D. Kreiter, Reliability, in Assessment in health professions education, R. Yudkowsky, Y.S. Park, and S.M. Downing, Editors. 2019, Routledge: London.

[29] Hassan, S. and R. Hod, Use of item analysis to improve the quality of single best answer multiple choice question in summative assessment of undergraduate medical students in malaysia. Education in Medicine Journal, 2017. 9(3): p. 33-43.

[30] Green, S.B. and M.S. Thompson, *Structural equation modeling in clinical psychology research*, in *Handbook of research methods in clinical psychology*, M.C. Roberts and S.S. Ilardi, Editors. 2008, Wiley-Blackwell. p. 138-175.

[31] Mahjabeen, W., et al., *Difficulty index, discrimination index and distractor efficiency in multiple choice questions.* Annals of PIMS-Shaheed Zulfiqar Ali Bhutto Medical University, 2017. **13**(4): p. 310-315.

[32] Mehta, G. and V. Mokhasi, *Item analysis of multiple choice questions-an assessment of the assessment tool.* Int J Health Sci Res, 2014. **4**(7): p. 197-202.

[33] Tarrant, M., J. Ware, and A.M. Mohammed, *An assessment of functioning and non-functioning distractors in multiple-choice questions: A descriptive analysis.* BMC Medical Education, 2009. **9**(1): p. 40.

[34] Puthiaparampil, T. and M. Rahman, *How important is distractor efficiency for grading best answer questions?* BMC medical education, 2021. **21**(1): p. 1-6.

[35] Gajjar, S., et al., *Item and test analysis to identify quality multiple choice questions (mcqs) from an assessment of medical students of ahmedabad, gujarat.*

Indian journal of community medicine: official publication of Indian Association of Preventive & Social Medicine, 2014. **39**(1): p. 17.

[36] Kumar, D., et al., *Item analysis of multiple choice questions: A quality assurance test for an assessment tool.* Medical Journal Armed Forces India, 2021. **77**: p. S85-S89.

[37] Date, A.P., et al., *Item analysis as tool to validate multiple choice question bank in pharmacology.* International Journal of Basic & Clinical Pharmacology, 2019. **8**(9): p. 1999-2003.

[38] Abdalla, M.E., *What does item analysis tell us? Factors affecting the reliability of multiple choice questions (mcqs).* Gezira Journal of Health Sciences, 2011. 7(2).

[39] Fozzard, N., et al., *Analysis of mcq and distractor use in a large first year health faculty foundation program: Assessing the effects of changing from five to four options.* BMC Med Educ, 2018. **18**(1): p. 252.

[40] Sajjad, M., S. Iltaf, and R.A. Khan, Nonfunctional distractor analysis: An indicator for quality of multiple choice questions. Pak J Med Sci, 2020. 36(5): p. 982-986.

[41] Haladyna, T.M., S.M. Downing, and M.C. Rodriguez, *A review of multiple-choice item-writing guidelines for classroom assessment.* Applied measurement in education, 2002. **15**(3): p. 309-333.

[42] Swanson, D.B., K.Z. Holtzman, and K. Allbee, *Measurement characteristics of content-parallel single-best-answer and extended-matching questions in relation to number and source of options.* Academic Medicine, 2008. **83**(10): p. S21-S24.

[43] Frary, R.B., *More multiple-choice item writing do's and don'ts.* Practical Assessment, Research, Evaluation, 1994. **4**(1): p. 11.

[44] Abdulghani, H.M., et al., *The relationship between non-functioning distractors and item difficulty of multiple choice questions: A descriptive analysis.* Journal of Health Specialties, 2014. **2**(4): p. 148.

[45] Alhummayani, F.M., *Evaluation of the multiple-choice question item analysis of the sixth year undergraduate orthodontic tests at the faculty of dentistry, king abdulaziz university, saudi arabia.* Egyptian Orthodontic Journal, 2020. **57**(June 2020): p. 1-18.

[46] Licona-Chávez, A.L. and L.R. Velázquez-Liaño, *Quality assessment of a multiple choice test through psychometric properties.* MedEdPublish, 2020. **9**.

[47] Hassan, S., *Item analysis, reliability statistics and standard error of measurement to improve the quality and impact of multiple choice questions in undergraduate medical education in faculty of medicine at unisza.* Malaysian Journal of Public Health Medicine, 2016. **16**(3): p. 7-15.

[48] Hingorjo, M.R. and F. Jaleel, *Analysis of one-best mcqs: The difficulty index, discrimination index and distractor efficiency.* J Pak Med Assoc, 2012. **62**(2): p. 142-7.

[49] Lord, F.M., *The relation of the reliability of multiple-choice tests to the distribution of item difficulties.* Psychometrika, 1952. **17**(2): p. 181-194.

[50] Uddin, I., et al., *Item analysis of multiple choice questions in pharmacology.* J Saidu Med Coll Swat, 2020. **10**(2): p. 128-131.

[51] Kim, M.-K., et al., *Incorporation of bloom's taxonomy into multiple-choice examination questions for a pharmacotherapeutics course.* American journal of pharmaceutical education, 2012. **76**(6).

[52] Nevid, J.S. and N. McClelland, *Using action verbs as learning outcomes: Applying bloom's taxonomy in measuring instructional objectives in introductory psychology.* Journal of Education and Training Studies, 2013. **1**(2): p. 19-24.

[53] Elfaki, O., K. Bahamdan, and S. Al-Humayed, *Evaluating the quality of multiple-choice questions used for final exams at the department of internal medicine, college of medicine, king khalid university.* Sudan Med Monit, 2015. **10**: p. 123-27.

[54] Oermann, M.H. and K.B. Gaberson, *Evaluation and testing in nursing education*. 6 ed. 2019, New York: Springer Publishing Company.

[55] Bukvova, H., K. Figl, and G. Neumann, *Improving the quality of multiple-choice exams by providing feedback from item analysis.*

[56] Kaur M, Singla S, Mahajan R. Item analysis of in use multiple choice questions in pharmacology. International Journal of Applied and Basic Medical Research. 2016;6(3): 170-173.

[57] Bhat SK, Prasad KHL. Item analysis and optimizing multiple-choice questions for a viable question bank in ophthalmology: A cross-sectional study. Indian J Ophthalmol. 2021;69(2):343-6.

[58] Rogausch, A., R. Hofer, and R. Krebs, *Rarely selected distractors in high stakes medical multiple-choice examinations and their recognition by item authors: A simulation and survey.* BMC Medical Education, 2010. **10**(1): p. 1-9.

[59] Wood, D.A. and D.C. Adkins, *Test construction: Development and interpretation of achievement tests*. 1960: CE Merrill Books.

[60] Wiersma, W. and S.G. Jurs, *Educational measurement and testingallyn & bacon*. 1990, Boston. 415.

[61] Matlock-Hetzel, S., *Basic concepts in item and test analysis.* 1997.

[62] Sim, S.-M. and R.I. Rasiah, *Relationship between item difficulty and discrimination indices in true/false-type multiple choice questions of a para-clinical multidisciplinary paper.* Annals-Academy of Medicine Singapore, 2006. **35**(2): p. 67.

[63] Ramzan, M., et al., *Item analysis of multiple-choice questions at the department of community medicine, wah medical college, pakistan.* Life and Science, 2020. **1**(2): p. 4-4.

[64] Setiyana, R., *Analysis of summative tests for english.* English Education Journal, 2016. 7(4): p. 433-447.

[65] Oermann, M.H. and K.B. Gaberson, *Evaluation and testing in nursing education*. 2016: Springer Publishing Company.

[66] Aljehani, D.K., et al., *Relationship of text length of multiple-choice questions on item psychometric properties–a retrospective study.* Saudi Journal for Health Sciences, 2020. **9**(2): p. 84.

[67] Henrysson, S., *Gathering, analyzing, and using data on test items*, in *Educational measurement*, R.L. Thorndike, Editor. 1971, American Council on Education: Washington DC. p. 141.

[68] Maulina, N. and R. Novirianthy, *Item analysis and peer-review evaluation of specific health problems and applied research block examination.* Jurnal Pendidikan Kedokteran Indonesia: The Indonesian Journal of Medical Education, 2020. **9**(2): p. 131-137.

Chapter 10

Redefining Surgical Skill Acquisition

Vaikunthan Rajaratnam, Norana Abdul Rahman, Chaoyan Dong and Hannah Jia Hui Ng

Abstract

There have been reduced opportunities for surgical skill acquisition due to the COVID-19 pandemic and the regulated training hours. Despite these challenges, self-regulated learning allows trainees to learn continuously, and motor skills development can be augmented through mental practice and motor imagery. The aim of this chapter is to introduce the theoretical concepts in skill acquisition and the role of mental and deliberate practice as an alternative for skill training. A case study is presented using a design and development framework for producing an online basic micro suturing training resource based on self-regulated learning. This case study demonstrates the use of the ADDIE instructional design model and Mayer's multimedia theory guidelines, for creating online instructional resources. The methodological approach of a design and developmental framework to create an educationally sound online training module for micro suturing which has significant utility in hand surgery is discussed in this chapter. The tools described in this chapter are translatable to any psychomotor skills development in medical education.

Keywords: micro suturing, mental script, mental practice, motor imagery, deliberate practice

1. Introduction

The transformative changes occurring in the technology, political and economic landscape has not spared medical education (ME), which is further compounded by the ever-increasing knowledge and skills in medicine. The last few decades have seen an increasing expectation in the efficient utilisation of resources in ME. Despite all these changes and investments, doctors who are fit to practice competently in the community remain a challenge – lacking in the soft skills of medical practice and the hard skills of knowledge and procedural skills. It has been documented that ME has failed to meet the community's needs altogether [1]. There is a call by all transdisciplinary stakeholders for value for money, universal access, and increased quality of care, and this has impacted the medical education field, including suggestions to adopt a transdisciplinary and transnational approach to designing and delivering competency-based medical education. This requires an alignment and integration of medical education to quality of care to patients and populations with a sense of accountability founded on social justice [2].

Surgery as a specialty is dependent on psychomotor skills and has traditionally followed a mentor-apprenticeship model where experienced surgeons train the learners in the work environment [3] to produce surgeons who are competent in specific motor skills within a stipulated time. Learners need to aspire to excellence in the interest of their patients [4]. The traditional surgical training models, including mentoring, role-modelling, and one-to-one supervision, produce skilled and competent surgeons. However, this mode of teaching is vanishing due to time constraints and the heavy burden of service commitment to meet the needs of the community [5, 6]. The emphasis on service efficiency has curtailed on-the-job teaching and exposure to live patients in the current hospital environments. Innovative strategies have been adopted to make the programmes more flexible and efficient, more trainee-oriented, incorporating innovations like simulation technology, competency-based assessments, online learning, and resources, emphasizing teamwork, professionalism, communications, and quality patient care [7]. The aim of a surgical training is to produce competent surgeons skilled and safe, who fulfill the community's needs [8–11].

2. Theoretical models for surgical motor skill acquisition

Advancement in surgical education research sheds light on the understanding of competency and assessment, in the sense that competency cannot be assumed when trainees can perform parts of a task or individual surgical skills, as many complex tasks require the integration of many skills. Literature showed that surgical trainees at both undergraduate [12] and postgraduate levels [13] do not feel competent or ready to operate independently at the end of their training. Competence is not equal to excellence. Due to the lack of time and opportunities to practice, the learning process focuses on competence rather than excellence [14]. For surgical motor skill acquisition, the following four theoretical models are commonly used (**Table 1**) - Fitts and Posner's 3-Stage Model of Motor Skills Acquisition, Bandura's Theory of Social Learning, Ericsson's Deliberate Practice Model, and Motor Simulation Theory of Jeannerod.

Mental practice (MP) is "the cognitive rehearsal of a task in the absence of overt physical movement" [19]. It has successfully improved psychomotor performance to enhance skill and performance in sports and music [20, 21]. Mental imagery (MI) has been shown to activate similar neural processes to those used in the actual performance of a given skill [22, 23]. MP has been used lately as an alternative strategy in surgical training. The current literature shows the successful use of MP in surgical training or enhancing surgical performance, but lacks methodological details for the development of educational resources incorporating MP.

Theory	Summary
Fitts and Posner's 3-Stage Theory of Motor Skill Acquisition [15]	Motor skill acquisition goes through 3 stages, i.e., cognitive or learning stage, associative or motor behaviour stage, and autonomous or expert stage.
Bandura's Theory of Social Learning [16]	Based on observational learning and modelling: attention, internalisation or retention, reproduction, and motivation
Ericsson's Deliberate Practice Model [17]	Deliberate practice in motivated individuals with regular reinforcement and feedback to support learning
Motor Simulation Theory of Jeannerod [18]	Cognitive rehearsal of a task in the absence of overt physical movement using script-based mental rehearsal

Table 1.
Summary of surgical training theories.

In summary, the current body of knowledge on psychomotor skill acquisition to an expert level [24, 25] requires:

- observation of the skill demonstrated by an expert
- internalisation with motor imagery
- mental practice and repetition
- physical deliberate practice

The current model of surgical training programmes for motor skill acquisition focuses on the direct supervision of the expert in the operating room, providing direct observation, guidance, and feedback, ensuring compliance to the pre-operative plan. Graduated responsibility and progression in surgical performance are allowed based on the level of surgical performance and adherence to patient safety [26]. The emphasis has been the development of competencies which is a minimum level of skill to be demonstrated, rather than mastery associated with a higher level of proficiency. Competency requires much less training than mastery and is facilitated by the very structured and focused training. Hence, to overcome the reduced opportunity to learn and practice in the operating room, low fidelity bench models, basic surgical skills, surgical laboratory practice, and higher fidelity human cadaver models to live animal model practice have been utilised [27]. From simulation to gaming and robotics, technology has also become the enabler in surgical training [28, 29]. These strategies have implications in cost-effectiveness and universal accessibility, as they require resources - both physical and trainee/trainer time, as they are synchronous platforms for learning [30]. However, the current model is singularly deficient in that there is no universally accessible opportunity to practice the surgical procedure outside of the operating theatre and without access to physical simulators.

Based on the review of these theoretical frameworks, we propose a model for the expert acquisition of motor skills in **Figure 1**. This model incorporates the theoretical framework of Fitts and Posner, Bandura, Ericsson, and Jeannerod, and operationalises the steps described in the theories of skill acquisition and

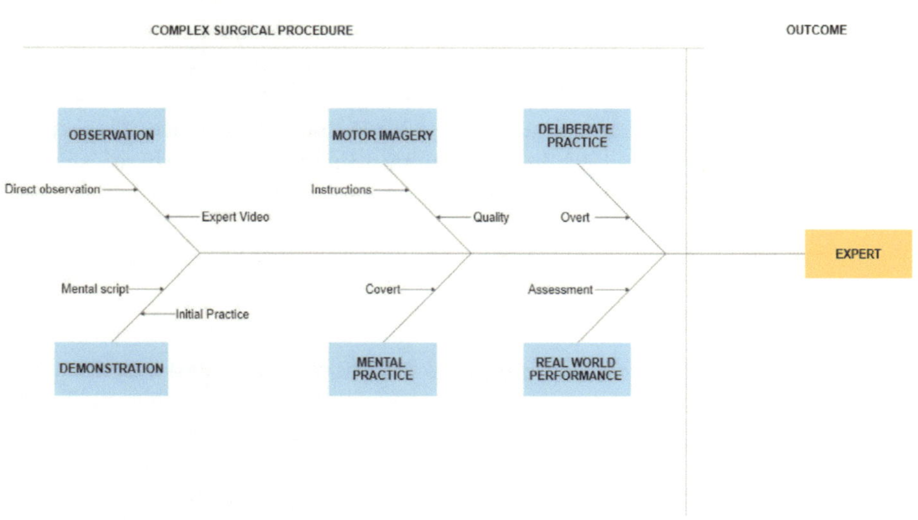

Figure 1.
An integrated model for surgical skill acquisition.

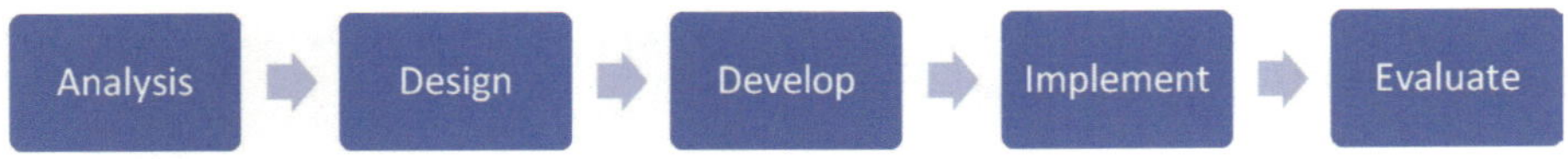

Figure 2.
ADDIE instructional design model.

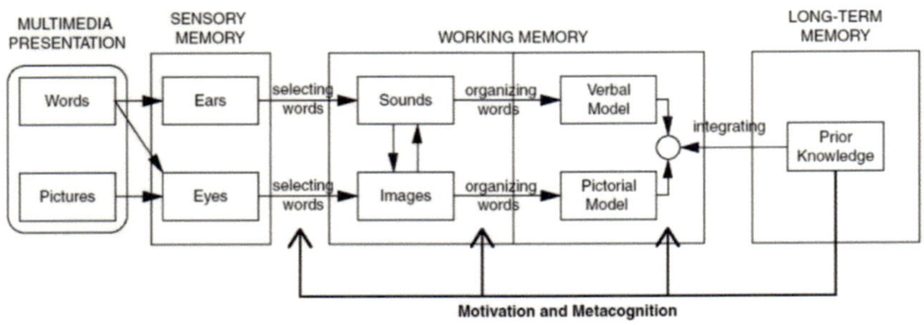

Figure 3.
Mayer's cognitive theory of multimedia learning.

mastery [15–18]. The observation of expert performance, with an introduction and performance of the task by the trainee, followed by mental practice with motor imagery augmented with deliberate practice, will need further authentication and validation.

More importantly, this model highlights the importance of applying instructional design models to create instructional materials and programmes for surgical skill acquisition. Instructional design (ID), the science of instruction, provides a systematic and evidence-based methodology for creating instructional materials for effective teaching. The various models and techniques have been used in surgical training [31–33].

A commonly used ID model for designing learning programmes is the Analysis, Design, Development, Implementation, and Evaluation (ADDIE) model in **Figure 2** [34] coupled with Mayer's cognitive theory of multimedia learning [35] in **Figure 3**. They can provide the framework for designing training programmes and materials for skill acquisition, which promotes mental simulation with deliberate practice in surgery training. Mayer's multimedia learning theory defines principles using texts, images, and audio to improve knowledge and skills acquisition. The theory explains how people learn through multiple sensory stimuli rather than a single channel such as texts, and empirical evidence showed that adding images and videos to words improves learning outcomes [36]. In addition, multimedia learning theories indicate best practices in designing multimedia teaching materials [37].

3. Our proposed model

The execution of the model – our proposed tool shown in **Figure 4** describes the use of a design and development research framework to produce instructional materials incorporating mental and deliberate practice. It describes the use of the expert review panel and in-depth interviews to identify the key tasks of complex surgical procedures from the expert's perspective. Incorporating a think-aloud/verbal walkthrough of the index motor skill by experts, followed by content and task analysis [38], allows for creating a detailed mental script to be incorporated into the instructional materials.

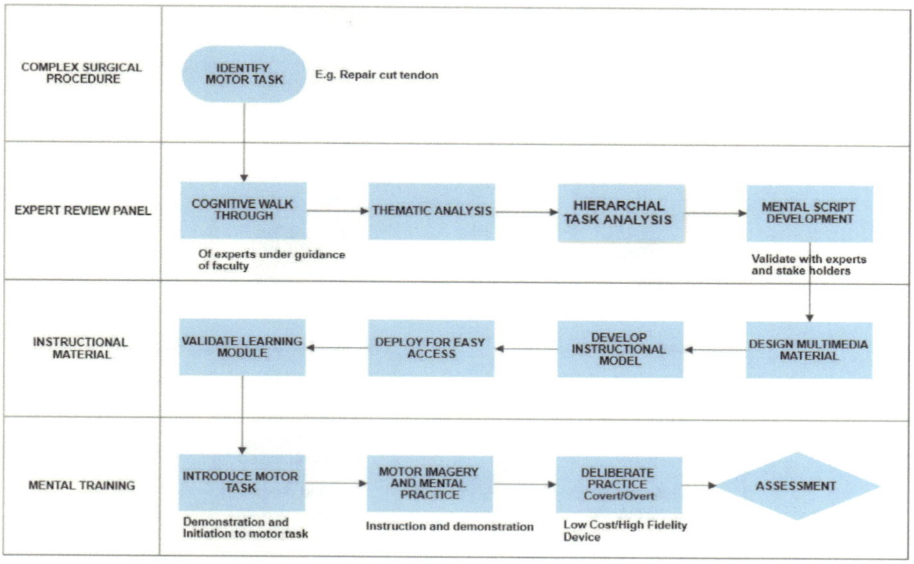

Figure 4.
Execution of model to create a training programme for a surgical skill.

The beginning of the model entails designing an instructional video, which includes the live demonstration of surgical procedures by an expert surgeon. The production of an instructional video of the master surgeon performing the procedure based on the task and subtask involved in the procedure will require the framework of multimedia instructional production [35]. In addition, the video will need the narration of the mental script produced from the methodology described in **Figure 4**. This will enable the trainee to perform mental practice and augmented with deliberate practice using low-cost practice models designed and developed by the master surgeons.

The ADDIE model is used to perform a content, task, and subtask analysis of the procedure with expert surgeons, which will aid in creating the storyboard, and designing the instructional video. For example, in tendon repair, a cognitive walkthrough is conducted with an expert surgeon, and the instructions and reflections, inclusive of kinaesthetic cues, are recorded and analysed verbatim to create a mental script validated by the master surgeon. This will be used as the narration for an expert instructional video showing the master performing the tendon repair. The instructional material – the video will then be validated by master surgeons. A low-cost practice model is needed for deliberate practice such as chicken or sheep tendon for tendon repair training. Combining the video and mental practice using the mental script allows the trainees to learn from expert surgeons anytime, anywhere, and improve with deliberate practice using the chicken/sheep practice model. Once they are ready, they are then assessed in the operating room for real-world performance to verify retention and transfer of skills in tendon repair surgery.

This new model that incorporates motor imagery and mental practice, augmented with deliberate practice, will provide an alternative training path for expert performance in surgical procedures. The tools to design and develop the instructional materials (expert instructional videos and mental scripts) with task and content analysis is founded on sound instructional design principles. It will, however, require further validation.

Current surgical training resources have been using various instructional mediums from text and multimedia materials, focusing on the step-by-step procedure

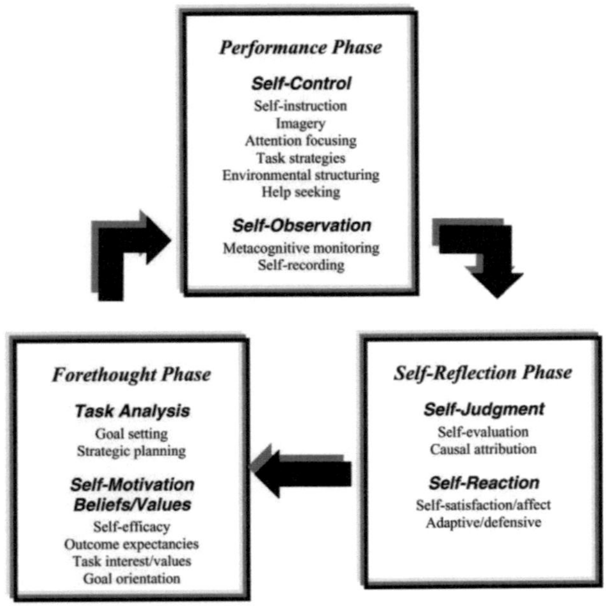

Figure 5.
Phases and sub-processes of Self-Regulated Learning (SRL).

for performing motor tasks. These need now to be expanded to incorporate mental scripts for each standard procedure in surgery.

The theoretical framework for continuous learning is self-regulated learning (SRL) (**Figure 5**). SRL perceives learning as "an activity that students do for themselves in a proactive way". It is a process by which the learner plans, monitors, and evaluates his learning to achieve learning objectives based on his developed strategies [39].

This model and tool that we proposed was executed in a study that used the design and development research framework dedicated to creating new knowledge and validating existing practice in instructional design. In this case study we aimed to demonstrate how to design, develop, and evaluate an online instructional module on micro suturing guided by Mayer's multimedia learning theory and incorporated a mental script for the mental practice of micro suturing.

4. Development of the online module to teach micro suturing skills

Using the tool for surgical skill training as a guide (as seen in **Figure 4**), the key tasks for micro suturing were identified and were listed as the expected learning outcomes with clearly stated essential tasks and competency levels. An expert review panel was identified and invited to perform a think-aloud cognitive walkthrough of these key skills. We conducted content and task analysis with the results and developed a detailed mental script for micro suturing. The mental script was incorporated into the instructional materials of the online module. The development of the online module was based on the framework of multimedia learning of the surgical procedure [37]. This online module consisted of instructional videos of the expert surgeons' live demonstration of micro suturing, with the concurrent narration of the mental script.

The participants in the experimental phase used this online module to practice. Combining the video and the mental script allowed the participants to learn from expert surgeons anytime and anywhere. In addition, this online module was augmented with deliberate practice using the low-cost rubber glove practice model.

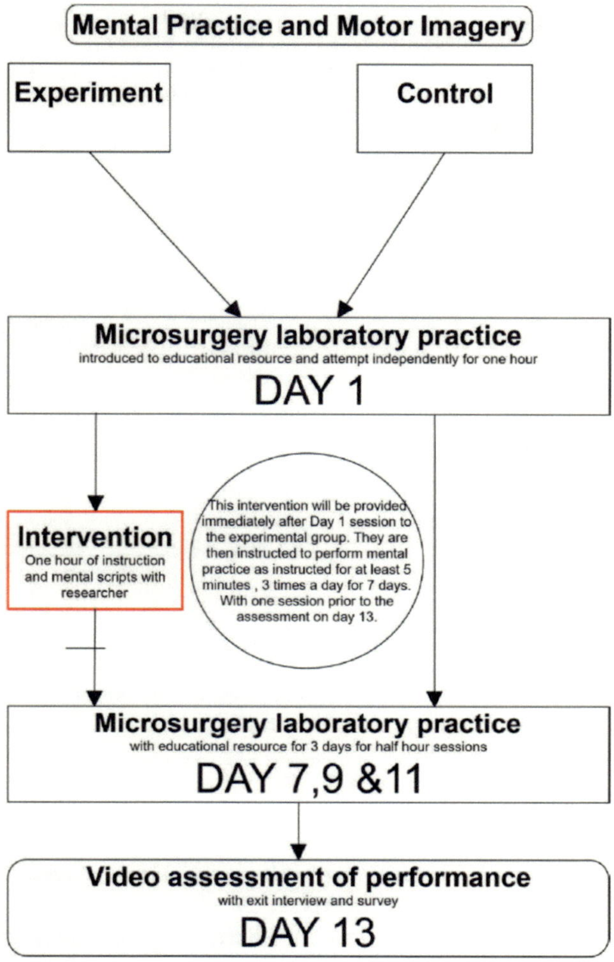

Figure 6.
Diagram of the pilot experiment using the learning module for micro suturing.

The online module allowed trainees to observe expert performance, followed by mental practice with motor imagery, and then deliberate practice to reach the mastery level, as summarised in the tool for developing instructional materials in **Figure 4**. The training module created was then evaluated in a pilot study using an experimental design (**Figure 6**).

5. Evaluation of the online module to teach micro suturing skills

To evaluate the online module, this case study used the design process in **Table 2**. It includes the evaluation on (1) the effectiveness of the module against the existing training programmes, (2) ease of use for this module, (3) the usability.

This pilot study evaluated the new training module by comparing it with reading the manual and observing the experts performing the surgery. Participants were volunteer medical students via opportunistic sampling from two medical schools in Singapore. All participants had completed an introductory suturing course and had not performed micro suturing procedures before the study. None had prior exposure to mental practice strategies in any domains. The exclusion criteria included non-consent, failure to understand and comply with new training techniques, and

Objectives	Questions	Methods	Variables	Analysis	Conclusions
To evaluate the effectiveness of this module against the existing training programmes	Does the online module provide the opportunity for authentic practice of surgical skills?	Experimental study Randomised after participant selection	Performance, effectiveness, and efficiency. SMaRT, MIQ, time taken to complete the task	Performance	Endorse module with MIMP
To evaluate the ease of learning of this module	Does the module allow for ease of learning basic micro suturing	Survey	Cognitive load (NASA-TLX)	Cognitive load (NASA-TLX)	Recommend MIMP incorporation in the program
To evaluate the usability of learning of the new module	Is the module usable in the real world	Survey	Usability attributes (SUS)	Usability analysis with SUS	Recommend use of MIMP in module

MIMP (Motor Imagery and Mental Practice); SUS (System Usability Scale); NASA-TLX (NASA Task Load Index); MIQ (Mental Imagery Questionnaire); SMaRT (Stanford Microsurgery and Resident Training Scale Instrument).

Table 2.
Research design matrix.

failure to meet the inclusion criteria. A sample size of 11 was chosen based on previous studies and available resources for this study.

As seen in **Table 3** below, five experienced hand surgeons (more than five years in practice as consultants/specialists) were recruited via purposeful sampling as an expert for the review process. The panel was also involved in creating the mental script and developing the training module.

5.1 Analysis of key tasks

A quantitative analysis of the commonly performed procedures was conducted from a previous study [40]. The expert panel used this to determine the index procedure (micro suturing) for this research and the motor skills with various tasks

Surgeon	Age	Sex	Years of Practice
1	62	M	35
2	46	M	13
3	40	M	7
4	47	M	17
5	68	M	41
Mean	52.6		22.6
Range	40–68		7–41

Table 3.
Expert review panel demographics.

and subtasks required to perform micro suturing [40]. For this study, the procedure of nerve grafts and repair was chosen by the expert panel as the index procedure. The basic operative motor skill required to perform this nerve repair surgery is performing micro suturing using the microscope with an 8/0 needle with a diameter of 150 microns (0.15 mm). Mental script development was done as per **Figure 4** of the conceptual framework.

5.2 Design and development of the model

A storyboard was used to create the expert video modeling artefact from the previous step. A video recording of an expert performing micro suturing in the rubber glove model was incorporated into a whole learning module. The various steps and the sequencing resulted from the analysis of the mental script, which was developed earlier, and the mental script was also used as the narration for the video [41].

5.3 Implement

The primary author used the authoring tool Rise 360 to create the e-learning module. Rise 360 is part of the Articulate suite of eLearning authoring software. The module was then exported as an eLearning object and deployed onto a Learning Management System for universal access and distribution [42]. Finally, participants in the evaluation phase were provided the link to the online module (https://tinyurl.com/MIMPSURGERY).

5.4 Evaluation of the pilot experiment

There were 11 participants in both the experimental and control group, with one participant dropping out in each group, leaving 10 participants per group. The control group had an average age of 23.9 years (range 22–26), with 50% male and female. The experimental group had an average age of 23.1 years (range 21–30), with 70% male and 30% female.

The time taken to complete five micro sutures in the control and experimental groups was not statistically significant ($p = 0.77$). The NASA-TLX scores between the control and experimental group were also not statistically significant ($p = 0.60$).

The experimental group's overall performance was significantly higher than the control group ($p = 0.004$).

Both groups had an average "good" grading for the SUS scores (**Table 4**), indicating that the online module for micro suturing has good usability.

	Control (n = 10)	Experiment (n = 10)	p-value
Average time to complete ± SD (minutes)	12.97 ± 7.11	11.85 ± 2.06	0.77
Median time to complete (minutes, range)	10.38 (range 6.50 to 29.17)	11.83 (range 9.40 to 13.92)	
SMaRT scale scores (mean ± SD)	3.9 ± 0.47	4.54 ± 0.37	0.004
NASA-TLX (mean ± SD)	61.14 ± 24.99	59.14 ± 25.63	0.60
MIQ scores (mean ± SD)	4.88 ± 1.19	5.46 ± 1.03	0.021
SUS scores (mean ± SD)	74.25 ± 13.8	71.5 ±18.0	0.68

Table 4.
Results of the pilot study.

The Cronbach's alpha for the SUS scale for the ten questions was computed to be 0.78, indicating acceptable reliability.

Based on the MIQ scores, the experimental group scored significantly higher than the control group in the aspects of mental imagery ($p = 0.021$).

6. Discussion

In this chapter we have explored the theoretical basis for surgical psychomotor skill development. We describe a model based on the educational theories and a tool to facilitate production of instructional resources and activities for this. We describe a study to evaluate the product created from the tool for its effectiveness in developing skills in a group of novices. It has shown that using a Design and Development Research approach and using the ADDIE model, subject matter experts can design and develop authentic and validated learning materials for motor skills training. We document the methodology to produce evidence-based instructional videos for surgery. This chapter elaborates on the processes involved in the creation of these learning resources, the use of specific protocols to understand the key components of a psychomotor skill from the experts; the use of the verbal protocol, and the hierarchical task analysis and its use to create a mental script to aid in the acquisition of surgical skills by the trainees. The findings of this study demonstrate the need for a new medium of instructional materials to be developed in the key and index clinical procedures in all the medical specialties requiring procedural skills. Incorporating detailed mental scripts for the surgical procedures and the methodologies to produce them need to be developed among faculty members. Most faculty members should be able to produce short, high-quality educational videos using the process described in this study. This will allow for motor imagery and mental practice to be practised by all surgical trainees to facilitate mastery in the current environment of reduced practice and motor skill learning opportunities. Deliberate practice is now universally accepted as one of the strategies for the expert performance of motor skills and has been proven effective in surgical training.

Faculty members need to be familiar with the methodology of creating mental scripts and the use of instructional design models to create multimedia instructional materials inclusive of the instructional videos by experts. The implication is for medical educators to apply instructional design and technology models to guide education curricula development. As the model described in this research and the process of creating the instructional materials and activities are translatable to other health professional education that requires the acquisition of motor skills, the findings of this research can therefore be adapted for use in other disciplines. The recommended strategy should incorporate mental skills training, i.e., the motor imagery and mental practice for the learners, and the faculty development programme for all health professionals. The faculty must be trained in the design and development of instructional videos and mental scripts. Every index procedure in surgical skill training should have the following:

1. Expert instructional video of the procedure

2. A mental script incorporating kinaesthetic cues

3. Narration of the mental script incorporated into the video

4. Inexpensive and easily accessible practice models for deliberate practice.

Though the model needs further external validation, this model and its methodology and approach to developing the individual scripts for motor imagery and mental practice will redefine surgical training. Considering the constraints of obtaining the opportunity to observe, practice, and perform in a work environment and the universal lack of accessibility to the alternative high-technology medical simulators, the trainee needs a model that will allow for deliberate practice anywhere at any time.

7. Limitations

The ability to imagine a motor task and generate that mental image and maintain it while doing deliberate practice was difficult to assess. The use of the motor imagery questionnaire (MIQ) to measure this ability was simplistic. A qualitative approach, such as interview or focus group discussions with participants, would have produced much richer and more authentic data on the quality of motor imagery and the use of a focus group of experts and novices for script validation. Also, the compliance of self-directed use of the mental script for motor imagery was difficult to control and measure.

In the experimental part of the study, the main challenge was to prevent the control group from indirectly practicing motor imagery and mental practice. This was built into the study by excluding sports and musical performers in the control group [43]. The adherence of the experimental group to the instructions on mental practice before the deliberate practice sessions could not be verified. The small sample size of the participants is an obvious limiting factor, as generalizability is not possible with such a small size.

The role of confounding factors such as periods of rest before task performance, different levels of innate fine motor skills, subconscious use of motor imagery, and practice in the control group were not considered in this research. This research was confined to a laboratory and a very structured and small motor task. The generalisability of these results to more complex motor tasks has yet to be determined. This study also did not look at the other competencies required of a master surgeon, including but not confined to diagnostics and decision making, team development, and communication skills.

8. Conclusion

We recommend that mental script development should be incorporated into the curriculum for faculty development. Learners should be instructed on motor imagery and mental practice techniques as part of the core skills training, like suturing and dissection. Furthermore, instructional design and technological competency should be incorporated into the curriculum for faculty development to develop instructional sound materials. Lastly, design and development research methodology should be incorporated into the faculty development programme to encourage design and developmental research in medical education research.

The case study described the methodological approach to design and develop a training module for skill acquisition for surgical training programmes, utilizing a design and developmental research framework. This study has addressed some of the challenges of surgical education and has described a model based on sound educational theories to design and develop training programmes. This will help health professional educators to design practical and relevant modules to facilitate procedural training moving forward. In summary, this study shows that instructional materials for standardised procedures should be guided by the design and development of a mental script. The tool that has been developed and described in this research provides the methodology for this.

9. Practice implications

Mental skill training for mental simulation should be incorporated into the surgical residency programme. Faculty members must be trained in the design and development of instructional videos and mental scripts. Every index procedure in procedural skill training should have the following:

1. Expert instructional video of the procedure
2. A mental script incorporating kinaesthetic cues
3. The narration of the mental script incorporated into the video
4. Inexpensive and easily accessible practice models for deliberate practice.

Conflict of interest

All authors have no conflicts of interest to declare.

Author details

Vaikunthan Rajaratnam[1*], Norana Abdul Rahman[2], Chaoyan Dong[3] and Hannah Jia Hui Ng[1]

1 Khoo Teck Puat Hospital, Singapore

2 MEDEDTECH, UK

3 Sengkang General Hospital, Singapore

*Address all correspondence to: vaikunthan@oum.edu.my

References

[1] Frenk J, Chen L, Bhutta ZA, Cohen J, Crisp N, Evans T, et al. Health professionals for a new century: transforming education to strengthen health systems in an interdependent world. Lancet. 2010 Dec 4;376(9756): 1923-58.

[2] Caverzagie KJ, Nousiainen MT, Ferguson PC, Cate O ten, Ross S, Harris KA, et al. Overarching challenges to the implementation of competency-based medical education. Med Teach. 2017 Jun 3;39(6):588-93.

[3] Gallagher AG, O'Sullivan GC. Fundamentals of Surgical Simulation [Internet]. London: Springer London; 2012 [cited 2016 May 29]. Available from: http://link.springer.com/10.1007/978-0-85729-763-1

[4] Tooke, J. Aspiring to excellence. Findings and final recommendations of the independent inquiry into modernising medical careers. London: MMC Inquiry.; 2008.

[5] Chung RS, Verghese J, Diaz J, Eisenstat M. One-on-One Mentor–Resident Rotation for Improving Continuity of Care in a Surgical Training Program. J Surg Res. 1997 May 1;69(2): 359-61.

[6] Souba WW. Mentoring young academic surgeons, our most precious asset. J Surg Res. 1999 Apr;82(2):113-20.

[7] Lin J, Reddy RM. Teaching, Mentorship, and Coaching in Surgical Education. Thorac Surg Clin. 2019 Aug 1;29(3):311-20.

[8] Dudrick SJ. Evolution of surgical education through the 20th Century into the 21st Century. Cir Cir. 2011;79(1): 16-35.

[9] Eckleberry-Hunt J, Tucciarone J. The Challenges and Opportunities of Teaching "Generation Y". J Grad Med Educ. 2011 Dec 1;3(4):458-61.

[10] Holmboe ES, Batalden P. Achieving the Desired Transformation: Thoughts on Next Steps for Outcomes-Based Medical Education. Acad Med. 2015 Sep;90(9):1215-23.

[11] Parsons BA, Blencowe NS, Hollowood AD, Grant JR. Surgical Training: The Impact of Changes in Curriculum and Experience. J Surg Educ. 2011 Jan 1;68(1):44-51.

[12] Hayes P. Newly Qualified Doctors' Views of Medical School Training and Its Adequacy in Making Them "Fit for Purpose" as First Year Doctors. Open Access Libr J. 2016 Sep 30;3(9):1-20.

[13] Elfenbein DM. Have We Created a Crisis in Confidence for General Surgery Residents? A Systematic Review and Qualitative Discourse Analysis. JAMA Surg. 2016 Dec 1;151(12):1166-75.

[14] Daniels AH, DiGiovanni CW. Is Subspecialty Fellowship Training Emerging as a Necessary Component of Contemporary Orthopaedic Surgery Education? J Grad Med Educ. 2014 Jun;6(2):218-21.

[15] Fitts PM, Posner MI. Human Performance. Brooks/Cole Publishing Company; 1967. 186 p.

[16] Bandura A. Social Learning Theory. 2nd Edition. Englewood Cliffs, N.J. : Prentice Hall, ©1977.; 1977. 247 p. (Prentice-Hall series in social learning theory.).

[17] Ericsson KA. Deliberate practice and the acquisition and maintenance of expert performance in medicine and related domains. Acad Med J Assoc Am Med Coll. 2004 Oct;79(10 Suppl): S70-81.

[18] Jeannerod M. Mental imagery in the motor context. Neuropsychologia. 1995 Nov 1;33(11):1419-32.

[19] Rosales A, Roy M, Li J, Safdie F, Rosenthal RJ. Introduction to Systematic Approach and Mental Training. In: Rosenthal RJ, Rosales A, Lo Menzo E, Dip FD, editors. Mental Conditioning to Perform Common Operations in General Surgery Training: A Systematic Approach to Expediting Skill Acquisition and Maintaining Dexterity in Performance [Internet]. Cham: Springer International Publishing; 2020 [cited 2020 May 5]. p. 9-10. Available from: https://doi.org/10.1007/978-3-319-91164-9_2

[20] Driskell JE, Copper C, Moran A. Does mental practice enhance performance? J Appl Psychol. 1994;79(4):481-92.

[21] Martin KA, Moritz SE, Hall CR. Imagery use in sport: A literature review and applied model. Sport Psychol. 1999;13(3):245-68.

[22] Pearson J, Naselaris T, Holmes EA, Kosslyn SM. Mental Imagery: Functional Mechanisms and Clinical Applications. Trends Cogn Sci. 2015 Oct;19(10):590-602.

[23] Wohldmann EL, Healy AF, Bourne Jr. LE. A mental practice superiority effect: Less retroactive interference and more transfer than physical practice. J Exp Psychol Learn Mem Cogn. 2008; 34(4):823-33.

[24] Schuster C, Hilfiker R, Amft O, Scheidhauer A, Andrews B, Butler J, et al. Best practice for motor imagery: a systematic literature review on motor imagery training elements in five different disciplines. BMC Med. 2011 Jun 17;9(1):75.

[25] Frank C, Land WM, Popp C, Schack T. Mental Representation and Mental Practice: Experimental Investigation on the Functional Links between Motor Memory and Motor Imagery. PLoS ONE [Internet]. 2014 Apr 17 [cited 2020 May 7];9(4). Available from: https://www.ncbi.nlm.nih.gov/pmc/articles/PMC3990621/

[26] Rashid P. Surgical education and adult learning: Integrating theory into practice. F1000Research [Internet]. 2017 Feb 14 [cited 2020 Feb 23];6. Available from: https://www.ncbi.nlm.nih.gov/pmc/articles/PMC5345767/

[27] Javid P, Aydın A, Mohanna P-N, Dasgupta P, Ahmed K. Current status of simulation and training models in microsurgery: A systematic review. Microsurgery. 2019;39(7):655-68.

[28] Evans CH, Schenarts KD. Evolving Educational Techniques in Surgical Training. Surg Clin. 2016 Feb 1;96(1): 71-88.

[29] Kerr RS. Surgery in the 2020s: Implications of advancing technology for patients and the workforce. Future Heal J. 2020 Feb 1;7(1):46-9.

[30] Singh M, Ziolkowski N, Ramachandran S, Myers SR, Ghanem AM. Development of a Five-Day Basic Microsurgery Simulation Training Course: A Cost Analysis. Arch Plast Surg. 2014;41(3):213.

[31] Camillan Huang. Designing high-quality interactive multimedia learning modules. Comput Med Imaging Graph. 29:223-33.

[32] Muhammad S. Application of Cognitive Theory of Multimedia Learning in Undergraduate Surgery Course. Int J Surg Res Pract [Internet]. 2018 Apr 30 [cited 2020 Feb 29];5(1). Available from: https://www.clinmedjournals.org/articles/ijsrp/international-journal-of-surgery-research-and-practice-ijsrp-5-065.php?jid=ijsrp

[33] Yue C, Kim J, Ogawa R, Stark E, Kim S. Applying the cognitive theory of multimedia learning: an analysis of

medical animations. Med Educ. 2013;47(4):375-87.

[34] Khalil MK, Elkhider IA. Applying learning theories and instructional design models for effective instruction. Adv Physiol Educ. 2016 Apr 11;40(2): 147-56.

[35] Mayer RE. Multimedia Learning [Internet]. 2nd ed. Cambridge, England: Cambridge University Press; 2009 [cited 2020 Jul 8]. Available from: https://www.cambridge.org/core/books/multimedia-learning/7A62F072A71289E1E262980CB026A3F9

[36] Mayer RE. How multimedia can improve learning and instruction. In: The Cambridge handbook of cognition and education. New York, NY, US: Cambridge University Press; 2019. p. 460-79.

[37] Mayer RE. Applying the science of learning to medical education. Med Educ. 2010;44(6):543-9.

[38] Ericsson KA. Protocol analysis and expert thought: Concurrent verbalizations of thinking during experts' performance on representative tasks. Camb Handb Expert Expert Perform. 2006;223-42.

[39] Safsouf Y, Mansouri K, Poirier F. A New Model of Learner Experience in Online Learning Environments. In: Rocha Á, Serrhini M, editors. Information Systems and Technologies to Support Learning. Cham: Springer International Publishing; 2019. p. 29-38. (Smart Innovation, Systems and Technologies).

[40] Sim WP, Ng HJH, Tan S, Bajaj SL, Rajaratnam V. Scope of Hand Surgery Using Surgeon Administered Local/Regional Anaesthesia. Ann Plast Surg. 2019 Sep;83(3):278-84.

[41] Jarvill M, Kelly S, Krebs H. Effect of Expert Role Modeling on Skill Performance in Simulation. Clin Simul Nurs. 2018 Nov 1;24:25-9.

[42] Orsborn G. Use of rapid e-learning authoring tools in higher education. Whitireia Nurs Health J. 2017;(24):47.

[43] Sevdalis N, Moran A, Arora S. Mental Imagery and Mental Practice Applications in Surgery: State of the Art and Future Directions. In: Multisensory Imagery [Internet]. Springer, New York, NY; 2013 [cited 2018 Jan 1]. p. 343-63. Available from: https://link.springer.com/chapter/10.1007/978-1-4614-5879-1_18

Chapter 11

How to Improve Hospital Flows in the Context of the COVID Pandemic

Paul-Eric Dossou, Luiza Foreste and Eric Misumi

Abstract

In healthcare systems, the adoption of logistics 4.0 main technologies in the processes flows is essential to avoid unnecessary movements and manual work performed by people who could be performing tasks that require logical reasoning. In the context of the COVID pandemic, the adoption of new technologies to replace people in manual processes had become even more usual. This paper aims to demonstrate through simulation, the opportunities of improvement with lean manufacturing concepts and industry 4.0 technologies the hospital flows. After describing the problem and the need of improvements in hospital logistics, a literature review with concepts of Industry 4.0, Lean Manufacturing, and Logistics 4.0 will be presented. The hybrid approach used in the development of a decision aid tool that combines real data and methods of machine learning and problem-solving will be then, an example will be given for illustrating the concepts and methods elaborated.

Keywords: Healthcare logistics, Industry 4.0, Lean manufacturing, Robotics, Digital twin, Decision aided system, Artificial intelligence

1. Introduction

The term Logistics 4.0 comes from the concept of Industry 4.0, which has as main objective to optimize the production process of a factory by using new technologies (IoT, cobot, AIV, decision aided tools, etc.) and organization models (6 Sigma, lean manufacturing, etc.). Nowadays, it is possible to find several scientific and practical sources that prove the efficiency and benefits of the Industry 4.0 and Logistics 4.0 application in the production environment. However, within the health field, such as hospitals and pharmacies, these applications still have many opportunities to be explored. Indeed, the healthcare environment must reapply optimization existing concepts.

In 2020, European countries as much as the others in the world has discover the COVID pandemic, with a high impact on hospitals organization and the appearance of many logistics and safety problems. For instance, the management of patient flow and how to heal the sick with safety for nurses and hospital workers have to be solved. The good medicines dispatching in all hospital services is also a problem to optimize. The safety patient meal preparation and distribution could also be presented as a point to improve. The requisite but dangerous collection, distribution, washing of cloths in the frame of Covid pandemic are also problems to solve. These deficiencies became even more relevant to be overcome. This is due to two main reasons. The first one is the low availability of time and number of employees in healthcare systems. The second reason is the way the virus spreads, that is through contact among people.

Having a real need and a problem to be solved, this project carried out a study showing how the Logistics 4.0 concepts can be implemented in a way to both optimize the process and contribute to the fight against the pandemic. The study will show how the implementation of logistics 4.0 could decrease the number of unnecessary contacts and consequently reduce the number of contaminated people inside hospitals. Indeed, the implementation of new technologies is crucial for healthcare professionals to be able to focus on the high demand of patients instead of wasting time on manual tasks.

The study presents a literature that contains the main methods and new technologies in the field of Industry 4.0, Lean Manufacturing, Logistics 4.0, and Healthcare 4.0 that can be used to solve the indicated problems. Then, concepts and methodology developed for solving these problems will be exposed. The elaborated general approach based on Case-based reasoning and generalization reasoning will contribute to the definition of a hospital flows reference model. Indeed, the general structure of the decision aided tool, based on artificial intelligence and being developed for helping hospitals in the process of logistics optimization will be shown. And finally, an example will be presented for illustrating how these concepts could be applied to improve hospital logistics in the frame of logistics 4.0, named here Healthcare Logistics 4.0.

2. Literature review

The literature review of this paper aims to democratize and centralize the main concepts and new technologies used in the development of the project. Industry 4.0 concepts have been presented through Cyber-Physical Systems, IoTs, big data analytics, Artificial Intelligence (AI). With the focus on studying logistics within hospitals, research was conducted in the fields of Logistics 4.0 and Healthcare 4.0 to connect the two concepts. Finally, research was carried out into the methods used to optimize processes such as Lean Manufacturing and Lean Healthcare. Hence the chapter has a summary of each of the topics that were necessary to develop the tool and concepts presented in this article.

2.1 Industry 4.0

Based on some values and known as the fourth industrial revolution (**Figure 1**), industry 4.0 is a term that emerged in Germany in the 2011 edition of the Hanover Fair, seen as a tech strategy for 2020, and remarkably based on the development of cyber systems. Modern industrial systems are complex systems that include physical, software, and networking elements into so-called cyber-physical systems [1].

Cyber-physical systems are considered as the heart and the base of the 4.0 industry [2]. The Internet of things and the Internet of services, allow to define "intelligent manufacturing", which together with the production planning and control should play a key role within the 4.0 Industry [3, 4]. By using the Internet, Industry 4.0 matches products, services, production, and optimization to build a process based on data recorded by cyber-physical systems, without the need to involve a human being [3].

The context of Industry 4.0 is influenced by the intelligent capabilities of five basic technologies (Internet of Things, Cyber-physical Systems, Big Data and Analytics, Artificial Intelligence, and Additive Manufacturing), which have greatly stimulated the development of intelligent manufacturing [2, 4]. As a preferred

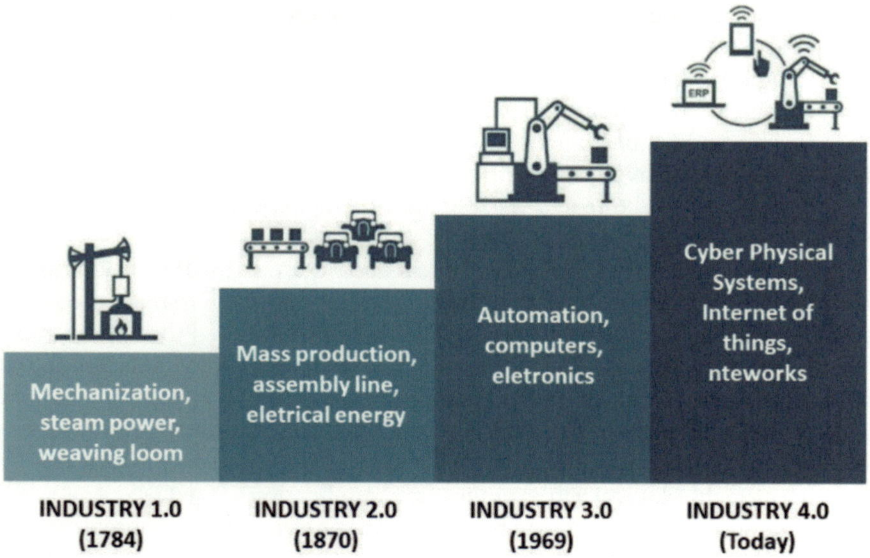

Figure 1.
Four industrial revolutions.

means of such integration, Cyber-physical systems, and digital twins (DT) have gained great attention from researchers and industry professionals [2]. Indeed, robot, cobot, mobile robot, intelligent machines, immersive realities, IoTs represent machines and tools that could increase the efficiency of the industry4.0 concepts.

Artificial intelligence (AI) methods and tools such as expert systems, machine learning, deep learning, multi-agent systems are used for supporting Industry 4.0 concepts implementation in the company digital transformation through modeling, simulation, or decision support systems. These methods are also used for the same reasons in the frame of healthcare. For instance, Case-based reasoning (CBR) and multi-agent systems concepts are exploited in [5] for predicting risk in surgery in a non-determinist context. Case-based reasoning process is described as a cycle of four processes: Retrieve the most similar cases, Reuse the cases for solving a new problem, Revise the proposed solution, and Retain the new solution as a new case [6, 7]. This cycle is generally used in medical classification, prediction, and diagnosis problems. These concepts are adapted to hospital processes transformation and could be combined with multi-agent systems (MAS). MAS are defined as a composition of autonomous entities that interact with to certain rules in a specific environment. For instance, MAS could be used for solving problems such as the ecological and epidemiological analysis of infectious diseases [8]. In this kind of combination MAS could generate risk situation that will be compared to old cases by the CBR system for solving problems [5]. This hybrid system philosophy is also adapted for solving hospital logistics flow problems. Indeed, a decision aided system that will measure the state of healthcare logistics digital transformation could be elaborated by using expert systems theory and architecture. As described in [9], expert systems are used for supporting different application domains such as ontologies elaborated for modeling and managing the knowledge about drugs and patients [10] which flows (in this paper case) must be optimized in healthcare logistics.

2.2 Logistics 4.0

Logistics 4.0 is a relatively new term, directly linked to Industry 4.0. The development of Industry 4.0 was based on digitalization and automation, and that for Logistics 4.0 presents not only enormous challenges but also opportunities to increase efficiency [11]. Indeed, before the advent of Industry 4.0, the concept of intelligent logistics was previously introduced to represent a technology-driven approach to the management of material flows within and outside the factory limits [12]. The concept of Logistics 4.0 means a set of solutions aimed at improving logistics processes, avoiding errors and disruptions in transport and storage processes, thanks to the continuous exchange of data between the players in the logistics system [13].

Logistics 4.0 is a combination of technical and organizational solutions aimed at improving material and information flows and adjusting them to meet the requirements of Industry 4.0 solutions. Therefore, logistics is intended to support manufacturing processes, whereby, as they evolve towards intelligent and autonomous solutions, logistics must follow this change [13].

Due to the fact that the Industry 4.0 concept is considerably affected by the use of new technologies, logistics 4.0 has been intuitively perceived from the perspective of technological achievements and applications (e.g. GPS, WMS, TMS, RFID, CPFR, etc.) [14]. In addition to the explanations mentioned above, modern companies make use of dedicated technologies such as goggles, gates, forklifts, and automatic vehicles, or even intelligent carriers. The objective of this concept is to increase the efficiency and performance of the members of the supply chain [15].

It has been assumed that the new technologies and tools are determining factors for the realization of Logistics 4.0 and that they can be used as evaluation criteria for the implementation level [14]. Through the implementation of Logistics 4.0, many advantages can be noted, among them the lower cost in human work, the high standardization in logistics functions, and the use of new technologies in the equipment of logistics companies. The disadvantages are the high investment costs and the requirement to own the information technology supply network [15]. These concepts could be used in healthcare logistics for optimizing flows but also respecting Covid pandemic distancing attitudes and saving lives.

2.3 Healthcare 4.0

Healthcare industry has been assisting in saving and extending patients' lives through the progress of technologies adopted by healthcare professionals and through the transformations that the sector has undergone. In the health field, the practices and techniques have been developed from Healthcare 1.0 to Healthcare 4.0. In the context of Healthcare 1.0, there was a scarcity of resources and the efforts were primary since the approach was doctor centric. As the information technology field and medical technologies advanced, it was possible to replace manual records with electronic healthcare records (EHR), what has been termed Healthcare 2.0. Healthcare 3.0 had, as the main characteristic of the patient-centric approach, developed new and effective treatment methods through data processing systems and computational methods. In this context, EHR was used to help doctors to get important information faster. Healthcare 4.0 corresponds to the integration of new technologies, such as Cloud Computing, Internet of Things, Fog Computing and Telehealthcare, to facilitate the doctor-patient interface through data portability. Strong communication interface and the ability to share data enable doctors to make well-informed decisions and increase the quality of healthcare around the world [16, 17].

The adoption of Industry 4.0 main technologies, such as the Internet of Things, Cloud and Fog Computing, and Big Data analytics, has revolutionized the healthcare sector, changing the way to provide traditional products and services. IoT is supposed to integrate the virtual and physical world through interconnected devices and platforms. The Internet of Health Things (IoHT) has as main objective, the tracking of patient medical conditions and the anticipation of critical situations through the combination of connected devices. The Internet of Medical Things aims to create a personal hub connecting implantable and wearable devices to a personal smartphone. Cloud, Fog and Mobile Edge Computing represent a huge part of Healthcare 4.0 to simplify health processes, facilitate the adoption of healthcare best practices, and inspire the adoption of more innovations. The healthcare sector can benefit from the capacity of management of a huge amount of data demonstrated by Cloud and Fog Computing. Big data and analytics are largely used in the healthcare sector, not only to store and treat patient data but also to collect enterprise data, allowing to implement studies that cover beyond the health domain (biological and medical aspects) [18] and to analyze them in detail for taking good decisions and aiding doctors in the patient support.

The implementation of Industry 4.0 core principles in the healthcare sector is far from optimal, despite the great importance of its main technologies isolated. The problem lies in the fact that a successful implementation of Healthcare 4.0 implies transformations of technical and sociocultural aspects inside the hospitals. The main barriers are associated with the development of an incorporated IT infrastructure aligned with the hospital's strategy. This issue is proven that healthcare has been the slowest sector to adopt information technologies. To mitigate this problem, the focus must change from design and implementation processes to the end-user experience with solutions already implemented, i.e., more prototypes must be tested [19, 20]. Indeed, this transformation has to be linked with the global healthcare logistics organization.

2.4 Lean manufacturing and lean healthcare

In recent times, the enterprise environment requires the implementation of the Lean Manufacturing approach to create added value with optimal resource utilization. Aiming to present the Toyota Work Philosophy, the term 'Lean' first appeared in the 90s. The bases of this philosophy are waste elimination and value creation. Waste can be defined as all processes that do not create any added value. Seven types of Mudas (tasks with no added value) were developed: overproduction, wait, transport, stock, unnecessary activity, defects, and motion. The overproduction is the task that generates the most losses [21].

To implement the Lean philosophy, several tools and techniques were developed to reduce/eliminate waste. The use of the tool VSM (Value Stream Mapping) enables the decision making of the Lean through the analysis of a deterministic and static value chain observation. VSM helps to distinguish the non-waste and waste processes [22]. The implementation of the Lean Manufacturing approach is realized in three main stages: pre-implementation stage (lean readiness), implementation stage (lean approach), and post-implementation stage (results) [23].

Aiming at increasing process efficiency and mitigating non-added value processes, Lean Manufacturing methods have been extensively implemented in healthcare institutions [24]. The main uses of Lean in this context are to eliminate duplicate and unnecessary procedures, such as collecting patient information several times, unnecessary patient displacement, excessive waiting by patients for appointments, and uncoordinated processes. Despite the wide application of lean assumptions in hospitals and clinics, the prospected results are not achieved [23]. The significant number of failures can be explained by 3 main factors:

- Absence of adaptation: it is essential to adapt lean concepts to knowledge-intensive service sectors such as healthcare. This transition is not always clear, which causes a higher probability of failures [23].

- Lack of readiness: the unawareness about the Lean Manufacturing approach by most of the employees added to the inefficient training systems are the main bottlenecks encountered for an efficient lean implementation. The main problems in lean implementation projects are caused by a lack of corporate culture and change management [23].

- Lack of systemic approach: the Lean approach is widely used for specific problems, without taking into consideration all the processes [23].

With this purpose and to help the production process in SMEs (Small and Medium Enterprises), a methodology and a framework has been developed with the aim of contributing to the implementation process of industry 4.0 and logistics 4.0, with the focus on sustainability aspects [4, 24]. The next section presents concepts and methodology that could firstly be used for transforming digitally the hospitals and increasing their flow performance, and secondly be integrated in the process of both patient and hospital staff lives saving in the context of covid pandemic.

3. Concepts and methodology

Based on industry 4.0, logistics 4.0, Healthcare 4.0 and lean manufacturing concepts presented above, a general framework, a global approach and a problem-solving method have been elaborated to insure the hospital digital transformation for respecting COVID pandemic constraints and optimizing hospital flows.

3.1 The generic framework

A general framework was developed in this study, correlating the methods, concepts and tools of Industry and Logistics 4.0 applying in the context of healthcare.

Based on sustainability, social and environmental criteria, the general framework for process optimization in hospitals has two main stages. With the main objective of having a good quality in the treatment of patients within the hospitals, the first stage has the patient at the center of all improvements. Then, the next stage will be to ensure the well-being, health, and productivity of health services, with the focus on increasing the efficiency of the hospital. Currently, this stage is even more relevant since the challenge of ensuring the health of nurses and doctors has become even more crucial due to the combat of the pandemic.

With this framework, the goal is to define a reference model for logistics in healthcare, aiming to achieve the following aspects: sustainability (health of professionals), social (quality in the treatment of patients) and environmental (optimization and reduction of costs of processes). The reference model will also serve as the basis for the decision-aided tool, which will be a model to be reached in the optimization of logistics in hospitals.

The **Figure 2** presents the general framework illustrating the progressive transformation of the hospital, in stages, for an optimization of logistics in hospitals.

3.2 The global approach

The **Figure 3** describes a global approach for implementing industry 4.0 and logistics 4.0 in the healthcare systems.

As shown in the figure above, the global approach has as its center the sustainability aspects for the implementation of the industry 4.0 and logistics 4.0 concepts. This approach uses new technologies such as cobots, mobile robots, IoTs, as

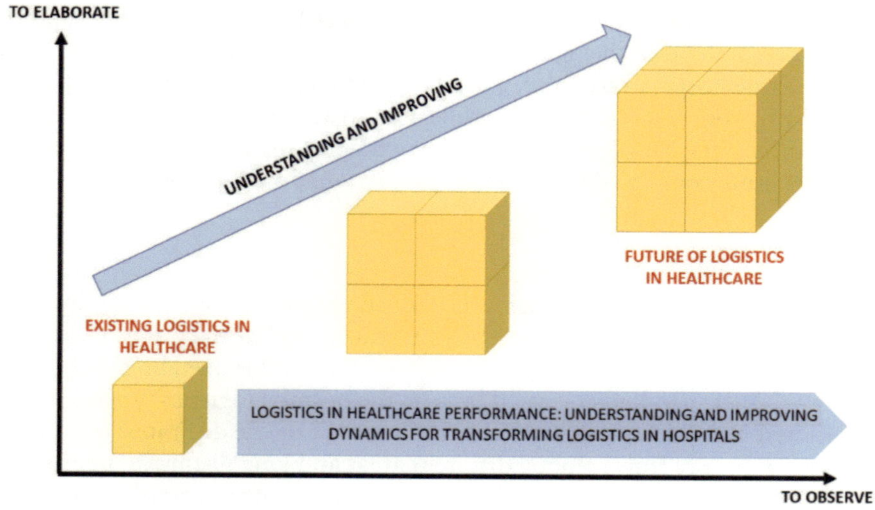

Figure 2.
Framework for healthcare logistics implementation.

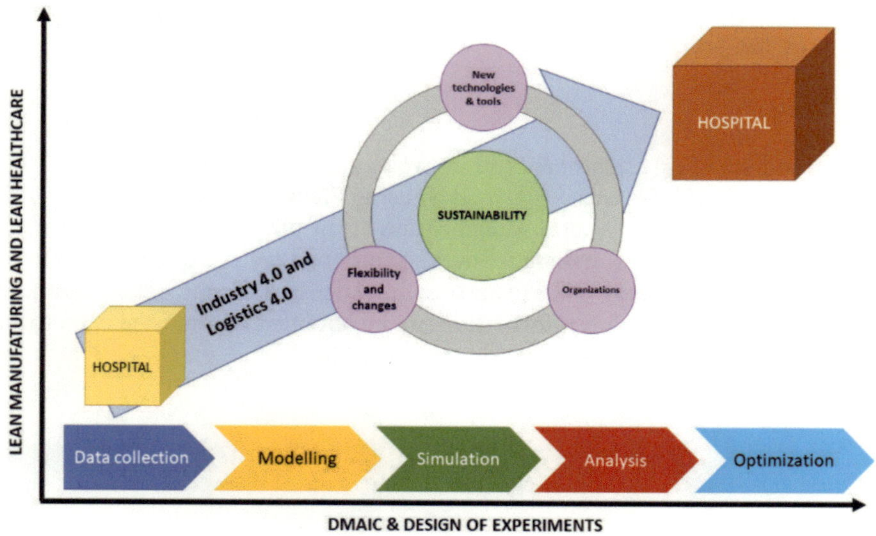

Figure 3.
Global approach for implementing industry 4.0 and logistics 4.0 in hospitals.

well as new organizations such as Blockchain for transforming digitally the hospital. Finally, it becomes necessary to be flexible to the changes to implement them. The global approach has the following steps:

- An initialization phase for acquiring the hospital global context and main data
- A modeling phase for representing the existing hospital organization
- A simulation phase for elaborating the hospital flows digital twin
- An analysis phase for detecting inconsistencies and points to improve
- A design phase for defining optimization scenarios by exploiting the elaborated reference model and the decision aided tool being developed for managing this transformation process.

This process has been followed in the definition of the reference model and the decision aided tool. From the modeling, the simulation, the analysis, and the design of a real existing hospital structure, generalization reasoning has been applied for defining the reference model that would be used in a hospital flows digital transformation in the COVID pandemic context. Then the transformation of the existing hospital structure could be done by using the reference model developed.

3.2.1 Modeling

To understand the logistical operation carried out inside the hospitals including the transportation of medicines carried out by the host pharmacy, it is necessary to collect information through data and interviews. Due to this need before the beginning of the COVID pandemic, several data on the hospital logistics process have been collected in two hospitals located in the south of the Ile de France region.

As these processes travel among different areas and long distances, in this article the focus is made on the medicine delivery processes and on the sterile medical devices. The **Figure 4** presents a complete flow of the medicine delivery processes.

To allow a clear analysis of the processes and with the interdepartmental locomotion the modeling of the processes was done following the BPMN methodology and BonitaSoft software. This methodology seeks to describe an organization's value chains and process in the form of a graphical representation.

3.2.2 Simulation

After understanding the process and its problems, a simulation (digital twin) of the hospital logistics flows was performed by using Flexsim software (**Figure 5**). This simulation, besides allowing better visualization of the process, provided us information on the transport time and distance data. Another advantage of the simulation was the possibility of changing the process to optimize it, bringing a clear comparison between before and after. This information can be obtained without the need to go to the field that during a pandemic period is not possible.

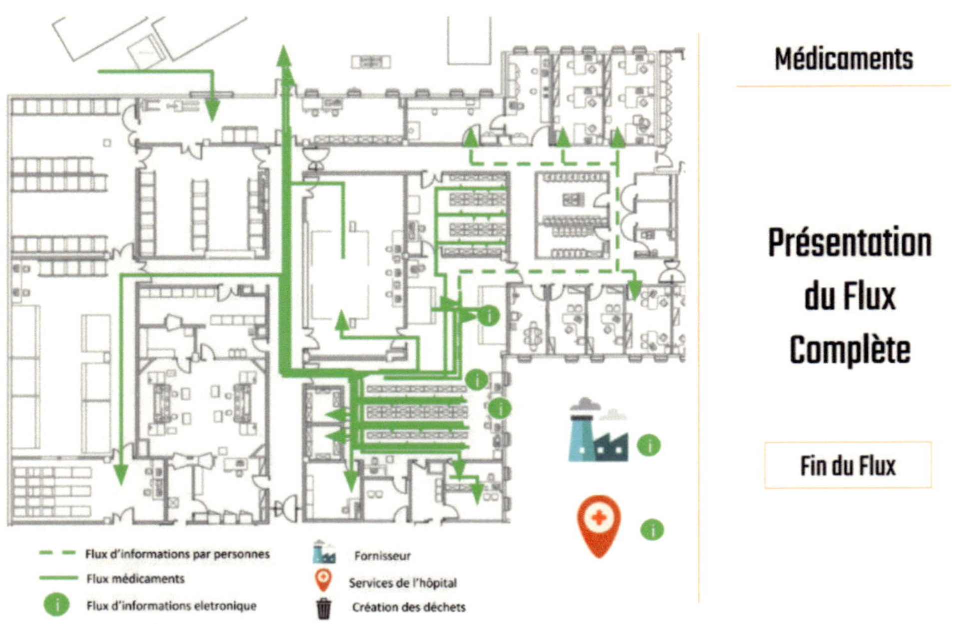

Figure 4.
Medicine delivery complete process flow.

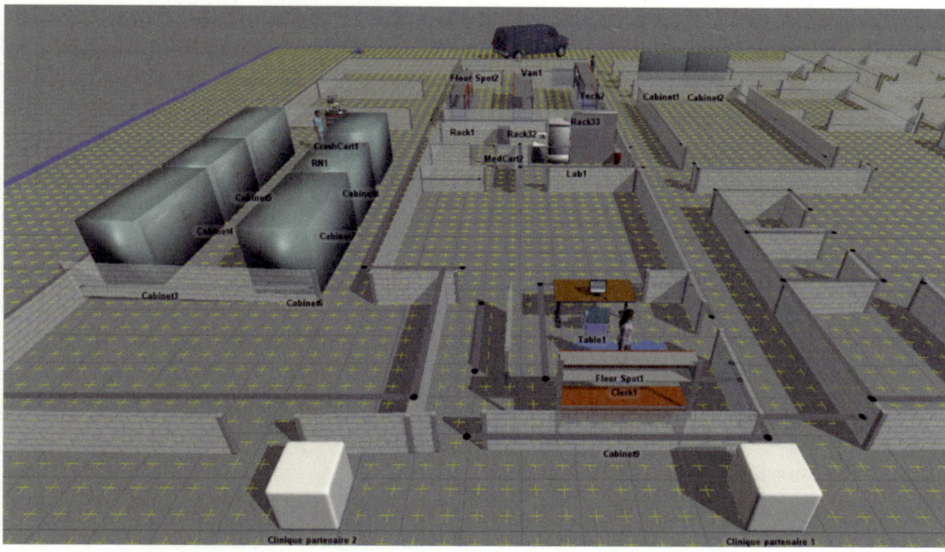

Figure 5.
Sterilization process of equipment - simulation using FlexSim software.

3.2.3 Analysis

The process description and its modeling were analyzed to detect inconsistencies and to find the possibilities of improvement. Inconsistencies at this stage have been found manually. But the advantage of the decision aided system being developed will be to contain rules able to detect all inconsistencies in any hospital system. An example of inconsistency could be found in the process of food dispatching. Indeed, the existing organization uses nurses, and caregivers for taking food from the hospital restaurant and bringing it to patients. One of the difficulties for managing the actual pandemic crisis is the nurse availability (lack of time). This transfer could also be made by other people, but it would increase the possibility of contamination. Other examples of required improvement are:

- The lack of a continuous flow
- Unnecessary transport
- Non-optimized logistics
- Lack of organization
- That any of the process could be replaced by machines
- That these same problems were found in most of the other processes analyzed.

3.2.4 Reference model

Through the use of the simulation software, each process studied during the previous phases was improved in order to propose most of the tools and digital technologies to increase the level of performance and security.

For this purpose, the digital flows of hospital logistics processes were simulated. First the processes were simulated separately and after implementing the optimization, they all were combined into a single simulation model. The objective of this model was to seek first the opportunities for improvement within the model, in which after stabilization it would be possible to bring them all together and make improvements to the combined logistics processes.

An example of improvement is the use of Automated Guided Vehicles (AGV) for the transportation of food from the hospital restaurant to the patients. Indeed, this action contributes to the loss of time by the nurses and caregivers.

3.3 The problem-solving method

The **Figure 6** presents the structure of the problem-solving method.

The first step of the problem-solving method is the hospital problem context acquisition. Main properties and data must be defined during this step. According to theory of systems, the description of the system will be done by finding properties associated.

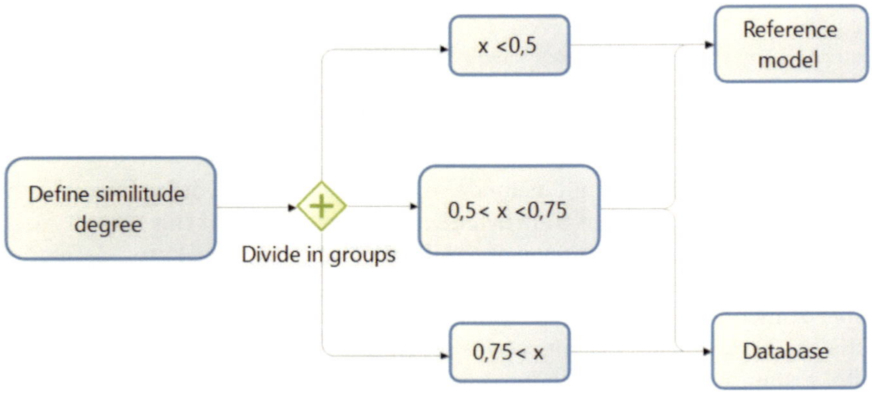

Figure 6.
Path of the problem-solving method.

Then, this problem will be compared to old cases contained in a capitalization database (use of case -based reasoning (CBR)). For this comparison a similitude degree will be defined. If this number is less than 0.5, it means that there are no efficient possible cases in the database.

Then, the main system transformation will be by using the reference model elaborated. If the number is between 0,5 and 0,75, both possibilities could be exploited. The cases found will be extracted from the database and the reference model will also be applied for transforming the system.

Then, if the degree is more than 0,75, only cases existing in the database will be presented to ensure the hospital flows transformation for solving problems. A decision-aided tool will be developed for managing the hospital flows digital transformation.

4. The decision aided tool

In this chapter the framework of the software is discussed, thus containing the architecture and the information flow. Finally, the application of the AGV (Automatic guided vehicle) in the optimization of hospital logistics is also illustrated. The tool has as functionalities to:

- Facilitate knowledge acquisition,
- Contribute to existing models and simulations elaboration
- Compare data with old cases
- Extract old corresponding cases or reference model
- Exploit the aided structure for elaborating the hospital flows expected digital transformation.

The decision aided tool will combine different artificial intelligence concepts (expert systems, machine learning, multi-agent systems) with reasoning such as CBR, generalization, and transformation.

4.1 Expert system and machine learning

To allow hospitals to optimize the internal logistic process, a decision-making tool is being developed. Combining the concepts of Industry 4.0, Logistics 4.0 adapting them in the context of healthcare. The tool being developed is based on the use of Artificial Intelligence utilizing machine learning tools and expert systems.

In this way, the decision aided system will be elaborated by having the ability to ratiocinate and learn in its own way. For this, Case-based reasoning (CBR) system will be combined with the multi-agent system, which makes it possible to achieve this specificity in the tool. With this, the system can suggest solutions to problems or give proposals for improvement, reusing or adapting the approaches developed in previous applications.

Then, machine learning, through the repetition of a behavior, will contribute to the decision-aided tool by generating new inputs and in this way progressively enriching the database.

4.2 Software framework

The software framework is divided in 3 main parts, which are, the information input, generation of the current process with the problems and possibilities of improvement, and finally the generation of the process optimized with the results of the optimization.

As the final objective of the tool is to enable an optimization of the internal logistics of the hospital, eliminating inconsistencies in the processes and reducing the non-value-added time, the inputs required by the tool will be:

- Location of the beginning and the end of each step of the process
- Number of workers
- Type of process
- Times per day and week
- Equipment used
- Duration of the process
- Upload layout in DWG format

With those inputs, the systems can through machine learning and expert systems, compare the data collected in hospitals with the referring hospital to achieve the ideal logistic model.

This ideal logistics model will be developed after applying Lean Manufacturing and Logistics 4.0 methodologies in several processes in different hospitals, and it will be progressively improved through machine learning.

After the analysis, the second stage of the tool will generate a series of data and the simulation relating to the process, giving the user a general idea about the logistics efficiency. The software will present the problems encountered and make suggestions for improvement to the user.

In the third and last step, after the selection of the improvements, the software will implement them in the process. For this, the system will again need to use machine learning and the expert system to make the changes and generate the data regarding the optimized process.

With this decision aided tool, the user will be able to test changes within the process and see what the results will be, facilitating the logistics optimization process within hospitals as it will reduce time and cost and increase the effectiveness.

4.3 Architecture of the software

The **Figure** 7 represents the architecture of the model, it aims to organize the components, modules, and information flow of the software in a visual way. Since the decision aid tool will have as functionalities, learn, and update its database in an automatic way, where several components will act, a structure was chosen where the database is centralized and combined with the tool manager.

This tool is composed of the following components:

- Database: Main data storage of the software, where it will contain the reference model, the imputed data, and the results.

- Tool manager: Module responsible for performing the interactions between the components.

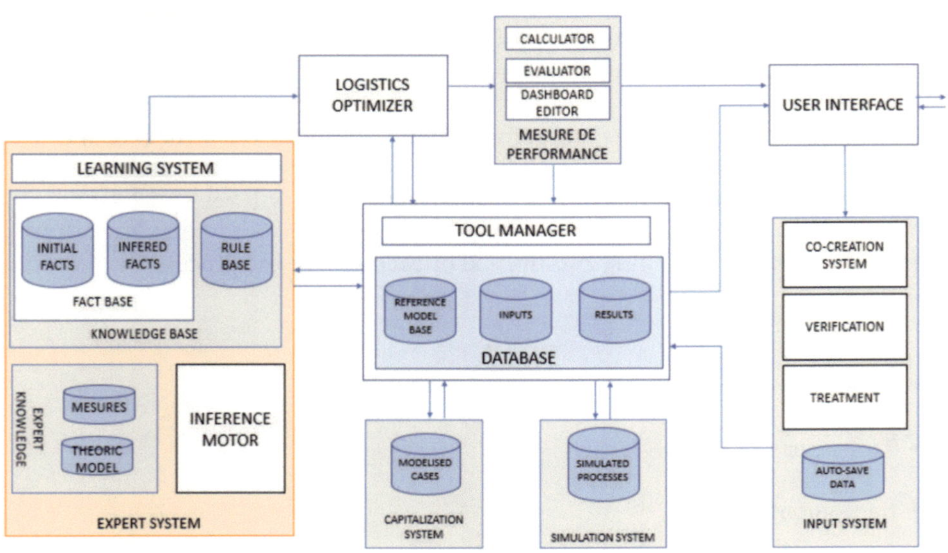

Figure 7.
Architecture of the software.

- The user interface: Component that carries out the interactions between the user and the tool, where he will be able to impute, modify the data as well as apply the improvements and see the results.
- Expert system: Place where the automatic learning of the system will be carried out, thus to be able to store data and to analyze the system and suggest the most appropriate improvements to the situation.
- Logistics optimizer: Module responsible for solving the problems found by the expert system.
- Measure of performance: It will perform the comparison between the two scenarios, current and optimized to measure the impacts of the changes.
- Capitalization system: Component that will be used as a storage location for the old cases and also perform the comparison between them and the current one.
- Simulation system: Module that will make the connection of the tool with the simulation software.
- Input system: Place responsible for verifying, treating, and storing automatically the information imputed by the user.

5. Illustration

This section focuses on two hospitals studies for defining their existing system finding inconsistencies and points to improving by applying the previous methodology and using adapted new technologies tools for increasing the hospitals performance. The first hospital had just integrated a new building and would like to use this opportunity for transforming digitally its logistics flow organization. The second hospital already started working with lean manufacturing for structuring its storage area and needs to reduce products dispatching and to optimize all logistics flows. The focus was made on six flows for the improvement: meals, patients, medicines, cloths, consumables, and wastes.

After the use of the methodology for defining the existing system, and finding non-added values and added values, a detailed digital transformation process has been applied on each hospital. New technologies and tools were defined for increasing the hospital flow performance. For instance, Automated Intelligent Vehicles have been chosen for transporting products and reducing waste time for nurses and caregivers. The Automated Intelligent Vehicles (AIVs) solution exemplifies how logistics applications 4.0 and lean manufacturing can contribute to help fighting against the pandemic through the personal health reduction of exposure to the virus. The **Figure 8** presents the result of the transport time optimization in the first hospital. This data concerns the dispatching flows and human non-values were identified. The integration of the AIV allows to reduce the duration of tasks but also serves as a gain of time for nurses and caregivers.

In the two hospitals studied in this paper for validating concepts elaborated, nurses and caregivers spent their times by managing the logistics and transportation of food, medicines, and materials. This situation contributes to the increase of contact between professionals, patients, and different departments, thus influencing the increase of exposure to the virus. Besides, with the need for more health

Activities	Actual duration	Optimized duration
Meal collection (minutes)	45	18,07
Waste collection (minutes)	135	53,58
Meal dispatching (minutes)	45	15,48
New laundry dispatching (minutes)	60	27,4
Urgency collection (minutes)	Not actually measured	45
Return of laundry, waste and meals (minutes)	120	41,98
Pharmacy flows (minutes)	60	13,11
Total (minutes)	465	214,62
Total (hours)	7,75	3,57
Difference (hours)	4;18	

Figure 8.
Non-added transport time optimization.

professionals, to support the flow of Covid patients, the more time they must contribute to the quality of care and not to the logistics, will increase their capacity to give people the right and well-done treatment.

The study in these two hospitals even before the pandemic showed that the number of patients was increasing in the hospitals, but no increase of nurses. The results of one hospital were about 2700 additional hours to be paid to the nurses. This situation has to be suppressed probably been increased by the covid pandemic. Then, the implementation of AIVs within hospital logistics will contribute to the following aspects:

- Ergonomics of health professionals
- More staff time for service
- Less movement between departments
- Medium- and long-term cost reduction
- Decreased exposure of employees to the virus

The **Figure 9** shows the model of AIVs studied in a second hospital located in the south of the Ile de France region. The referring hospital elaborated by exploiting data acquired in these two hospitals had 4 AIVs and delivered medicines and meals on 5 floors. These tools according to the digital twin developed were sufficient for ensuring all the products dispatching in each of these hospitals.

Applying the hospital logistics optimization system presented in this paper to the medicine distribution process presented in **Figure 4**, it was possible to find several possibilities of improvement. The most impacting was the application of the AIV system presented in this chapter since the process had 16 transport operators in which at least 8 could be replaced by AIVs and affected to more important tasks. Thus, it was possible to reduce 50% of the transport actions performed by nurses and caregivers, giving more energy and time for activities related to patient care.

In both hospital cases the desire to integrate new technologies and tools for optimizing all their flows and making their health personnel available for other tasks was high. These hospitals give data and information for defining reference models for healthcare logistics flow. The management of all these data and the diversity of

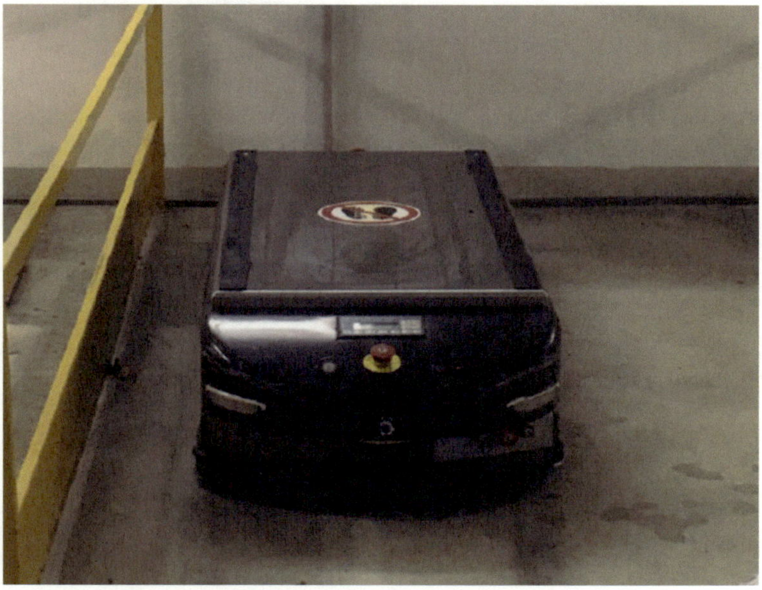

Figure 9.
Mobile robot (AIV).

decision to take, validate the need of a decision-aided tool for driving the digital transformation process in hospitals. The digital twins are being developed for each hospital and will participate to the improvement of the reference model for healthcare 4.0. The digital transformation of these hospital is growing up.

6. Conclusion

This project aim to show the importance of new technologies and sustainability in the digital transformation of a hospital in the Covid pandemic context. Considering the need to improve hospital logistics with the worsening of it, with the presence of the COVID pandemic, the article presents a generic model of optimization of hospital logistics, where first was presented a literature review containing the new technologies and tools of industry 4.0, logistics 4.0, Lean manufacturing and lean healthcare. After this step, the concepts and methods applied in the development of the project and containing the steps of a global approach have been presented. Finally, the decision aided tool designed to facilitate the logistics optimization process has been presented, containing its functionalities and architecture.

Many of the improvements presented in this article are already applied and consolidated as efficient technologies in the industrial field, but in the healthcare field it is still possible to reuse them to cause a great impact. Today, at such a critical moment for the healthcare field, the need to facilitate the optimization of hospital logistics has become even more relevant. As a result, the tools presented in this article will allow hospitals, doctors, nurses and patients to benefit from the results, thus reducing costs and increasing the time and quality of care.

The opportunity to validate concepts elaborated on two hospital transformations is an advantage for improving the methodology and tools that are proposed in this paper. Sustainability aspects in this healthcare logistics 4.0 concepts implementation concern social and societal dimensions but not sufficiently environmental transformation. This transformation such as waste valorization and reverse logistics, circular economy will be integrated in the study after the validation of the decision tool being developed.

Acknowledgements

This project is being realized by ICAM (Insitut Catholique des Arts et Métiers), a French engineering High school and FEI (Fundaçao Educacionnal Inaciana), a Brazilian University of business and engineering in collaboration with two hospitals of the south east of “Ile de France” region in France.

Notes/thanks/other declarations

Authors would like to thank the health personnel of both hospitals who do not hesitate to help them in this hospital transformation study.

Author details

Paul-Eric Dossou[1,2]*, Luiza Foreste[1] and Eric Misumi[1]

1 Icam, Site of Paris-Sénart, Lieusaint, France

2 University of Gustave Eiffel, AME, SPLOTT, Marne-La-Vallée, France

*Address all correspondence to: paul-eric.dossou@icam.fr

References

[1] Dossou, P.E., Pereira, R., Salama, C., Chang Junior, J. How to use lean manufacturing for improving a Healthcare logistics performance. Procedia Manufacturing, Elsevier, 51 (2020) 1657-1664. doi:10.1016/j.promfg.2020.10.231

[2] Tao F, Qi Q, Wang L, Nee AYC. Digital Twins and Cyber–Physical Systems toward Smart Manufacturing and Industry 4.0: Correlation and Comparison. Engineering. 2019;5(4):653-661. doi:10.1016/j.eng.2019.01.014

[3] Torbackia W, Kijewskaa K. Identifying Key Performance Indicators to be used in Logistics 4.0 and Industry 4.0 for the needs of sustainable municipal logistics by means of the DEMATEL method. 2018; 39: 534-543. doi:10.1016/j.trpro.2019.06.055

[4] Jordon K, Dossou P.E., Junior J. Using lean manufacturing and machine learning for improving medicines procurement and dispatching in a hospital. Procedia Manufacturing. 2019;38:1034-1041. doi:10.1016/j.promfg.2020.01.189

[5] Perez, P., Lang, C., Heinriet, J., Philippe, L., Auber, F., Risk Prediction in surgery using case-based reasoning and agent-based modelization, in Computers in Biology and Medicine, 128(2021) 104040, Elsevier.

[6] Aamodt, A., Plaza, E. (1994), Case-based reasoning: Foundational issues, methodological variations, and system approaches. AI Communications, 7(1), 39-59.

[7] Bentaiba-Lagrid, M. B., Bouzar-Benlabiod, L., Rubin, S. H., Buabana-Tebibel, T., Hanini, M. R., A case-based reasoning system for supervised classification problems in the medical field, in Expert Systems With Applications, 150 (2020) 113335, Elsevier.

[8] Roche, B., Guégan, J.F., Bousquet, F., Multi-agentsystems in epidemiology : a first step for computational biology in the study of vector-borne disease transmission, BMC Bioinf. 9 (1) (2008)435.

[9] Fiannaca, A., La Rosa, M., Rizzo, R., Urso, A., Gaglio, S., An expert system hybrid architecture to support experiment management, in Expert Systems with Applications, 41 (2014) 1609-1621, Elsevier.

[10] Chen, R.C., Huang, Y.H., Bau, C.T., Chen, S.M., A recommendation system based on domain ontology and SWRL for anti-diabetic drugs selection, Expert Systems with Applications, 39, 3995-4006, Elsevier, http://dx.doi.org/10.1016/j.eswa.2011.09.061.

[11] AKostrzewski M, Kosacka-Olejnik M, Werner-Lewandowska K. Assessment of innovativeness level for chosen solutions related to Logistics 4.0. Procedia Manufacturing. 2019;38:621-628. doi:10.1016/j.promfg.2020.01.080

[12] Cimini C, Lagorio A, Pirola F, Roberto Pinto. Exploring human factors in Logistics 4.0: empirical evidence from a case study. 2019;52(13):2183-2188. doi:10.1016/j.ifacol.2019.11.529.

[13] Oleśków-Szłapka J, Wojciechowski H, Domański R, Pawłowski G. Logistics 4.0 Maturity Levels Assessed Based on GDM (Grey Decision Model) and Artificial Intelligence in Logistics 4.0 -Trends and Future Perspective. Procedia Manufacturing. 2019;39:1734-1742. doi:10.1016/j.promfg.2020.01.266

[14] Werner-Lewandowska K, Kosacka-Olejnik M. Logistics 4.0 Maturity in Service Industry: Empirical Research Results. Procedia Manufacturing. 2019;38:1058-1065. doi:10.1016/j.promfg.2020.01.192

[15] Szymańska O, Adamczak M, Cyplik P. Logistics 4.0 - a new paradigm or set of known solutions? Accessed January 30, 2021. https://search-ebscohost-com.ezproxy.univ-catholille.fr/login.aspx?direct=true&db=edseur&AN=edseur.https%3a..www.europeana.eu.item.205..nnrxR98%3futm.source%3dapi%26utm.medium%3dapi%26utm.campaign%3dYuvuWBeCa&lang=fr&site=eds-live&scope=site

[16] Hathaliya JJ, Tanwar S. An exhaustive survey on security and privacy issues in Healthcare 4.0. Computer Communications. 2020;153:311-335. doi:10.1016/j.comcom.2020.02.018

[17] Kumari A, Tanwar S, Tyagi S, Kumar N. Fog computing for Healthcare 4.0 environment: Opportunities and challenges. Computers and Electrical Engineering. 2018;72:1-13. doi:10.1016/j.compeleceng.2018.08.015

[18] Aceto G, Persico V, Pescapé A. Industry 4.0 and Health: Internet of Things, Big Data, and Cloud Computing for Healthcare 4.0. Journal of Industrial Information Integration. 2020;18. doi:10.1016/j.jii.2020.100129

[19] Janya Chanchaichujit, Albert Tan, Fanwen Meng, Sarayoot Eaimkhong. Healthcare 4.0:Next Generation Processes with the Latest Technologies. 2019; doi:10.1007/978-981-13-8114-0

[20] Tortorella GL, Fogliatto FS, Espôsto KF, et al. Effects of contingencies on healthcare 4.0 technologies adoption and barriers in emerging economies. Technological Forecasting & Social Change. 2020;156. doi:10.1016/j.techfore.2020.120048

[21] Cortes H, Daaboul J, Le Duigou J, Eynard B, Strategic Lean Management: Integration of operational Performance Indicators for strategic Lean management. 2016; 49(12): 65-70. doi:10.1016/j.ifacol.2016.07.551.

[22] Narayanamurthy G, Gurumurthy A, Subramanian N, Moser R. Assessing the readiness to implement lean in healthcare institutions – A case study. International Journal of Production Economics. 2018;197:123-142. doi:10.1016/j.ijpe.2017.12.028

[23] Narayanamurthy G, Gurumurthy A. Is the hospital lean? A mathematical model for assessing the implementation of lean thinking in healthcare institutions. Operations Research for Health Care. 2018;18:84-98. doi:10.1016/j.orhc.2017.05.002

[24] DOSSOU, P.E. Impact of Sustainability on the supply chain 4.0 performance. Procedia Manufacturing, [s. l.], v. 17, p. 452-459, 2018. DOI 10.1016/j.promfg.2018.10.069.

Chapter 12

Emotional Intelligence and Leadership Development: Implications for Family Medicine Residency Programs

Seul Jee Ha, Sridhar Reddy Patlolla and Thomas Robert Wojda

Abstract

High-level emotional Intelligence (EI) and leadership skills are crucial for physicians to prioritize responsibilities and successfully interact with numerous stakeholders in an every-increasingly complex healthcare system. Although recent research has shown an association between emotional intelligence and leadership, few studies have examined this relationship among family and primary care physicians. Family physicians play an essential role in the evaluation and treatment of illnesses as well as health and wellness promotion. These providers are often the first point of contact with the patient and the use of emotional intelligence and development of leadership abilities of primary care physicians are vital to the maintenance, sustainability, and optimization of a medical organization. Furthermore, high- level emotional intelligence and sharpened leadership skills may aid the patient-provider relationship and dealings with coworkers. This chapter explores key themes of EI and physician leadership as it pertains to Family Medicine Residency.

Keywords: emotional intelligence, family medicine, leadership, self-awareness, burnout

1. Introduction

Medical organizations are under pressure from consumer and regulatory demands to reduce costs and boost quality and value. Patient-centered medical homes, accountable care organizations, and various other advances will have substantial influence on the future of the US health care system. These modern paradigms involve high-level cooperation among physicians and various stakeholders. Unfortunately, physicians have often been judged by their inability to effectively collaborate. What's more comparatively little consideration has been given to collaboration as it pertains to traditional physician education and career advancement [1]. The reasons behind sub-optimal collaboration are multifactorial; however they may be more broadly divided into personal and structural reasons. On a personal level, it may be that physicians traditionally reveled in self-sufficiency.

Also, persons attracted to and selected for medical careers may have been customarily independent, self-directed, and assured [2]. Because physicians basked in autonomy, they may have inadvertently propagated a culture that prioritizes individuality. Subsequently, today healthcare systems are repeatedly designed like silos, which further undercut teamwork [1, 3–5]. Consequently, any effective health network must concentrate on a move from a philosophy that the physician is the sole provider to one that fosters and promotes strong relationships and effective communication [2]. Strong physician leadership is vital to the implementation and success of this shift.

Emotional intelligence (EI) is the ability to perceive and express emotion, assimilate emotion in thought, understand and reason with emotion, and regulate emotion in the self and others [6]. It has been considered an essential leadership proficiency [7]. In medicine, its applicability may range from the boardroom to the patient's bedside [7, 8]. There are various representations of different evaluative methods for EI. One of the more mainstream depictions includes self-awareness, self-regulation, social awareness, and relationship management (**Figure 1**) [9]. The cells are further populated by component competencies that define EI (**Figure 1 legend**) [10].

EI, rather than being something one is born with, is a set of skills that can be improved upon to boost performance [11, 12]. This is in stark contrast to hard to define views of professionalism or leadership as an EI template is clear, teachable, and allows for an honest assessment of where one is and where one needs to be in regards to development. Ample evidence supports the importance of EI as a key leadership competency in business [13–15]. Conversely, far less attention has been paid to EI as it pertains to health care.

The remainder of this chapter will focus on EI and its implications on Graduate Medical Education (GME) specifically Family Medicine Residency. The chapter will examine the association between EI and leadership traits among family physicians as well as the effects of different EI implementation strategies such as coaching, Balint Seminars, advisor and focus groups, and their impact on physician trainees as well as further commentary on future best practices.

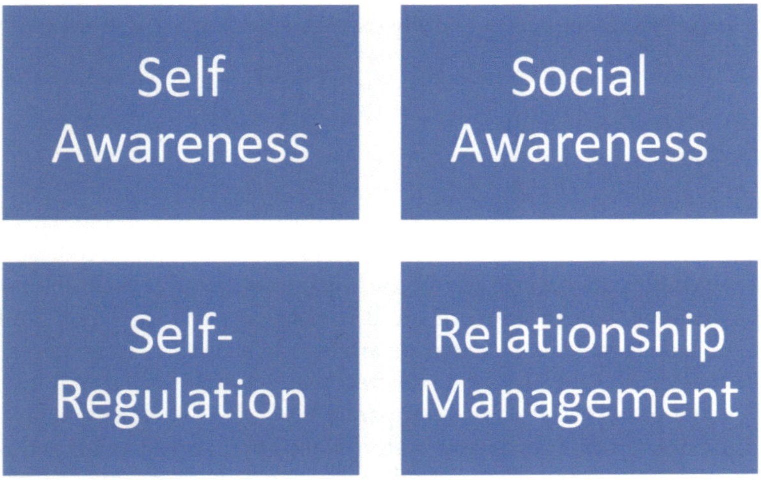

Figure 1.
*Four components of emotional intelligence. *Further divided into competencies self-awareness: Emotional self-awareness, accurate self-awareness, self-confidence; social awareness: Empathy, organizational awareness, service orientation; self-management: Self-control, trust-worthiness, conscientiousness, adaptability, achievement orientation, initiative; social skills: Influence, leadership, developing others, communication, change catalyst, conflict management, building bonds, team work and collaboration.*

2. Emotional intelligence and leadership traits among family physicians

Emotional intelligence and leadership traits are intimately linked [16–18]. A common thread that weaves these explorations is the idea that leaders with high EI are more effective in management than those with low EI [17, 19]. Leadership traits may be illustrated on an organizational and personal level (**Figure 2**) [16, 20].

EI requires self-discipline, self-efficacy, self-evaluation, and self-criticism, which enhances leadership and job fulfillment [21–23]. What's more, through the enrichment of strong relationships with their patient's and colleagues, any physician may be considered a leader. Therefore, it behooves the physician to foster these aptitudes to deliver excellent care [16]. Moreover, physicians' EI has bearings on their interactions and relationships with patients. Although it is crucial to exhibit competence in medicine, insufficient EI may hinder the ability to fully understand the complexities of a patient's being during their evaluation and treatment. In fact! Compared to physicians with higher EI those will low EI are less likely to foster empathic connections with their patients and appreciate or make out their emotions [23, 24]. EI may facilitate the patient–doctor rapport [22–24]. It shapes judgments concerning patient management, encourages self-control in demanding circumstances, and the avoidance of emotionally charged behaviors and decisions. Physicians who can identify and manage their emotions can remain calm when faced with patients who are under stress, anxious, or trigger the provider in some way. EI will allow the physician to convey their thoughts and feelings empathically and without judgment to the patient, which affords the most advantageous care [25].

EI plays a part in the physicians' ability to acclimate well with other people, optimize team-based care, and respond appropriately to external pressures. Health-care providers with noticeable levels of EI may drive forward institutional missions. Besides the personal and relational aspect of EI, there may also be administrative benefits. For example, it may lower hospital costs by reducing burnout, medical errors, and litigation [23–25].

Family physicians are indispensable health-care workers who evaluate, treat, and manage acute and chronic diseases, promote health and wellness, and enhance the well-being of patients and communities through the application of the therapeutic relationship. Because family physicians may be a patient's first and potentially only contact with a healthcare provider, the development of EI for primary

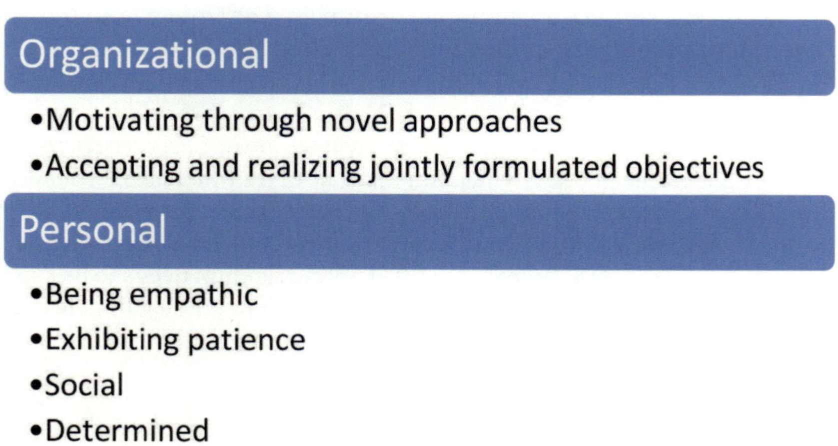

Figure 2.
Organizational and personal examples of leadership traits.

care physicians is essential to the healthcare system. What's more, a high level of EI in family physicians may help in team-based care [22, 25].

A study by Coskun et al. aimed to determine the association of different variables and *trait emotional intelligence* (TEI). TEI consists of four basic factors that include: well-being, self-control, emotionality, and sociability [26]. This was a descriptive population-based study conducted from September 2013 to December 2014. The total population comprised 20,185 family physicians working at family healthcare centers across the seven regions of Turkey [27]. Women scored higher than did men for well-being, emotionality, and global TEI, which reflect similar GME outcomes. For instance, female medical students have exhibited significantly higher EI, empathy, and utilization of emotions than their male counterparts [28]. Society and environment may play a crucial role in the way women construct their personal and business lives. In this study, the sex differences gap was not particularly large, which may point to a shift in societal sex roles. Still, higher EI and leadership skills promote empathic communication, trust, and positive interactions between physicians and patients regardless of sex; therefore, both female and male physicians may benefit from training related to improving EI and leadership. Additionally, significant differences were found in well-being, self-control, and emotionality according to age and health-care experience. There may be a positive correlation between EI and experience, which hints that EI raises as a person advances through their career [24]. It may also be that as people age they are more likely to gravitate toward emotions that give them joy and avoid negative emotions if possible [23, 24]. Inexperienced physicians may struggle to adapt to their new role, thus displaying decreased EI. Fascinatingly, leadership traits of family physicians have not shown to vary significantly based on age or years of experience. Although it may be assumed that advanced age and years of experience would be associated with increased leadership traits, these variables appear to exert an insignificant effect on leadership styles in general [29]. Tenure has no effect on leadership ability either [18]. It may well be that age and experience optimize results with leadership experience.

According to Goleman, the most effective leaders are those who possess emotional intelligence [21]. Emotional understanding, emotional management, empathy, social flexibility, and adaptability are essential for individual growth and development as well as indispensable for societal regulation in the work setting [30]. Whereas low EI may lead to less effective teamwork, diminished work satisfaction, and heightened anxiety among physicians, higher EI preserves good physician–patient relationships, superior teamwork and communication skills, healthier stress management, and top-quality commitment and leadership [18, 20, 23, 31]. Personal well-being, empathy, teamwork, and leadership skills are all staples to a physician's work [17–20].

Youthful physicians with less experience may have lower EI scores compared to older, more experienced ones, which implies that EI may increase throughout training. GME programs that integrate EI and leadership competencies allow for students to attain these skills earlier and perhaps most importantly provides a platform to generate meaningful results [19]. This curriculum needs to be supplemented by coaching, mentorship, or other directives to ensure sustainable change in self-awareness and emotional intelligence among physicians.

3. Coaching emotional intelligence

The Accreditation Council for Graduate Medical Education (ACGME) mandates that residents be taught and assessed in six general competencies, which include:

patient care, medical knowledge, practice-based learning and improvement, interpersonal and communication skills, professionalism, and systems-based practices [32]. EI has been proposed for teaching interpersonal and communication skills as well as professionalism [33]. EI contains the skill to carry out precise interpretation on the subject of feelings and the aptitude to exercise emotions and emotional knowledge to boost thought [34]. Moreover, abundant positive correlations that link EI with desirable outcomes exist (**Table 1**) [35].

Although much is known about the numerous positive impacts EI may have, there is still much to elucidate in regards to proper implementation, maintenance, and enhancement of EI skills. In a quasi-experimental design, with an intervention and control group composed of one class each of family medicine residents researchers assessed the Emotional and Social Competence Inventory (ESCI), a 360-degree EI self and peer reported survey for 12 EI competencies (**Table 2**) to determine if coaching would enhance emotional intelligence [36].

Unfortunately, there was no significant difference in ESCI scores in the intervention versus control group. Interestingly, teamwork significantly declined. Regrettably, a drop in aspects of EI during training is not unique. Specifically, Wagner et al. found a decline in self-reported medical student EI scores [37]. A deterioration in humanitarianism, enthusiasm and idealism experienced by medical students has also been ascribed to the fall of EI throughout training [38].

Despite the lack of significance, this study was plagued by implementation barriers, which are important to understand. First, no faculty were given protected time for coaching. Second, resident's comments suggested that increasing EI was not a priority for them at this juncture in their training. Third, resident's EI scores were already relatively high; therefore additional time spent may not have been felt to be justified. Finally, there remains a lack of validity of ESCI for the medical community.

It is vital that if EI is to be tested and enhanced in a residency program that it be implemented properly. For example, EI coaching should have built-in protected time. It may be beneficial for residents toward the end of training when they appear to be less stressed and more focused on future goals. Alternatively, in view of its time-intensive make-up, EI training could selectively center on residents with low EI ratings. Post-residency it may be provided as continuing medical education for stress management, remediation of deficiencies, or advanced training.

It should be stressed that EI coaching requires a high level of trainee engagement and commitment. This course may include cognitive behavioral assignments between coaching sessions. An EI training session may include a trainee's initial statement of ideal career goals along with a guided review of EI survey results.

Leadership Success
Employee Self-Esteem
Job Satisfaction
Job Commitment
Teamwork
Customer Satisfaction
Decreased Turnover
Less Work/Family Conflict

Table 1.
Positive outcomes associated with emotional intelligence.

Trait	Definition
Emotional self-awareness	Recognizing one's emotions and their effects
Emotional self-control	Keeping disruptive emotions and impulses in check
Adaptability	Flexibility in handling change
Achievement Orientation	Striving to improve or meeting a standard of excellence
Positive Outlook	Persistence in pursuing goals despite obstacles, setbacks
Empathy	Sensing others' feelings/perspectives, taking active interest
Organizational Awareness	Reading group's emotional currents and power relationships
Coach and Mentor	Sensing other's development needs and bolstering their abilities
Inspirational Leadership	Inspiring and guiding individuals and groups
Influence	Wielding effective tactics for persuasion
Conflict Management	Negotiating and resolving disagreements
Teamwork	Working with others toward shared goal, creating group synergy

**ESCI norms apply to other ratings only and are based on a North American sample of workers all ages and job levels. Achievement orientation is the highest rated competence in the norms, and self-awareness the lowest [36].*

Table 2.
Emotional intelligence competency definitions.

The coach could then emphasize EI strengths of the trainee while simultaneously employing schemes to build upon areas of improvement for the trainee. The trainee and coach would then set performance goals, negotiate assignments, time frames, frequency of coaching sessions, and add or modify selected goals based upon progress.

EI has been proclaimed fundamental for leaders who are coping with change management [39]. This skill is all the more important as it relates to physicians and the current health care landscape. Even so, much work remains to be done to provide clear-cut proof that investment in EI training is warranted. A reasonable next phase would be to substantiate approaches that consistently boost physician EI. Advantages and disadvantages to implementation are shown (**Table 3**).

Potential research ought to emphasize the elaboration of an expedient reasonably priced 360-degree EI instrument for physicians. Ideally, this would be enhanced by providing established external validity measures that further correlate medical outcomes, patient satisfaction, and physician satisfaction. Multi-institution collaboration may possibly evaluate EI development in distinctive training paradigms and fields of practice. Perhaps longitudinal research will explore EI development post training, specifically in relation to physician impairment or disruptive behavior. If EI tools demonstrate sustained value in the domains of physician selection, education, training, and remediation, they may well become more generalizable and important to the medical community as a whole.

Advantages	Disadvantages
Validated 360-degree assessment instruments	Time and labor intensive
Access to well-developed training models	Expense
Published norms	Lack of physician norms

Table 3.
Potential advantages and disadvantages to emotional intelligence training.

4. Emotional intelligence, feelings, responses, and burnout

Hungarian-born British psychoanalyst Michael Balint pioneered Balint groups among practicing physicians in the 1950s to explore the doctor–patient relationship [40]. Balint groups help make physicians aware of their blind spots during their interactions with patients as well as use their feelings and responses to patients as instruments to better comprehend the physician–patient relationship [41]. These seminars consist of longitudinal experiential learning over a period of time as well as a group of residents who periodically meet and are accompanied by two Balint leaders. A case that bothers one of the residents is presented, which is followed by a discussion from the point of view of the patient, doctor, and their relationship with the caveat that medical care not be discussed [42–44]. After, Balint leaders help the residents in the expansion, consideration, and illumination of their thoughts and feelings related to the case from both the patient and physician's perspective. Examples of benefits and detriments to these sessions are found (**Table 4**) [45–47].

Given Balint training is closely linked with the ability to understand and regulate emotions, a quasi-experimental observational study aimed to measure the effects of Balint seminars on EI and burnout among internal medicine residents [48]. Bi-weekly Balint seminars were delivered throughout the academic year. Two major outcomes were measured using validated instruments: EI using the Mayer Salovey and Caruso Emotional Intelligence Test (MSCEIT) and burnout using the Maslach Burnout Inventory (MBI). The MSCEIT, based on a four-branch model of EI, is the most comprehensive measure of EI as an ability [49]. The MBI is the gold standard for measuring burnout [50]. Depictions of these instruments are found in **Figures 3–5** respectively. A total of 20 Balint seminars were delivered; however on average, residents attended six sessions. The total post-Balint EI score improved among women versus men. Many residents showed severe burnout levels on at least one of the three domains of burnout at baseline; however, Balint seminars did not have any effect on any of the burnout domains even when accounting for gender, attendance or training level.

Evidence suggests no predetermined gender differences in EI ability among medical residents according to specialty [51]. Nevertheless, Balint seminar results may be affected by gender, learning style, and training year. Indeed, Balint interventions may be more effective among women than men [52]. The openness of women to such educational activities could explain why the female residents improve their EI. Also despite lack of statistical significance in this study, EI still improved in a small number of trainees, which could be due to various learning styles, personality and level of training. Criticisms of Balint seminars include a lack of focus on problem solving and firm structure that may not meet residents' developmental needs [53]. Different levels of training may explain the non-uniform effectiveness of this intervention [54].

Pros	Cons
Communication skills and professionalism	Time Consuming
Awareness of feelings/values, develop appropriate treatment based on psychological needs of patient	Significant Resources required
Positive effects on self-efficacy, burnout and job satisfaction, breaking bad news, empathy	Measurable outcomes still controversial

Table 4.
Pros and cons of Balint group.

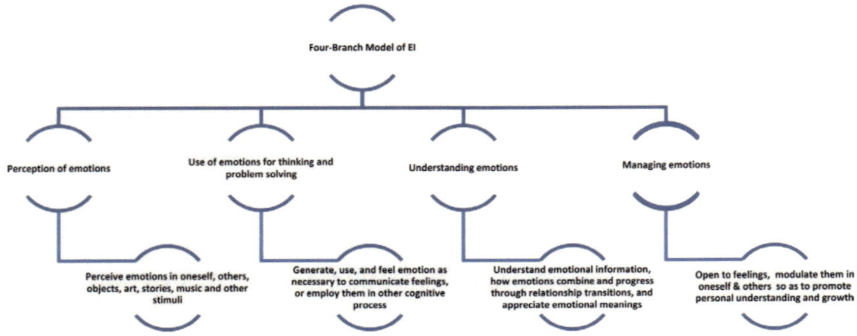

Figure 3.
Four-branch model of emotional intelligence.

Score	Meaning
<69	Develop
70-89	Low average score
100-109	High average score
110-119	Competent
120-129	Strength
>130	Significant Strength

Figure 4.
*Scoring system of Mayer Salovey and Caruso emotional intelligence test (MSCEIT). *The MSCEIT provides 15 main scores: Total EIQ score, two area scores, four branch scores, and eight task scores. It can be scored using both the consensus and expert scoring methods. There are guidelines on how to interpret the score. The average MSCEIT score is 100 with a standard deviation of 115. There are 7 score ranges based on empirical percentiles.*

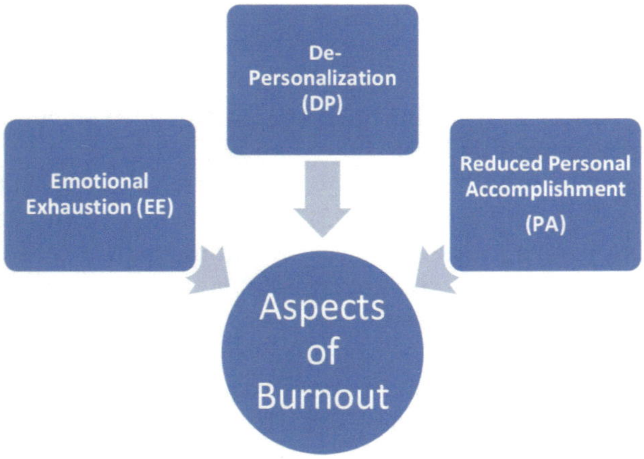

Figure 5.
Aspects of burnout according to Maslach burnout inventory.

Finally, EI measurement immediately post-intervention may be suboptimal. In two studies, the influence of an EI educational intervention was only measurable as a delayed positive effect several months after the intervention [55, 56]. Therefore, interventions to improve EI and decrease burnout levels may have more long term effects that may not immediately come to light.

5. Emotional intelligence, wellness, and cultural transformation

Physician burnout remains a sobering affair [57, 58]. It may be particularly egregious in medical residency [59]. Family medicine, internal medicine, and emergency medicine residents may be at particularly high risk given they are often on the "front lines" of care [60]. The side effects of burnout may include: unethical and bad-mannered behavior [61], patient-care mistakes [60, 62], and physicians quitting their practice [63, 64].

The benefits of cultivating psychosocial proficiencies in medical learners may include mitigation of contempt, anxiety, and improvement in clinical ability [65]. It may also further reduce grave medical oversights as well as better-quality bonds with contemporaries and patients [66]. Rather than focusing on the diagnosis and treatment of emotional fatigue and depersonalization among residents, there has been a more recent push in the direction of the formation of a scholastic philosophy of wellness [67]. An alternative residency culture has been proposed as a framework [68]. **Figure 6** is a schematic representation of an emotionally intelligent learning community [69].

With physician burnout a grave concern and a scarcity of evidence on successful tactics to diminish it during residency, an intervention to lower burnout through an emphasis on wellness, safety, and interpersonal skills in a family medicine program was proposed. In a mixed-methods case study that utilized results from three quantitative self-reported instruments for well-being, along with content analysis of transcripts from 20 focus groups and 33 resident advising sessions described experiences of family medicine residents in a single site enrolled between July 2007 and June 2012 [69].

In this intervention, no statistically significant quantitative differences in the well-being of residents compared with the family medicine faculty and staff was discovered; however residents in general recognized the nurturing culture of the program. While individuals' commentaries about experiences during residency were unique, analysis revealed six recurrent themes (**Figure 7**). Although well-being scores for residents and the community did not change during the intervention, resident feedback over the five years showed they acknowledged purpose of the curriculum changes, recognized the new curricular practices, and respected the importance of physical and emotional wellness.

It should be pointed out that not every learner will embrace the innovations of emotional intelligence, leadership-development, or other form of wellness curriculum and some may even have utter contempt for the methodology. Still, even being able to articulate this disdain creates a culture of safety and helps dissipate the "culture of silence" that is all too often pervasive in academic medicine [70].

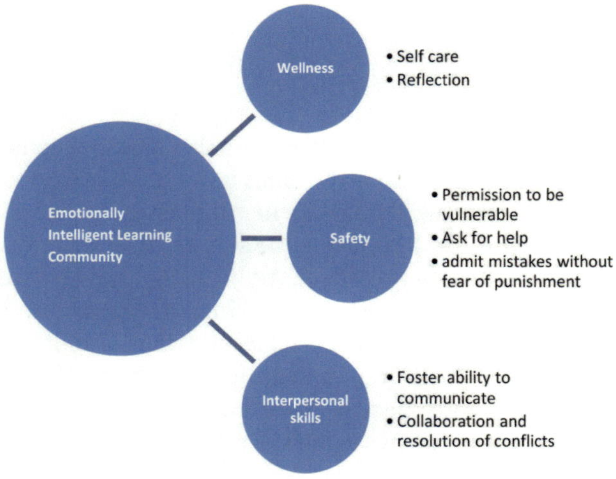

Figure 6.
Representation of an emotionally intelligent learning community.

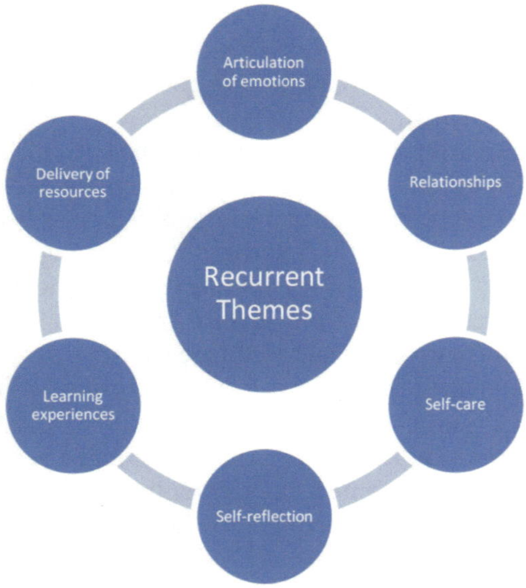

Figure 7.
Six recurrent themes of an emotionally intelligent learning community.

What's more, scholastic culture change utilized by a program that focuses on EI may provide ample time and space for residents to reflect on what it means to be a doctor without any modifications to the day-to-day clinical obligations of the residents. Lastly these interventions may help regulate resident's feelings as they move between different stress levels throughout their training [71].

It has been difficult to find interventions that reduce burnout during residency. Limited evidence supports duty hour reductions, a revised grading system, mindfulness training, and self-development groups to prevent burnout in medical students and residents [72]. An electronic reflective writing portfolio has been created as a professional identity development tool, which provides opportunities for residents to explore work-life balance, resiliency, and burnout prevention [73]. There are calls for GME to reform the way medicine is taught and to place more emphasis on the heart and mind of a clinician [74]. Future research should include multisite studies and control sites with less emphasis on well-being as well as studies that follow residents into practice to determine if long-term benefits exist.

6. Conclusion

In summation, there remains a scarcity of valuable research about EI in family medicine residency that obviously welcomes more consideration. Studies are needed to further address each of the themes that emerged in this chapter. Certainly, increased focus must be given to the standardization and applicability of EI measurement in healthcare providers. Additionally, the benefits and shortcomings of the instruments that have been used in health care studies such as the Emotional Competence Inventory, Mayer-Salovery-Caruso Emotional Intelligence Test, or specially designed 360-degree evaluations must be further explored. Likewise, greater attention must be paid to the particular components of EI, the most optimal time to focus on them during the training period, and how enhancing these competencies may shape the career trajectory of physicians. A real discussion must take place if all physicians should receive formal emotional intelligence and leadership development training, or if it should be only for those who are specifically recruited or express an interest. Finally long-term outcomes of EI training on family physician, patient, and hospital systems are needed. Solutions to these enquires will command extraordinary leadership to solve imminent healthcare challenges.

Author details

Seul Jee Ha[1], Sridhar Reddy Patlolla[2] and Thomas Robert Wojda[3]*

1 Department of Family Medicine-Warren Campus, St. Luke's University Health Network, United States

2 Department of Internal Medicine, Suburban Community Hospital, United States

3 Department of Family Medicine, Conemaugh Memorial Medical Center, United States

*Address all correspondence to: trwojda@gmail.com

References

[1] Stoller, J., *Can physicians collaborate? An examination of organization development in health care.* OD PRACTITIONER, 2004. **36**(3): p. 19-24.

[2] Gabbard, G.O., *The role of compulsiveness in the normal physician.* Jama, 1985. **254**(20): p. 2926-2929.

[3] Weisbord, M.R., *Organizational diagnosis: A workbook of theory and practice*, in *Organizational diagnosis: a workbook of theory and practice*. 1978. p. 180-180.

[4] Weil, T.P., *Difficulties in consummating a meaningful hospital-physician collaboration.* J Med Pract Manage, 2012. **28**(1): p. 47-50.

[5] Brenner, D.A., *2012 Association of American Physicians Presidential Address Next-generation academic medicine.* The Journal of clinical investigation, 2012. **122**(11): p. 4280-4282.

[6] Geher, G. and K.L. Renstrom, *Measurement issues in emotional intelligence research.* 2004.

[7] Lobas, J.G., *Leadership in academic medicine: capabilities and conditions for organizational success.* The American journal of medicine, 2006. **119**(7): p. 617-621.

[8] Bohmer, R.M., *Leading clinicians and clinicians leading.* The New England journal of medicine, 2013. **368**(16): p. 1468.

[9] Boyatzis, R., A. McKee, and D. Goleman, *Primal leadership: Learning to lead with emotional intelligence*. 2003: McGraw-Hill.

[10] Boyatzis, R.E., *Transforming qualitative information: Thematic analysis and code development*. 1998: sage.

[11] Kouzes, J.M., B.Z. Posner, and J. Bozarth, *Strengthening Credibility: A Leader's Workbook*. Vol. 233. 2011: John Wiley & Sons.

[12] Posner, B.Z. and J.M. Kouzes, *Development and validation of the leadership practices inventory.* Educational and psychological measurement, 1988. **48**(2): p. 483-496.

[13] Dulewicz, V. and M. Higgs, *Emotional intelligence–A review and evaluation study.* Journal of managerial Psychology, 2000.

[14] Van Rooy, D.L. and C. Viswesvaran, *Emotional intelligence: A meta-analytic investigation of predictive validity and nomological net.* Journal of vocational Behavior, 2004. **65**(1): p. 71-95.

[15] Alon, I. and J.M. Higgins, *Global leadership success through emotional and cultural intelligences.* Business horizons, 2005. **48**(6): p. 501-512.

[16] Chaudry, J., et al., *Physician leadership: the competencies of change.* Journal of Surgical Education, 2008. **65**(3): p. 213-220.

[17] Stoller, J.K., C.A. Taylor, and C.F. Farver, *Emotional intelligence competencies provide a developmental curriculum for medical training.* Medical teacher, 2013. **35**(3): p. 243-247.

[18] Siegling, A., C. Nielsen, and K. Petrides, *Trait emotional intelligence and leadership in a European multinational company.* Personality and Individual Differences, 2014. **65**: p. 65-68.

[19] Johnson, D.R., *Emotional intelligence as a crucial component to medical education.* International Journal of Medical Education, 2015. **6**: p. 179.

[20] i Solà, G.J., et al., *Self-perception of leadership styles and behaviour in primary health care.* BMC health services research, 2016. **16**(1): p. 1-9.

[21] Goleman, D., *Working with emotional intelligence*. 1998: Bantam.

[22] Kirby, R., *Emotional intelligence and medicine.* Trends in Urology & Men's Health, 2016. 7(3): p. 30-31.

[23] Weng, H.C., et al., *Associations between emotional intelligence and doctor burnout, job satisfaction and patient satisfaction.* Medical education, 2011. **45**(8): p. 835-842.

[24] Weng, H.C., et al., *Doctors' emotional intelligence and the patient–doctor relationship.* Medical education, 2008. **42**(7): p. 703-711.

[25] Hammerly, M.E., L. Harmon, and S.D. Schwaitzberg, *Good to great: using 360-degree feedback to improve physician emotional intelligence.* Journal of Healthcare Management, 2014. **59**(5): p. 354-366.

[26] Petrides, K.V. and A. Furnham, *Trait emotional intelligence: Psychometric investigation with reference to established trait taxonomies.* European journal of personality, 2001. **15**(6): p. 425-448.

[27] Coskun, O., et al., *Emotional intelligence and leadership traits among family physicians.* Postgraduate medicine, 2018. **130**(7): p. 644-649.

[28] Austin, E.J., et al., *A preliminary study of emotional intelligence, empathy and exam performance in first year medical students.* Personality and Individual Differences, 2005. **39**(8): p. 1395-1405.

[29] Zilembo, M. and L. Monterosso, *Nursing students' perceptions of desirable leadership qualities in nurse preceptors: A descriptive survey.* Contemporary Nurse, 2008. **27**(2): p. 194-206.

[30] McCALLIN, A. and A. Bamford, *Interdisciplinary teamwork: is the influence of emotional intelligence fully appreciated?* Journal of nursing management, 2007. **15**(4): p. 386-391.

[31] Mintz, L.J. and J.K. Stoller, *A systematic review of physician leadership and emotional intelligence.* Journal of Graduate Medical Education, 2014. **6**(1): p. 21-31.

[32] Education, A.C.f.G.M., *Accreditation Council for Graduate Medical Education (ACGME) outcome project*. 2005.

[33] Grewal, D. and H.A. Davidson, *Emotional intelligence and graduate medical education.* JAmA, 2008. **300**(10): p. 1200-1202.

[34] Mayer, J.D., R.D. Roberts, and S.G. Barsade, *Human abilities: Emotional intelligence.* Annu. Rev. Psychol., 2008. **59**: p. 507-536.

[35] Jordan, P.J., N.M. Ashkanasy, and K.W. Ascough, *Emotional intelligence in organizational behavior and industrial-organizational psychology.* 2007.

[36] Webb, A.R., Young R.A, and Baumer J.G. *Emotional intelligence and the ACGME competencies.* Journal of graduate medical education, 2010. **2**(4): p. 508-512.

[37] Wagner, P., et al., *Emotional intel-44. ligence changes during medical school.* Teaching and Learning in Medicine, 2005. **17**(4): p. 391-395.

[38] Stratton, T.D., J.A. Saunders, and C.L. Elam, *Changes in medical students' emotional intelligence: An exploratory study.* Teaching and learning in medicine, 2008. **20**(3): p. 279-284.

[39] McEnrue, M.P., K.S. Groves, and W. Shen, *Emotional intelligence training: Evidence regarding its efficacy for developing leaders.* Leadership Review, 2010. **10**: p. 3.

[40] Balint, E., *The possibilities of patient-centered medicine.* The Journal of the Royal College of General Practitioners, 1969. **17**(82): p. 269.

[41] Lustig, M., *Balint groups: An Australasian perspective for psychiatrists.* Australasian Psychiatry, 2016. **24**(1): p. 30-33.

[42] Diaz, V.A., et al., *Balint Groups in Family Medicine Residency Programs.* Family medicine, 2015. **47**(5): p. 367-372.

[43] Horder, J., *The first Balint group.* The British Journal of General Practice, 2001. **51**(473): p. 1038.

[44] Johnson, A.H., et al., *The current status of Balint groups in US family practice residencies: a 10-year follow-up study, 1990-2000.* FAMILY MEDICINE-KANSAS CITY-, 2001. **33**(9): p. 672-677.

[45] Lichtenstein, A., et al., *Mapping the Balint groups to the Accreditation Council for Graduate Medical Education family medicine competencies.* The International Journal of Psychiatry in Medicine, 2018. **53**(1-2): p. 47-58.

[46] Kjeldmand, D. and I. Holmström, *Balint groups as a means to increase job satisfaction and prevent burnout among general practitioners.* The Annals of Family Medicine, 2008. **6**(2): p. 138-145.

[47] Van Roy, K., S. Vanheule, and R. Inslegers, *Research on Balint groups: a literature review.* Patient education and counseling, 2015. **98**(6): p. 685-694.

[48] Antoun, J., et al., *Effect of Balint seminars training on emotional intelligence and burnout among internal medicine residents.* Health Education Journal, 2020. **79**(7): p. 802-811.

[49] Cartwright, S. and C. Pappas, *Emotional intelligence, its measurement and implications for the workplace.* International Journal of Management Reviews, 2008. **10**(2): p. 149-171.

[50] Maslach, C., M.P. Leiter, and W. Schaufeli, *Measuring burnout.* The Oxford handbook of organizational well being, 2008.

[51] McKinley, S.K., et al., *Are there gender differences in the emotional intelligence of resident physicians?* Journal of surgical education, 2014. **71**(6): p. e33-e40.

[52] Cherry, M.G., et al., *What impact do structured educational sessions to increase emotional intelligence have on medical students? BEME Guide No. 17.* Medical teacher, 2012. **34**(1): p. 11-19.

[53] Smith, M. and G. Anandarajah, *Mutiny on the balint: Balancing resident developmental needs with the balint process.* FAMILY MEDICINE-KANSAS CITY-, 2007. **39**(7): p. 495.

[54] Lewis, N.J., et al., *Emotional intelligence medical education: measuring the unmeasurable?* Advances in Health Sciences Education, 2005. **10**(4): p. 339-355.

[55] Gorgas, D.L., et al., *Teaching emotional intelligence: a control group study of a brief educational intervention for emergency medicine residents.* Western journal of emergency medicine, 2015. **16**(6): p. 899.

[56] Rabinowitz, S., T. Kushnir, and J. Ribak, *Preventing burnout: increasing professional self efficacy in primary care nurses in a Balint Group.* Aaohn Journal, 1996. **44**(1): p. 28-32.

[57] Billings, M.E., et al., *The effect of the hidden curriculum on resident burnout and cynicism.* Journal of graduate medical education, 2011. **3**(4): p. 503.

[58] Maslach, C. and M. Leiter, *The thruth about burnout*. 1997, San Francisco: Jossey-Bass.

[59] Dyrbye, L.N., et al., *Burnout among US medical students, residents, and early career physicians relative to the general US*

population. Academic medicine, 2014. **89**(3): p. 443-451.

[60] Shanafelt, T.D., et al., *Burnout and satisfaction with work-life balance among US physicians relative to the general US population.* Archives of internal medicine, 2012. **172**(18): p. 1377-1385.

[61] Leape, L.L., et al., *Perspective: a culture of respect, part 2: creating a culture of respect.* Academic medicine, 2012. **87**(7): p. 853-858.

[62] Wallace, J.E., J.B. Lemaire, and W.A. Ghali, *Physician wellness: a missing quality indicator.* The Lancet, 2009. **374**(9702): p. 1714-1721.

[63] Bodenheimer, T.S. and M.D. Smith, *Primary care: proposed solutions to the physician shortage without training more physicians.* Health Affairs, 2013. **32**(11): p. 1881-1886.

[64] Linzer, M., et al., *Organizational climate, stress, and error in primary care: the MEMO study.* Advances in patient safety: from research to implementation, 2005. **1**: p. 65-77.

[65] Dunn, L.B., A. Iglewicz, and C. Moutier, *A conceptual model of medical student well-being: promoting resilience and preventing burnout.* Academic Psychiatry, 2008. **32**(1): p. 44-53.

[66] Haidet, P. and H.F. Stein, *The role of the student-teacher relationship in the formation of physicians.* Journal of General Internal Medicine, 2006. **21**(1): p. 16-20.

[67] Eckleberry-Hunt, J., et al., *Changing the conversation from burnout to wellness: physician well-being in residency training programs.* Journal of Graduate Medical Education, 2009. **1**(2): p. 225.

[68] Cohen-Katz, J.L., W.L. Miller, and J.M. Borkan, *Building a culture of resident well-being: Creating self-reflection, community, & positive identity in family practice residency education.* Families, Systems, & Health, 2003. **21**(3): p. 293.

[69] Cohen-Katz, J., et al., *Developing emotional intelligence in the clinical learning environment: a case study in cultural transformation.* Journal of graduate medical education, 2016. **8**(5): p. 692.

[70] Dankoski, M.E., J. Bickel, and M.E. Gusic, *Discussing the undiscussable with the powerful: why and how faculty must learn to counteract organizational silence.* Academic Medicine, 2014. **89**(12): p. 1610-1613.

[71] Addison, R.B., *Covering-over and over-reflecting during residency training: using personal and professional development groups to integrate dysfunctional modes of being*, in *Becoming a family physician*. 1989, Springer. p. 87-110.

[72] Williams, D., et al., *Efficacy of burnout interventions in the medical education pipeline.* Academic Psychiatry, 2015. **39**(1): p. 47-54.

[73] Wald, H.S., et al., *Professional identity formation in medical education for humanistic, resilient physicians: pedagogic strategies for bridging theory to practice.* Academic Medicine, 2015. **90**(6): p. 753-760.

[74] Irby, D.M., M. Cooke, and B.C. O'Brien, *Calls for reform of medical education by the Carnegie Foundation for the Advancement of Teaching: 1910 and 2010.* Academic Medicine, 2010. **85**(2): p. 220-227.

Chapter 13

Making Soft Skills a Part of the Curriculum of Healthcare Studies

Niva Dolev, Lior Naamati-Schneider and Adaya Meirovich

Abstract

In recent decades, it has been increasingly recognized that soft skills play an important role in healthcare education and must be developed alongside other professional skills. Furthermore, the contribution of emotional intelligence (EI) to the ability to adapt to the changing environment of the 21st century has been widely agreed upon. Yet, despite these findings, social–emotional intelligence (SEI) and related skills skills are not widely developed in healthcare education settings, and if at all, only in a limited way. The present chapter presents a model and a methodological tool (SE-SD) for the development of social–emotional skills (SEI) as part of existing healthcare curricula, applying a broad view of the healthcare professions and associated skills. Soft, social–emotional, skills are positioned as a relevant and integral part of healthcare courses, thereby avoiding the need for significant changes in existing curricula. The SEI development process is implemented in three stages: preparation, action and assessment. The tool allows learners to embark on a self-directed, yet supervised, learning and development process, and can be applied to a single course or through the entire study program. The incorporation of a soft skill development process into healthcare education programs could help health systems to adapt and to cope better with the challenges of the 21st century, both present and future.

Keywords: Soft skills, medical education, emotional intelligence, innovation in teaching

1. Introduction

In the last decades, healthcare systems in the Western world have been undergoing constant, profound, local and global changes. These changes present new challenges to health systems and require them to adapt to the new and dynamic era of the 21st century.

Macro-level changes and consequent challenges include the digital revolution [1, 2]; the need to work with, and alongside, technological innovations and artificial intelligence (AI) [3]; frequent reforms and changes to regulations (citation removed for blinding); an increase in life expectancy and other demographic changes; and the need to address all of these changes with limited resources and in face of increasing competition within health care organizations [4].

Micro-level challenges include changes in patients' consumerist approach and in patients' access to information, as well as changes in the power relations between patients and care- givers, and the entry of younger generations (Generations Y and Z) into the workplace.

In order to address these challenges and effectively carry out these systemic changes and prepare healthcare students and professionals to additional current and future changes, healthcare personnel need to adopt a wide range of new skills, and healthcare systems need to find effective ways to disseminate these skills among present and future employees [5].

1.1 Social-emotional skills and healthcare professions

Faced with the need to change and modify healthcare systems, one crucial set of skills that has been predominantly referred to is "soft skills". The term describes skills that are not strictly cognitive or technical [6] and ones that include both intra-personal and interpersonal competencies [7]. Thus, many of the soft skills which are now referred to as "critical skills" or "core skills", are included in the concept of Emotional Intelligence (EI).

In its essence, EI involves an optimal combination of emotion and thought and consists of one's ability to identify, use, understand and manage feelings in oneself and in others [8, 9]. Several models have proposed a set of emotional and social skills and competencies that are related to emotionally intelligent behaviors and outcomes in various fields, and which can be actively developed [10–12]. Such skills typically include self-awareness, awareness of others (empathy), emotional management (self-regulation) and interpersonal communication.

In recent years, a broad body of research has highlighted the contribution of EI and social–emotional skills to areas such as physical and psychological health; interpersonal relationships; and effectiveness and success in academic studies and in a wide range of organizations, occupations and levels of employment [11, 13–15]. In particular, a large number of studies have emphasized the importance of SEI for coping with challenges of the 21st century [16].

In the field of medicine, social–emotional skills have been linked to success across a wide range of positions and roles [17]. Noted examples include links to effective performance under pressure, increased commitment to healthcare organizations, positive interpersonal communications, and effective teamwork among medical staff [18]. Additional studies have pointed out correlations between SEI and better doctor–patient relations [19], fewer medical lawsuits [20], empathic treatment [21], precision in medical diagnoses and consequently in treatment [22], lower levels of situation-related anxiety in patients [23], higher levels of patient responsiveness to treatment, increased patient satisfaction and higher patient trust in healthcare staff [24]. Yet despite the clear benefits offered by social–emotional skills in the healthcare professions, the social–emotional skills of medical students have often been noted to be similar or even lower than those of the average population [25], and at times were even noted to decrease during their studies [26].

Consequently, there has been a call to develop social–emotional intelligence among medical students, nursing students and medical management students [27]. Nevertheless, to date, and despite a growing understanding of the importance of social–emotional skills to medical professions, the development of these skills has only captured a limited place in medical school curricula and in the training of healthcare staff.

1.2 Teaching social-emotional skills: academic and professional training

Until recently, both admissions to healthcare education programs and subsequent academic success were defined primarily on the basis of superior cognitive abilities. Traditional teaching, learning and assessment processes focused on knowledge and on cognitive abilities (citation removed for blinding).

However, in recent years, it has been increasingly recognized that cognitive and professional abilities are not sufficient criteria for success in medical schools and in the medical profession. Consequently, several hospitals have begun incorporating social–emotional skill development efforts as part of ongoing training for their medical teams [28]. Several medical schools have also introduced admission measures that examine candidates' personal and interpersonal abilities [29] as well as courses for social–emotional skill development [30]. Nevertheless, such efforts are still limited, due to time and overload constraints and to a lingering, mainly cognitive, focus. This paper will introduce the theoretical and methodological underpinning of a novel tool for the development of social–emotional skills, suitable for use among medical students and staff.

2. The Social-Emotional Skill Development Tool (SE-SD)

In order to integrate the development of social–emotional skills into existing academic and training curricula in a wide field of subjects, a unique Social–Emotional Skill Development tool (SE-SD) that is based on guidelines for effective practices in social–emotional development (e.g. [31, 32]) has been recently developed. This tool is highly suited for healthcare education systems, in particular in light of the above-noted time constraints and the challenges imposed by a predominantly cognitive focus [2, 33].

The SE-SD tool offers a broad perspective on the field of healthcare education and addresses the need for non-cognitive social–emotional skills in the field. In addition, it aims to complement and to work in synergy with existing training tools and to support other professional skills. It can be further viewed more broadly as a method and pedagogy for integrating the development of social–emotional skills in healthcare training. By doing so, it is expected to enable students to cope with a changing healthcare reality and thrive in it.

2.1 The social-emotional skill development tool: underlying principles

The SE-SD tool is based on eight underlying principles:

2.1.1 An inclusive theoretical framework

The theoretical framework at the basis of the SE-SD tool is the well-established Bar-On [11] model of Emotional–Social Intelligence. This framework, which addresses both behaviors and outcomes, has been noted to be especially suitable for educational settings [34, 35] and has been employed successfully in the medical arena [36–38]. It allows for a holistic and inclusive development approach that has been noted especially effective in SEI trainings [39]. Similar to the Bar-On framework and associated tool (EQ-i), the SE-SD tool includes ten skills, nine such as emotional self-awareness and expression, self-regulation, empathy and interpersonal relations, social responsibility, flexibility, stress-tolerance, optimism and self-regard from the original Bar-On model (**Figure 1**) [11], with the addition of Growth Mindset. All linked to different aspects of various healthcare professions [25]. The SE-SD skills are arranged in 4 major clusters: intrapersonal, inter-personal, adaptability and stress-management, to which the well-being indicator of the original model has been added.

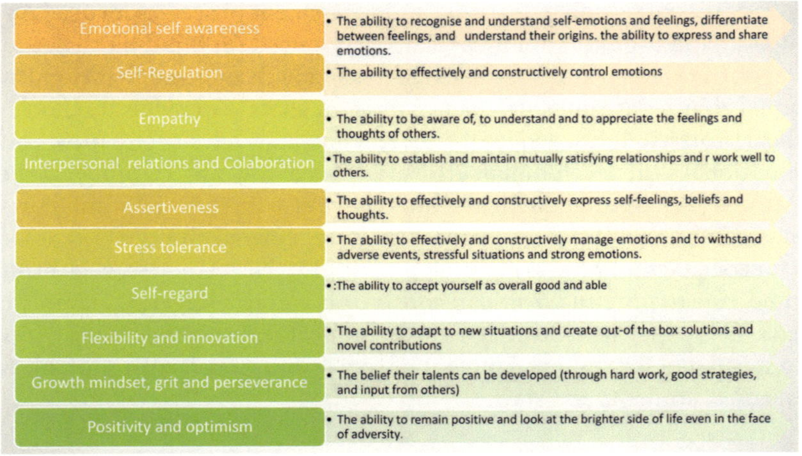
Emotional self awareness
• The ability to recognise and understand self-emotions and feelings, differentiate between feelings, and understand their origins. the ability to express and share emotions.
Self-Regulation
• The ability to effectively and constructively control emotions
Empathy
• The ability to be aware of, to understand and to appreciate the feelings and thoughts of others.
Interpersonal relations and Colaboration
• The ability to establish and maintain mutually satisfying relationships and r work well to others.
Assertiveness
• The ability to effectively and constructively express self-feelings, beliefs and thoughts.
Stress tolerance
• The ability to effectively and constructively manage emotions and to withstand adverse events, stressful situations and strong emotions.
Self-regard
• :The ability to accept yourself as overall good and able
Flexibility and innovation
• The ability to adapt to new situations and create out-of the box solutions and novel contributions
Growth mindset, grit and perseverance
• The belief their talents can be developed (through hard work, good strategies, and input from others)
Positivity and optimism
• The ability to remain positive and look at the brighter side of life even in the face of adversity.

Figure 1.
List of essential soft skills for healthcare professions.

2.1.2 A wide variety of pedagogical methods

In line with the inclusive model at its basis and the wide variety of social–emotional skills it includes, the SE-SD tool addresses a offers a wide range of development assignments and a wide range of methodical tools (such as dedicated articles, video clips, short interviews, reflective questions, real-life experimentation, etc.). This variability is in line with earlier studies where the successful development of social–emotional skills was noted to include both cognitive and emotional components and to require varied and experiential methods [40].

2.1.3 A curriculum-integrated approach

It has been widely acknowledged that SEI development cannot be achieved by means of a single workshop [41–44] and requires an extensive, routinised, long-term effort that provides time for learning, practicing and achieving development [31]. A curriculum integrated approach allows for such extensive and long-term development efforts as well as for offering a contextual, rather than isolated, experience.

In line with these findings, the SE-SD tool has been designed to be integrated into existing course materials. This integrated approach helps students and instructors overcome time constraints as well as highlights the links between the targeted SEI skills and different aspects of the profession, making the development relevant and meaningful. Integration is achieved through two parallel processes: by linking specific social–emotional skills with the general course material; and through home assignments that target SEI development, are self-paced and are completed and evaluated at different points in time throughout the entire course.

2.1.4 A generic tool

Social–emotional skills have been noted to be relevant across a wide range of roles and positions in the field of healthcare [17].

Accordingly, the SE-SD tool, and in particular the assignments associated with each skill, were structured in a more general manner and therefore can be easily applied to a variety of subjects in the academic curriculum and can be integrated into a variety of healthcare academic courses, disciplines and academic levels.

2.1.5 Modularity

The SE-SD tool can be used in a modular and "spiral" manner in order to integrate a wide range of skills into different courses throughout the academic program. Such modularity is particularly suited to the development of social–emotional skills, a process noted to involve continuous and lifelong learning [45, 46] and in which links between skills exist [11]. Importantly, while the SE-SD tool can be used in isolation, as part of a single course or a number of courses, a multiyear, spiral SEI development program which corresponds with the desired graduate vision can enhance the overall effectiveness and sustainability of the SEI development process [31] and ultimately contribute to the quality of healthcare professionals.

The nature of healthcare studies supports such modularity as healthcare students may need to employ different SEI skills at different stages of their academic training (pre-clinical and clinical years for example).

Finally, assignments that form part of the SE-SD tool are constructed in a modular fashion, building up from theory to practice. This modular structure is built on the premise that theoretical knowledge provides a foundation for the development of SEI [44] and that effective social–emotional development should follow several steps: the acquisition of a theoretical basis; and an understanding of the concept of EI and the specific SEI skills as they are being targeted, achieved through theoretical assignments. These are followed by gaining understanding of the relevance of the targeted skills to the course material and to future practice through reflective assignments. Practical assignments then provide a step-by-step opportunity to develop and practice newly acquired skills. Ideally, these steps lead to changes in habits, attitudes and behaviors [31, 44].

2.1.6 A formative tool

The SE-SD tool focuses on the process of SEI development rather than on its outcomes. It is assumed that social–emotional development is an on-going lifelong process which takes place within relationships (in this case, with the course instructor). It has been demonstrated that relationships that are based on trust, guidance, support and formative feedbacks enhance SEI development [12, 32]. As an inseparable part of the SE-SD tool, therefore, evaluations and feedbacks from course instructors provide formative comments which students can use in order to continue to progress and to refine their development process. All these elements have been noted to enhance SEI development [47] and motivation levels [31].

Academic assignments that integrate the SE-SD tool are evaluated based on their degree of completion and on the students' level of understanding of several elements: the concept of EI, the specific SEI skills that are being acquired, and the relevance of these skills to the particular healthcare profession at the center of the course. During the active development stage, students are evaluated based on their level of engagement and reflection. The importance of reflective learning has been previously highlighted [44], noting that reflections on thoughts, feelings and behaviors that underlie attitudes and habits, both personal and of others, enhance the development of SEI competencies.

2.1.7 A self-directed and self-paced process

As emotions, thoughts, competencies, behaviors and habits are all unique to each individual, it is recommended that social–emotional development processes include a focus on individual social–emotional skills [12, 48]. To this end, the SE-SD tool allows students to follow their own individual development path at their own pace, to start the development process from their own individual starting point, to focus on their own specific goals and to self-assess their progress. Self-directed processes encourage participants to be personally accountable for their progress and involve them in planning, carrying out and evaluating their own learning experiences. These elements, in turn, were noted to enhance motivation, which is key to social–emotional training success [12].

In order to manage their self-directed learning, students receive "road maps" (either in a digital form or in print) that outline their assignments and set specific points in time for evaluations and feedbacks. The assignments are order-dependent, as each assignment builds on the previous one, and the order in which assignments are offered is pre-determined. While students can follow the development process at their own pace, they are instructed to avoid completing their assignments all at once. This time-paced approach maximizes the effectiveness of the learning process, allowing students time for reflection and practice and providing instructors with at least two opportunities, at two different points in time, to deliver evaluations and feedbacks to students.

2.1.8 A flexible and dynamic tool

The SE-SD tool is both flexible and adaptable. The tool's flexibility is manifested in the choice of SEI skills that are to be associated with a given course, in the links drawn between these skills and the course materials, in the number of assignments chosen from the selection offered and in the variety of these assignments. The tool offers further flexibility in terms of feedbacks and evaluations: instructors can limit themselves to the two formal evaluations (intermediate and final) that are provided as part of the tool, but may choose to provide additional informal and more frequent feedbacks. Furthermore, additional skills to those offered in the model can be added, consistent with the principles embedded in the tool: designing developmental activities and assignments that would support knowledge acquisition and enhance the understanding of these skills, determining the relevance of the added skill to a particular course, and identifying starting points and goals for each of the participants.

Taken together, these features of the SE-SD allow healthcare education systems to include social–emotional development as a strategic plan for preparing students and workers for a changing professional reality.

2.2 Inculcating the model: methodological considerations

Skill-development processes often follow a sequence of stages that have been recognized to contribute to effective development (e.g. [31, 41, 47]). These include: preparation (gaining students' commitment, identifying needs, and jointly designing a development program); action (implementing the program – introduction and development); and evaluation. In the case of the SE-SD tool and healthcare education settings, these stages have been adapted to meet the specific requirements of various healthcare professions (**Figure 2**).

2.2.1 Preparation

The preparation stage begins with the selection of an SEI skill to be developed during a given course. This skill, selected by the course instructor from a list of social–emotional skills offered in the tool (**Figure 1**), is chosen based on its degree of relevance to the course material and its suitability in terms of the students' academic level.

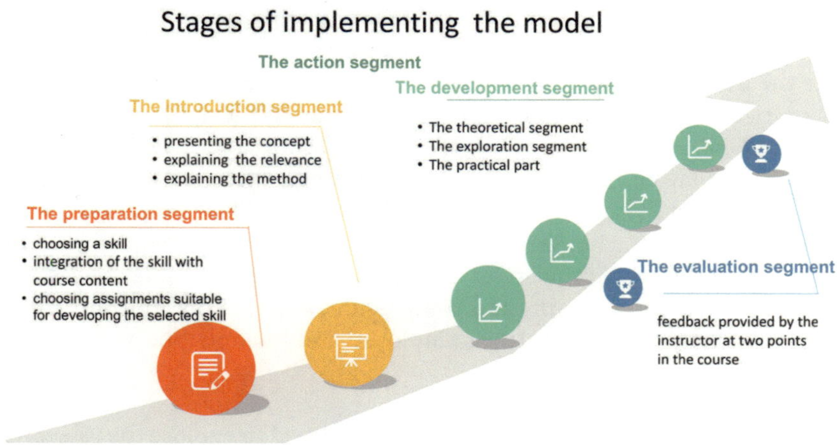

Figure 2.
Process of model implementation.

The course instructor then plans how to integrate the skill into the course material. For example, if integrated into a course that focuses on patient-caregiver relationships, the instructor may decide to discuss empathy as part of a segment that examines how to deliver difficult news to patients.

Lastly, the course instructor goes over the SE-SD assignment list and chooses assignments that correspond to the selected skill.

When a three-year process is involved, these steps are followed in group discussions where faculty members jointly decide on the skills to be introduced each year and the classes they most fit.

2.2.2 Action

The action stage includes two parts, introduction and development.

2.2.2.1 Introduction

This part of the action stage is designed to highlight the relevance and importance of SEI to the students and to promote motivation to participate in the EI development process. The course instructor begins by introducing the concept of social–emotional skills to the students, highlights the relevance of these skills to the course and notes their importance to students' overall growth and future careers in the 21st century.

Following these introductory remarks, the SE-SD model and tool are presented and the methods by which the development process will be incorporated into the course, both during class and by means of home assignments and their evaluation, are explained. The instructor notes the order by which the assignments are to be completed, the corresponding time frames, and the formative evaluation method by which they would be assessed.

2.2.2.2 Development

The development part of the action stage relies on individual home assignments that students are asked to carry out throughout the entire course. Students are instructed to complete the assignments in a pre-determined order and can only access subsequent assignments after completing the previous ones. In line with the structure of the SE-SD tool, the assignments include three hierarchical segments: Theoretical background, Exploration, and Practice.

- The theoretical background segment aims to provide the students with a solid theoretical basis for personal development. Students learn about the concept of EI and come to understand the targeted SEI skills and the mechanisms by which they may be employed. As part of this segment, students are encouraged to read relevant literature and to watch illustrative video presentations. For example, as part of a background segment on empathy, students may read a paper about the concept, watch a relevant video program, note the distinction between empathy, sympathy and compassion, and find out more about the mechanisms by which empathy is employed and its contribution to the health-care professions.

- During the exploration segment, students proceed to explore the relevance of targeted EI skills to various healthcare professions. By answering a set of guiding questions and/or conducting short interviews with professional in the field, students are able to identify the relevance of any given skill to their course material, to their chosen profession and to present and future life outcomes. Finally, they are asked to identify their own individual starting point with respect to the targeted skill and to define the corresponding goals. The SE-SD tool provides a set of guiding questions and/or a short questionnaire that support this exploration process. For example, in the case of empathy, students are asked to identify links between empathy and healthcare professions, use guiding questions to evaluate the gains they are likely to derive from enhanced empathy, and assess their starting point with regards to the development process using an empathy questionnaire.

- The practice segment involves students in a wide range of activities, all aimed at developing the targeted SEI skill. This is the longest segment of the three, in line with Boyatzis [12, 32] who noted the importance of experimenting with new behaviors for an effective social–emotional development process. The assignments that form the core of this segment are designed to develop cognitive, emotional and behavioral components of the targeted skill. For example, in the case of empathy, the students are asked to engage in empathic dialogues, take on another person's perspective (e.g. a patient or a team member), or examine case studies that center on interactions between patients and caregivers. The culminating assignment includes reflection and self-evaluation.

2.2.3 Evaluation

Finally, during the evaluation segment, students are provided with feedbacks and formative assessments that can help them further develop their social–emotional skills. These feedbacks and evaluations are provided by their course instructors at two points in time during each course: mid-term (which coincides with the goal-setting stage of the development process) and at the end of the course (after all assignments have been completed). These feedbacks are accompanied by self-evaluations.

As noted above, participant students are evaluated based on their level of commitment, efforts and engagement in the development process (as opposed to the level of development that has been achieved); their level of understanding of the targeted EI skill; and the level of personal and professional reflectiveness they demonstrate throughout the entire course.

Furthermore, beyond the mid-term and end-of-term evaluations, instructors can choose to provide additional evaluations and feedbacks in the course of the program, in accordance with available time resources.

3. Discussion

In light of the global changes and challenges that face many professionals in the 21st century, there is an increasing understanding that it is of primary importance to develop and foster social–emotional skills, also referred to as "soft skills", among workers in a wide range of fields. A prominent example is the field of healthcare. Skills that are likely to benefit healthcare professionals may include emotional self-awareness, self-regulation, empathy, and interpersonal relations. These, as well as other social–emotional skills, were noted to improve coping abilities, academic learning and professional effectiveness among both medical teams and healthcare management teams [49, 50].

The importance of social–emotional skills to medical staff and to healthcare systems and their currently limited place in medical school curricula, call for a proactive initiative on the part of academic institutions. Such an initiative should address needs and challenges, both current and future, that face healthcare professionals and can transform medical schools from knowledge providers to leaders of cultural and social changes.

Given the noted difficulties to integrate the development of social–emotional skills into existing curricula in the field of healthcare, we propose a novel and holistic SE-SD tool that integrates social–emotional learning into existing curricula while overcoming time and workload barriers.

Furthermore, the assignments that form part of the SE-SD tool are prepared and provided ahead of time by the tool designers, and therefore instructors do not require any prior expertise in the field of social–emotional learning in order to implement the tool as part of their courses.

Effective implementation of social–emotional skill development programs has been noted to benefit from a supportive climate. It is therefore highly recommended that faculty is included in the proposed social–emotional training process. Social–emotional training is expected to heighten faculty awareness of the importance of the process, increase their willingness to take risks as they implement the SE-SD model in their respective institutions, and enable them to model socially-emotionally behaviors and to 'walk the talk' [49]. All these were found to contribute to the development of social–emotional skills in students.

In addition to academic institutions which can take upon themselves to develop social–emotional skills in students and faculty, development of these skills should form an integral part of on-going professional training for both healthcare staff in post-academic settings. Such life-long learning will support earlier development efforts in academic institutions and will insure its sustainability.

Lastly, although research regarding the effectiveness of the SE-SD tool is still a work in progress, we believe that the use of integrative learning methodologies like the one described here would bring healthcare academic institutions and their graduates one step closer towards adapting to the 21st century and meeting its demands.

Author details

Niva Dolev[1], Lior Naamati-Schneider[2]* and Adaya Meirovich[2]

1 Department of Education and Community, Kinneret Academic College on the Sea of Galilee, Israel

2 Department of Management of Service Organizations, Health Track, Hadassah Academic College, Jerusalem, Israel

*Address all correspondence to: inaanati@yahoo.com

References

[1] Reis S. The doctor in the digital age competencies needed and a road map for their achievement [review]. Harefuah. 2019; 158(10): 648-653. Hebrew.

[2] Reis S, Visser A, Frankel R. Health information and communication technology in healthcare communication: the good, the bad, and the transformative. Patient Education and Counseling. 2013; 93 (3): 359-362. https:// DOI: 10.1016/j.pec.2013.10.007

[3] Ananiadou K, Claro M. 21st century skills and competences for new millennium learners in OECD countries. OECD Publishing. OECD Education Working Papers No. 41. 2009. http://dx.doi.org/10.1787/218525261154

[4] Naamati-Schneider, L. (2020), Strategic management as adaptation to changes in the ecosystems of public hospitals in Israel, Israel Journal of Health Policy Research, Vol. 9, Article 65. https://doi.org/10.1186/s13584-020-00424-y

[5] Naamati-Schneider, L. (2020b), "Public–private: unequal competition: Israeli public hospitals vs. the private health-care system following government reforms", International Journal of Organizational Analysis. https://doi.org/10.1108/IJOA-06-2020-2237

[6] Hurrell SA. Rethinking the soft skills deficit blame game: Employers, skills withdrawal and the reporting of soft skills gaps. Human Relations.2016; 69(3): 605-28. https://doi-org.mgs.hac.ac.il/10.1177/0018726715591636

[7] Dell' Aquila E, Marocco D, Ponticorvo M, di Ferdinando A, Schembri, M, Miglino O. (2016). Educational games for soft-skills training in digital environments. Switzerland: Springer, Cham. Chapter 1, Soft skills; 2016; (pp 1-18). https://doi.org/10.1007/978-3-319-06311-98. Mayer JD, Salovey P. What is emotional intelligence? (In Salovey P, Sluyter D. Eds.). Emotional development and emotional intelligence: educational implication. New York (NY): Basic Books; 1997; (pp. 3-31).

[8] Mayer JD, Salovey P, Caruso DR. Emotional intelligence: theory, findings, and implications. Psychological inquiry. 2004; 15(3): 197-215. https://doi-org.mgs.hac.ac.il/10.1207/s15327965pli1503_02

[9] Goleman D. Working with emotional intelligence. New York (NY): Bantam Books; 1998; (pp. 3-30).

[10] Bar-On R. The Bar-On model of emotional social intelligence (ESI). Psicothema. 2006; 18 (sup): 13-25. https://www.redalyc.org/articulo.oa?id=72709503

[11] Boyatzis RE. (2007). Developing emotional intelligence through coaching for leadership, professional and occupational excellence. In Bar-On R, Maree JG, Elias MJ. (Eds.), Educating people to be emotionally intelligent. Westport (CT): Praeger; 2007; (pp. 155-168).

[12] Levitats Z, Vigoda-Gadot E. Yours emotionally: how emotional intelligence infuses public service motivation and affects the job outcomes of public personnel. Public Administration. 2017; 95(3): 759-775 https://doi-org.mgs.hac.ac.il/10.1111/padm.12342

[13] Naseem K. Job Stress and Employee Creativity: The mediating role of Emotional Intelligence. International Journal of Management Excellence. 2017; 9(2): 1050-1058.

[14] Rode JC, Arthaud-Day M, Ramaswami A, Howes S. A time-lagged

study of emotional intelligence and salary. Journal of Vocational Behavior. 2017; 101: 77-89. https://doi.org/10.1016/j.jvb.2017.05.001

[15] Leberecht T. The new emotions of the new machine age: will AI and robots change how and what we can feel? Psychology Today. 2018. https://www.psychologytoday.com/us/blog/the-romance-work/201807/the-new-emotions-the-new-machine-age.

[16] Kasman DL, Fryer-Edwards K, Braddock CH. Educating for professionalism: trainees' emotional experiences on IM and pediatrics inpatient ward. Acad Med. 2003; 78(7): 730-741.

[17] McCallin A, Bamford A. Interdisciplinary teamwork: is the influence of emotional intelligence fully appreciated? J Nurs Manag. 2007; 15(4): 386-391. DOI: 10.1111/j.1365-2834.2007.00711.x

[18] Weng HC, Chen HC, Chen HJ, Lu K, Hung SY. Doctors' emotional intelligence and the patient-doctor relationship. Med Educ. 2008; 42 (7): 703-711. DOI: 10.1111/j.1365-2923.2008.03039.x

[19] Mendelson RA. Reduce risk of malpractice suits by forging patient relationships. AAP News. 2003; 22(6): 260.

[20] Austin EJ, Evans P, Magnus B, O'Hanlon KA. Preliminary study of empathy, emotional intelligence and examination performance in MBChB students. Med Educ. 2007; 41(7): 684-689. DOI: 10.1111/j.1365-2923.2007.02795.x

[21] Del Canale S, Louis DZ, Maio V, Wang X, Rossi G, Hojat M, Gonnella JS. The relationship between physician empathy and disease complications: an empirical study of primary care physicians and their diabetic patients in Parma, Italy. Academic Medicine. 2012; 87(9): 1243-1249. DOI: 0.1097/ACM.0b013e3182628fbf

[22] Nooryan K, Gasparyan, K, Sharif K, Zoladl M. Controlling anxiety in physicians and nurses working in intensive care units using emotional intelligence items as an anxiety management tool in Iran. Ing J Gen Med. 2012; 5: 5-10. DOI : 10.2147/IJGM.S25850

[23] Weng HC, Chen YS, Lin CS, Tu YK, Lin HH, Yu SW. Specialty differences in the association between health care climate and patient trust. Med Educ. 2011; 45(9): 905-912. https://doi-org/10.1111/j.1365-2923.2011.03984.x

[24] Stein SJ, Book HE. The EQ Edge - emotional intelligence and your success. Toronto (Canada): Stoddart Publishing; 2000; (pp. 9-210, 223-251).

[25] Meirovich A, Ber R, Moore M, Rotschild A. (2016). Student centered tutoring as a model for patient centeredness and empathy. Adv Med Educ Pract. 7:423-28. https://dx.doi.org/10.2147%2FAMEP.S107115

[26] Stoller JK, Taylor CA, Farver CF. Emotional intelligence competencies provide a developmental curriculum for medical training. Med Teach. 2013; 35(3): 243-247. https://doi-org.mgs.hac.ac.il/10.3109/0142159X.2012.737964

[27] Dolev N, Goldental N, Reuven-Lelong A, Tadmor T. 2019. The evaluation of emotional intelligence among medical students and its links with non-cognitive acceptance measures to medical school. Rambam Maimonides Med J. 10(2):e0010. https://dx.doi.org/10.5041%2FRMMJ.10365

[28] Razack S, Faremo S, Drolet F, Snell L, Wiseman J, Pickering J. Multiple mini-interviews versus traditional interviews: stakeholder acceptability comparison. Medical Education. 2009;

43: 993-1000.https://doi-org.mgs.hac.ac.il/10.1111/j.1365-2923.2009.03447.x

[29] Fletcher I, Leadbetter P, Curran A, OSullivan H. A pilot study assessing emotional intelligence training and communication skills with 3rd year medical students. Patient education and counseling. 2009: 76(3): 376-379. https://doi.org/10.1016/j.pec.2009.07.019

[30] Cherniss C, Goleman D, Emmerling R, Cowan K, Adler M. Bringing emotional intelligence into the workplace: A technical report. New Brunswick (NJ): Consortium for Research on Emotional Intelligence in Organizations, Rutgers University; 1998. http://www.eiconsortium.org/pdf/technical_report.pdf.

[31] Boyatzis RE. Developing emotional, social, and cognitive intelligence competencies in managers and leaders in educational settings. (In Hughes M, Thompson HL, Terrell JB. Eds.). Handbook for developing emotional and social intelligence: best practices, case studies, and strategies. San Francisco (CA): Pfeiffer; 2009; (pp. 359-378).

[32] Kelm Z, Womer J, Walter JK, Feudtner C. Interventions to cultivate physician empathy: a systematic review. BMC medical education.2014; 14(1): 219-229. https://doi.org/10.1186/1472-6920-14-219

[33] Haskett R. Emotional intelligence and teaching success in higher education [dissertation]. Bloomington: Indiana University; 2003.

[34] Drew TL. The relationship between emotional intelligence and student teacher performance [dissertation]. Lincoln, Nebraska: University of Nebraska; 2006. https://files.eric.ed.gov/fulltext/ED499558.pdf

[35] Dolev N, Leshem S. 2016. Teachers' emotional intelligence: the impact of training. International Journal of Emotional Education. 8(1): 75-94.

[36] Bamberger E, Genizi Y, Kerem N, Reuven-Lalung A, Dolev N, Srugo I, Rofe A. 2017. A pilot study of an emotional intelligence training intervention for a Pediatric team. Arch Dis Child. 102 (2):159-164.

[37] Ciarrochi J, Mayer JD. The key ingredients of emotional intelligence interventions: similarities and differences. (In Ciarrochi J, Mayer JD. Eds.). Applying emotional intelligence: A practitioners' guide. New York (NY): Psychology Press; 2007; (pp. 144-156).

[38] MHS. The Complete EQ-i 2.0 Experience Guidebook. MHS Publications. MHS. The complete EQ-i 2.0 experience guidebook. Toronto, Ontario, Canada: MHS Publications; 2011. http://bit.ly/2VVpyQm.

[39] Chapman BP. Emotional intelligence at midlife: a cross sectional investigation of factorial variance, social correlates, and relationships to established personality and ability taxonomies [dissertation]. Denton: University of North Texas; 2005. http://citeseerx.ist.psu.edu/viewdoc/download?doi=10.1.1.457.7940&rep=rep1&type=pdf

[40] Brackett MA, Patti J, Stern R, Rivers SE, Elbertson, NA, Chisholm C, Salovey P. A sustainable, skill-based approach to building emotionally literate schools. (In Hughes M, Thompson HL, Terrell JB. Eds.). Handbook for developing emotional and social intelligence: best practices, case studies, and strategies. San Francisco (CA): Pfeiffer; 2009; (pp. 329-358).

[41] Brackett MA, Salovey P. Measuring emotional intelligence with the Mayer-Salovey-Caruso emotional intelligence test (MSCEIT). Psicothema. 2006; 18 (supl): 34-41. http://www.unioviedo.es/

reunido/index.php/PST/article/viewFile/8417/8281

[42] Neale S, Spencer-Arnell L, Wilson L. Emotional intelligence coaching: improving performance for leaders, coaches and the individual. London: Kogan; 2009; (pp. 90-117).

[43] Delors J. Education for the 21st century. The Delors report. Paris: UNESCO; 1996.

[44] Tawil S, Cougoureux M. Revisiting learning: the treasure within-N 4-assessing the impact of the 1996 'Delors Report'. UNESCO; 2013.

[45] Cherniss C, Goleman D. (2001). Training for emotional intelligence: A model. (In Cherniss C, Goleman D. Eds.). The emotionally intelligent workplace: how to select for, measure, and improve emotional intelligence in individuals, groups, and organizations. San Francisco (CA): Jossey-Bass; 2001; (pp. 209-233).

[46] Wolfe CJ. The practice of emotional intelligence coaching in organizations: a hands-on guide to successful outcomes. (In Bar-On R, Maree JG, Elias MJ. Eds.). Educating People to Be Emotionally Intelligent. Westport (CT): Praeger; 2007; (pp. 169-182). https://scholar.google.com/scholar?q=Educating%20people%20to%20be%20emotionally%20intelligent

[47] Dolev N, Leshem S. 2017. Developing emotional intelligence competence among teachers. Teacher Development. 21(1): 21-39.

[48] Arora S, Ashrafian H, Davis R, Athanasiou T, Darzi A, Sevdalis N. Emotional intelligence in medicine: a systematic review through the context of the ACGME competencies. Med Educ. 2010: 44(8): 749-764. https://doi-org.mgs.hac.ac.il/10.1111/j.1365-2923.2010.03709.x

[49] McCown K, Jensen AL, Freedman J. The self-science approach to social-emotional learning. In R. Bar-On, J.D. Maree, & M.J. Elias (Eds.), Educating people to be emotionally intelligent. Westport (CT): Praeger; 2007; (pp. 109-122). https://scholar.google.com/scholar?q=Educating%20people%20to%20be%20emotionally%20intelligent

[50] Stoller JK. (2008). Developing physician-leaders: key competencies and available programs. J Health Adm Educ. 2008; 25(4):307-328.

Chapter 14

Smartphone and Surgery, Reality or Gadget?

Sassi Boughizane, Badra Bannour, Imen Bannour, Faten Hacheni, Imen Bannour, Marwa Masmoudi, Jalel Boughizane and Sabri Youssef

Abstract

Surgical care is an essential component of health care. This basic universal right is not available to everyone. Indeed, countries with low economic resources suffer from a lack of access to surgical care and the most developed countries will have to reduce the cost of health care to ensure the sustainability of provided care quality. New communication technologies have invaded the field of health and have led to the development of a new concept of mobile health. The purpose of this paper is to answer the following question: Can these new tools, and in particular the Smartphone, remedy, even partially, the lack of health care in poor countries and reduce the cost of health care in rich countries? New communication tools, led by the Smartphone, have the capacity to capture, store, retrieve and transmit data to provide instant and personalized information to individuals. This information could be a key element in health systems and can contribute to monitoring health status and improving patient safety and care quality. Mobile telephony via applications and connected objects can facilitate the pre-, intra- and post-operative management of patients. These mobile systems also facilitate the collection and transmission of data. This will allow better analysis of this data and will greatly pave the way to the introduction of artificial intelligence in medicine and surgery. The Smartphone can be used as an important tool for both, diagnosis care and surgical training. Surgeons must adapt their equipment to local resources while respecting safety standards. Covid-19 has put health systems around the world under severe strain. Decision-makers are being forced to make adjustments. The long-vaunted digital health is becoming a reality and a necessity. Healthcare authorities and strategy specialists face challenges in terms of disease prevention and therapy, as well as in terms of health economics and management.

Keywords: smartphone, surgery, mobile health, medical information

1. Introduction

Surgical care is an essential component of health care. This basic universal right is not available to everyone. Indeed, countries with low economic resources suffer from lack of access to surgical care and the most developed countries will have to reduce the cost of health care to ensure the sustainability of quality care provided.

It is estimated that two-thirds of the world's population do not have access to safe and affordable surgery and more than two billion people are unable to receive surgical care due to the lack of equipment and human resources. As a result, limited access to surgery kills nearly 17 million people each year. This is more than the number of deaths from HIV, TB and malaria combined [1, 2].

The economic inequalities on our planet are fully reflected in the field of health as 60% of surgical procedures are performed for only 15% of the world's population and only 6% of surgical procedures are performed for poor countries where one third of the world's population resides [3].

High-income countries have better indicators of quality and safety of care. However, this is associated with higher health care costs. The increase in health expenditure in developed countries is faster than the growth of the world economy. This seems to become unsustainable in the medium and long term.

New communication technologies have invaded the field of health and have been at the origin of the development of a new concept of mobile health. The purpose of this paper is to answer the following question: Can these new tools, and in particular the Smartphone, remedy, even partially, the lack of health care in poor countries and reduce the cost of health care in rich countries?

New communication tools, led only by the Smartphone, have the capacity to capture, store, retrieve and transmit data to provide instant and personalized information to individuals. This information could be a key element in health systems and can contribute to monitoring health status and improving patient safety and care quality.

Healthcare authorities and strategy specialists face challenges in terms of disease prevention and therapy, as well as in terms of health economics and management.

In addition, the Covid-19 global pandemic has suddenly put everything into question and put health systems around the world to the test. The long-vaunted digital health is becoming a reality.

2. Current state of surgery in the world

2.1 Surgical expenditure

High-income countries have excellent indicators of quality and safety of care [4], but this is associated with high health care costs in these countries.

The increase in health care expenditure in developed countries is faster than the growth of their economies. For example, in the United States of America, health expenditure has been increasing rapidly and in 2019 it accounted for 17% of gross domestic product [5].

For low-income countries, the situation is quite different. According to the Lancet Commission on Surgery, the cost of surgery and anesthesia causes "catastrophic" health care costs for 33 million people each year [6]. The problem lies mainly in the direct costs of surgical care, which are often high [7].

Given that, this burden has deleterious effects on health care systems worldwide, it has become necessary to search for solutions to reduce the cost of surgery.

2.2 Access to surgery

Despite the efforts made, at least half of the world's population lacks access to essential health services and does not enjoy the fundamental right to healthcare in practice. Striking urban–rural health inequities are still reported in many countries [8].

The Lancet Commission has established 6 key indicators for the strength of the surgical system in the world [9]:

1. Access to timely essential surgery.

2. Specialist surgical workforce density.

3. Surgical volume.

4. Perioperative mortality rate.

5. and 6. Risk of impoverishing and catastrophic expenditure on surgical management.

These indicators have revealed a perilous state of the surgical system worldwide that needs immediate improvement to achieve universal access to safe, affordable surgical and anesthesia care when needed.

It is estimated that 9 out of 10 people in low- and middle-income countries lack access to basic surgical care and that 143 million additional surgical interventions are needed each year to save lives and prevent disabilities [10].

It should also be noted that the inadequacy and uneven distribution of specialist surgical stuff has further compounded the disparity in access to care [11].

Therefore, the whole world and poor countries in particular need to develop policies to make surgical care easier to perform and learn.

2.3 Current status of minimally invasive surgery in the world

Traditionally, open surgical approaches have been the mainstay of surgical treatment, but in recent years the number of open surgeries has largely decreased in developed countries in favor of minimally invasive surgery in all surgical specialties [12].

Minimally invasive surgery has become the standard in many specialties and has overtaken traditional surgery in many cases.

Indeed, this type of surgery offers patients multiple benefits such as smaller incisions, faster recovery times, reduced adhesion rates, pain, morbidity, and postoperative length of stay, [13, 14]. It is therefore perfectly suitable for LMICs since, by reducing the length of hospital stays and speeding up recovery time, it reduces the total cost of surgery which is a major barrier to healthcare access for a significant population in these countries.

A major obstacle to assessing the adoption of this surgery worldwide is the lack of official data and publications in developing countries [2]. However, the limited published data from these countries indicate that the rates of laparoscopic surgery for gynecological indications are minimal and vary widely from hospital to hospital.

Published data from large referral hospitals in LMICs reported laparoscopic surgery rates for gynecological indications of less than 10% [15].

2.4 Obstacles to the adoption of minimally invasive surgery

The implementation and development of endoscopic surgery in LMICs is in fact confronted with multifactorial obstacles, the most important of which are insufficient investment in equipment and difficulties in accessing specific training [16]. Indeed, the lack of resources is the main obstacle. The low economic status in these countries makes it challenging to acquire and maintain endoscopic equipment, train surgeons and technicians and reinforce their capacity to perform endoscopic surgery. This explains the tendency to use endoscopy mainly as a diagnostic tool in developing countries [17].

There is a proportional relationship between a country's gross domestic product and the percentage and complexity of minimally invasive procedures performed [17].

The severe shortage of surgeons in low-income countries coupled with their heavy workload does not allow them to sub specialize; as a result, minimally invasive procedures are time-consuming and have the potential to lead to more significant complications [18].

This creates a self-inhibition that will make the learning curve much longer.

It has therefore become of paramount importance to facilitate and accelerate surgical training. The use of Smartphone seems to us to be an adequate solution [19, 20].

Surgery has traditionally been considered too expensive, complex and unprofitable. Indeed, surgery has never been included in primary health care, although surgical interventions are economically profitable in terms of saved lives and prevention of disabilities [21, 22].

The other hurdle is the socio-cultural barrier related to older surgeons' resistance to change and their reluctance to use new surgical technologies [16].

3. Concept of mobile health

According to WHO, e-health is the use of information and communication technologies (ICTs) to support health and health -related fields, including health care services, health surveillance, health literature and health education, knowledge and research [23].

In common parlance, e-health encompasses everything that is associated with the digitalization of health.

The adoption of IT tools in the field of health (e-health) has evolved throughout successive historic periods from medical records and professional messaging to telemedicine, online communities, mobile applications and connected objects, augmented reality and virtual reality, artificial intelligence and chat bots and, finally, the block chain technology [24].

Mobile health or m-health is a major component of connected health (e-health). Mobile health is defined as medical and public health practices that rely on mobile devices such as mobile phones, patient monitoring systems, personal digital assistants and other wireless devices [25].

This involves the integration of connected objects and mobile applications into the practice of medicine and the health system.

This concept has emerged from the exponential development of digital technologies in general and mobile wireless technologies in particular. Nowadays, these technologies are increasingly part of the daily life of both health professionals as well as patients. On the other hand, the world's health system is facing immense difficulties, mainly related to the increase in health expenditure and the disparity in access to care. As a result, mobile health has emerged as a promising solution to the current global health challenges.

4. Anatomy of a smartphone

A Smartphone is made up of many internal parts or components. There are differences between models and brands but the structure remains the same.

This technological jewel has several assets:

1. The wealth of its applications in number and performance

2. The increased performance of its connectivity

3. Highly sophisticated cameras

4. Sensors that turn the Smartphone into a multifunctional object

4.1 Smartphone applications

Today's Smartphone are a real revolution because of their ease of use and user-friendliness. These privileged interfaces provide applications that simplify software by making it more straightforward and accessible. The number of online health applications has grown exponentially [26].

Mobile health applications are divided into several categories:

- Remote monitoring applications.
  Remote monitoring apps help practitioners take care of patients even when they are at home [27].

- Clinical and diagnostic applications.
  Physicians can collect patient data, evaluate and share it. These apps allow practitioners to view lab results, check electronic health records or even perform digital imaging.

- Wellness apps:
  These monitor parameters such as heart rate and rhythm, diet, exercise and sleep [28].

- Clinical reference applications.
  These applications provide all the necessary information at your fingertips.

- Productivity applications.
  Productivity applications help to increase the efficiency of health care providers.

4.2 The smartphone's connectivities

4.2.1 Increasingly powerful connectivity

One of the main revolutions that the smartphone has brought to our daily lives is the ability to connect with anyone, anytime, and anywhere and with new high-speed communication standards constantly evolving, data transfer and sharing is becoming even faster. 5G, the 5th generation mobile network, promises many benefits, including much faster data transmission, Lower latency and high reliability.

4.2.2 Connected health objects

A connected object is an object that is connected to the Internet, capable of sending information in real time and interacting with its environment. A connected object is based on three essential things:

- Its ability to capture data through sensors of all types: speed, temperature, force, pressure, energy, location, power, volume, acoustics, distance, photometry, frequency, vibration, humidity, etc.

- Its capacity to provide data feedback to allow the visualization of information through specially designed dashboards.

- Its ability to inter-connect and interact to a greater or lesser extent with other objects, whether connected or not.

A connected object has two main functions:

- The collection of information from its environment, for example the user's heart rate.

- The triggering of an action based on the information collected and transmitted. For example, triggering an alarm in the event of a heart rate anomaly.

Examples of connected objects:

The weight is displayed directly on the scale and can also be displayed on the Smartphone via Bluetooth or Wi-Fi. The latter allows the saving and synchronization of measurements with a weight curve and also the transfer of data to a health professional (doctor/nutritionist).

Connected watches and bracelets placed around the wrist to record activity according to the sensors they contain (heart rate, GPS, accelerometer etc.). The recorded data is communicated to the Smartphone.

Connected mattresses, contain sleep and environmental sensors that collects and sends data to your Smartphone in order to determine your ideal sleeping temperature [29].

4.2.3 Connectivity and the internet of things

The Internet of Things is the set of objects connected to the Internet that generate data through specific sensors. What they have in common is that they are physical objects and transmit digital information as well as computations, remotely, through an application, often directed from a mobile device (phone, tablet, and computer) [24].

This allows data to be collected, sent and stored over a network without requiring human-to-human or human-to-computer interaction [30].

The application of the IoTconcept in the field of medicine and surgery has great potential. For example, the connection to various external sensors for diagnosis, monitoring and follow-up is a promising technological advance. The data collected from these different sensors constitute a valuable database that will be of great help during treatment. Communication between doctor and patient also takes on another dimension with these new modes of connectivity, making access to care easier.

Connected objects for medical purposes make it possible to monitor the patient's condition more frequently, more accurately and, therefore, better.

4.2.4 Connectivity and artificial intelligence

Artificial intelligence is a set of theories and techniques used to create machines capable of simulating human intelligence.

AI is applied to any activity that involves data collection, followed by decision making and taking action, the cycle repeating itself ad infinitum.

Use of AI in the medical field seems to be highly promising and the potential applications are endless. A medical device could, in theory, use the sum of the experiences of all medical images, of all surgeries if this data could be formatted and collected. It is through self-learning from real-life results that AI is becoming more and more powerful [24].

AI has been applied in various health fields including cancer research, cardiology, diabetes, mental health, etc.

4.3 Smartphone cameras

Smart phones are equipped with increasingly sophisticated cameras whose performance is equal to or better than that of professional cameras [31]. Some smart phones are equipped with high resolution cameras, even 4 K resolution, or three-dimensional cameras. Some professional films have been completely recorded by smart phones. Others have won awards [32].

The integration of microscopes into smart phones to visualize bio-components such as blood cells and micro-organisms has improved over time to the nanoscale level where nano particles, viruses and DNA can now be detected [33].

Smart phones may offer a viable solution for early diagnosis of skin diseases, specifically for remote screening and long-term monitoring of skin lesions [34].

4.3.1 The Smartphone's sensors

The Smartphone is equipped with a multitude of sensors:

- Some are intrinsic: these are the internal sensors.

- Others are integrated into the Smartphone: external sensors connected wirelessly or by cable.

4.3.1.1 Internal sensors of the smartphone

Smart phones embody a series of integrated sensors that allow them to interact with the outside world (movement, light, magnetic field ...): thus turning it into a real pocket laboratory.

In recent years, there has been a growing interest in the use of motion sensors embedded in smart phones such as accelerometers, gyroscopes and magnetometers, as well as location sensors such as GPS for real-time monitoring of physiological constants and activities of daily living.

4.3.1.2 External sensors

Nowadays, it is possible to attach several complementary electronic devices to the Smartphone, converting it into a multi diagnostic system depending on the nature of the attached device [35].

These technological solutions appear to be particularly cost-effective and attractive in resource-limited settings where access to diagnostics and care is not always possible.

Currently, many body organs can be monitored via smart phones.

For example, ultrasound probes can be directly connected to the Smartphone and seem to be a very interesting prospect for the future. Different probes are already available on the market for vascular, soft tissue, lung, abdominal and pelvic examination, FAST ultrasound... [36].

These handheld ultrasound probes have high diagnostic accuracy, sensitivity and specificity for basic anatomy and pathology and can be an acceptable and reproducible diagnostic tool with great potential for future applications particularly in low resource countries to increase access to ultrasound [37].

These connected objects can collect, store, process and transfer data or perform specific actions according to the information received. They carry out measurements in real time and can provide information on many parameters affecting health: weight, body temperature, pulse, blood pressure, breathing rate, heart rate, blood sugar level, sleep quality, etc. At the end of the object's connection is a computer or a Smartphone, a doctor or a call centre, a coaching centre, etc. aiming to create an alert system: any change in one of the parameters transmitted abruptly or reaching a previously set critical value prompts an intervention, special monitoring, advice or recommendations [24].

4.3.1.3 Biosensors

Biosensors are measuring instruments that integrate a biological element (enzyme, antibody, plant or animal cell, DNA fragment, lipid, etc.) and a physical transducer (electrode, optical fiber, etc.). The aim of biosensors is to detect characteristic markers of disease at an early stage in order to improve patient care. There are many potential applications. The most famous biosensor is the one used to analyze blood sugar levels in patients with diabetes [38].

The Smartphone is now a miniaturized computer system, to which several kinds of biosensors can be connected. A phone application can detect several biological agents using the data transmitted by the biosensor.

Currently, much work has focused on miniaturizing biosensors and bioelectronic devices, such as micro fabricated transducers and compact readout instruments, to achieve state-of-the-art, easy and reproducible real-time detection [33].

5. The smartphone in clinical evaluation and preoperative examination

We propose here the main applications of the Smartphone in preoperative care.

5.1 Cardiovascular analysis

Measurements of heart rate, blood pressure and even continuous monitoring have become possible [39].

One study compared finger-measured BP, using the OptiBP Smartphone application based on a pulse wave analysis algorithm, with BP measured via an arterial catheter. The difference in BP (mean ± standard deviation) between the two methods was within the norm. This may therefore become a valuable tool for detecting hypertension in various settings, such as pre-anesthetic assessment especially in low income countries [39].

A Chinese study done in 2021 proposed a new method of measuring heart rate variability using the Smartphone rear camera as a sensor. The fingertip video signals of 24 students were acquired using the rear camera of an HTC M8d Smartphone. ECG signals were recorded simultaneously as a reference. The results were comparable [40].

Some Smartphone-connected watches can perform a single-lead electrocardiogram (ECG) and detect atrial fibrillation. The clinical accuracy of the waveforms of these single-lead ECGs is still lower than a 12-lead ECG. But there is evidence, for example, that the Apple watch produces accurate ECGs in healthy adults with moderate to high agreement of baseline ECG intervals [41].

A study evaluating the efficacy of Cardio-Rhythm was conducted in 1013 patients with T2DM and hypertension: Atrial fibrillation was diagnosed in 28 patients (2.76%). The diagnostic sensitivity of CardioRhythm was 92.9% and was higher than that of a clinical score algorithm Alive Corautomated Algorithm (71.4%) [42].

5.2 Respiratory status

Smart phones can monitor and transmit arterial oxygen saturation (SpO2) data. The validity and reliability of a Smartphone oximeter has been validated by several studies [39, 43].

5.3 Measurement of hemoglobin level

- Non-invasive Hb measurement: HemaApp.

The HemaApp is an application to detect the hemoglobin level in the blood by color analysis using the HemaApp camera flash. By passing the light from the phone's camera flash through the patient's finger, HemaApp analyses the color of the patient's blood to estimate hemoglobin levels.

The FDA has approved it in the US as a non-invasive hemoglobin measurement tool [44].

- External sensors connected to the Smartphone to measure hemoglobin levels:

Automated external sensors linked to the Smartphone are able to quantitatively measure, without chemical reactions, the concentration of hemoglobin ([Hb]) in whole blood samples [45].

5.4 Measuring blood glucose

The conventional method of measuring blood glucose requires several pieces of equipment such as a glucometer, a test strip, a needle, an alcohol swab and gloves. This method of measurement is uncomfortable for the patient, especially if several measurements have to be performed every day.

To make the measurement more convenient and less invasive, researchers have developed a method based on colorimetric and electrochemical techniques to determine the glucose level using a Smartphone. This is called photo-plethysmography (PPG), a non-invasive, low-cost technique that measures the volumetric variation of blood in the arteries.

The principle of the proposed non-invasive technique is to record a short video (20 s–50 s) of the subject's fingertip using a commercial Smartphone camera. This video is then converted into images containing RGB channel information of different wavelengths. Because the wavelengths of the transmitted light (red, blue and green) are different, each penetrates the tissue differently: Red light has a longer wavelength than green or blue, and therefore penetrates deeper into the tissue. By integrating this image data (RGB channel), a PPG signal is generated from the recorded video.

Using these PPG signals acquired from the Smartphone and the corresponding glucose levels acquired with a glucose meter, linear regression models for glucose level prediction are created, allowing each PPG measurement to be assigned a blood glucose level. (Blood Glucose Level Regression for Smartphone PPG Signals Using Machine Learning Tanvir).

5.5 Hyperbilirubinemia

Other applications have been developed to detect hyperbilirubinemia based on the degree of absorption of the blue light emitted by the Smartphone flash. The image of the skin taken with this flash is compared to a color spectrum to classify it as icteric or non-icteric skin. The results are comparable to modern transcutaneous bilirubinometers [46].

5.6 Examples of connected medical devices

Several connected medical devices have been marketed in recent years such as stethoscopes, blood pressure monitors, ECGs, etc. [29].

The company EKO introduced on the market one of the first connected smart stethoscopes, capable of detecting heart murmurs with a sensitivity and specificity of 87% [47, 48].

There are many connected ECGs available on the market. Thanks to their connectivity with a Smartphone, sharing recordings is now easy between patients and doctors [49]. The principle consists in placing two fingers of each hand on the device and the result is displayed directly on the Smartphone.

Several studies have shown that these connected ECGs are capable of detecting atrial fibrillation in the ambulatory setting [50].

6. The smartphone in the operating theater

6.1 Estimation of blood loss in the operating room

Accurate assessment of blood loss is an important aspect of surgical management. Blood loss is usually assessed by visual estimation of the amount of blood in suction cartridges, surgical sponges and surgical drapes, which makes it very subjective.

An application has been recently developed to make this assessment more objective. It uses the Smartphone camera to capture images of surgical fields and then uses image analysis algorithms and cloud-based machine learning to accurately estimate the amount of hemoglobin (Hb) blood loss in real time on soaked surgical fields [51].

Another more relevant application developed by the same author allows the assessment of blood loss by estimating the hemoglobin level [52].

6.2 Location of tumor lesions

6.2.1 In neurosurgery

Operating theaters are equipped with microscopes to provide a good standard of care. However, in developing countries, microscopes are not always available. An adaptation of the Smartphone camera has been used as a valid alternative to the microscope. In a hospital in West Africa: using a simple tin can, a Smartphone shell and a rod attached to the bed, a Smartphone holder was created. This device provided surgeons with a magnification tool and a source of light in the surgical field. This simple "Smartphone-based exoscopy" allowed surgeons to obtain adequate magnification during brain surgery. This device has made it possible to overcome the lack of microscopes or surgical magnifying glasses, and can be useful in countries with limited resources [53].

6.2.2 Use of augmented reality to localize tumor lesions

Accurate localization of intracranial lesions before surgery is important, but sometimes difficult. Modern navigation systems are very useful, but expensive.

A low-cost solution for locating brain lesions and their surface projections in augmented reality has been described by a Chinese team. They used an iPhone to partially achieve this goal and assessed its accuracy and feasibility in a clinical neurosurgical setting.

This low-cost, iPhone-assisted, image-based augmented reality solution is technically feasible and useful for the localization of certain intracranial lesions, in particular superficial supratentorial intracranial lesions of medium size [54].

6.3 The smart scope

Another technological revolution should be mentioned: endoscopes Smartphone cameras, or otherwise called "Smart-Scopes".

In this case the Smartphone replaces the endoscopic camera and monitor by using its own camera and screen. The endoscope is coupled to the Smartphone camera and a removable light source completes the device. The Smartphone will be protected by a transparent sterile bag. The result is another laparoscopic surgical device called the smartscope that offers portable, cable-free, low-cost laparoscopic visualization.

Since the Smartphone used will mainly provide its camera to the surgical device: the higher the quality of the camera (4 K and 3D), the better the image of the surgical site. The size of the Smartphone is not important since the image obtained is immediately casted via Wi-Fi on a larger monitor. The image transfer is instantaneous and keeps the native resolutions.

The part that adapts the Smartphone to the endoscope can be made from an old, unusable camera head or purchased new. Different models are available on the market; some are specific to certain smart phones.

Removable camera sources are available on the market. Their disadvantage is that they have a limited life span.

The main advantage of this system is that it does not require any wiring. The image obtained on the Smartphone screen can be directly casted via Wi-Fi on a large monitor. It is a stand-alone system that completely dispenses with expensive laparoscopic columns. The surgeon holds the device and stands behind the Smartphone to watch the screen.

Real-time transmission of the image can be done through media streaming devices (such as Chromecast and Airplay). The device is plugged into the HDMI port of a TV and communicates, via Wi-Fi connection, with another Internet-connected device (computer, Smartphone, tablet, etc.), in order to display the received multimedia content on the TV [55].

The Smartphone therefore benefits from the power of the new cameras fitted to high-quality smart phones. As their cameras are constantly evolving, they allow high-definition images with true-to-life colors to be obtained. 4 k cameras are now available in many smart phones at much more affordable prices than 4 k-ultra HD laparoscopic columns.

The only limitation to this system is the limited duration of the removable light source.

The feasibility of this system is no longer in question. The smart scope has been used in various specialties: gynecology, urology, gastrology, otorhinolaryngology, etc.

In gynecology, a Greek team was able to create and test this device and proved its effectiveness in various surgical procedures. Thus it was possible to operate on ruptured ectopic pregnancies with hemoperitoneum, adnexal torsion, tubo-ovarian abscesses. This device has also made it possible to carry out diagnostic laparoscopy of ovarian cancer, enabling the extension and condition of the abdominal cavity to be assessed and biopsies of the mass to be performed. Image quality, resolution and acquisition were excellent, and the surgeons who performed the procedures reported no diagnostic problems with the new system [55].

Extrapolating the same principle, other basic surgeries such as appendectomy or cholecystectomy could be carried out without the need for a costly laparoscopic column.

In otolaryngology a Smartphone-based endoscopic device has also proven its clinical value and performance: The Smartphone system has shown an acceptable level of clarity for an ENT specialist to distinguish between healthy and diseased or damaged tissue regions via the Smartphone screen. By connecting to a wireless headset, the Smartphone-based endoscope system could even superimpose an endoscopic image on a real-world view [56].

In urology, a Smartphone coupled with a rigid endoscope can replace a cystoscope. It can be used in the emergency department for diagnostic procedures. As the system is fully self-contained and portable, it will make old, cumbersome and time-consuming procedures more efficient and cost-effective.

The 1951 USAF resolution test pattern was used to evaluate the image obtained from the smartscope. The results were found to be comparable to conventional cystoscopy for the rigid cystoscope [57].

The cost is approximately 50 to 70 times less than that of a standard high definition endoscopic camera [58]. Other devices replacing the usual laparoscopic surgical equipment have been developed and are constantly being improved. Optimization and validation of these systems is needed in terms of safety, as most of these devices are still in the experimental stage, but they have already proven to be of enormous benefit in developing countries: they are inexpensive and very easily reproducible. These devices have already been tested in basic laparoscopic surgeries: cholecystectomy, appendectomy, tubal ligation... [59].

The main advantages of the smart scope are:

- Cost: it costs 70 times less than the standard HD endoscopic camera [58].

The endoscope system with LED light source costs around $45 with the cost of a Smartphone with a good camera estimated at $1000 versus conventional video endoscopy with a standard camera and XL light source which costs $45000 [60].

Ease of use and availability:

- This system allows simple procedures: salpingectomies, adnexal detorsions, abscess drainage, tubal ligation....

- Facilitates access to endoscopic surgery, which remains limited in some regions: This device could save surgeons' time and save patients in hospitals where resources are not available. In some hospitals that have only one laparoscopic column, two surgical emergencies that require immediate interventions could not be managed at the same time due to the lack of resources. This surgical Smart-scope allows to ensure the same chances in terms of access to care.

- Facilitates the sharing of peroperative videos in real time through the internet, case presentation and discussion with colleagues.
- The ability to use the properties of the smartphone e.g. to zoom in on images.
- The possibility to access HD, 4 K and 3D quality images.

The only disadvantage of the smartscope is the limited duration of the removable light source.

7. The smartphone in postoperative care

The fields of application of the Smartphone in postoperative care are limitless, among which we can cite.

7.1 Monitoring of hemodynamic and vital constants

Several systems enable the delivery of mobile health monitoring services for outpatients and/or those outside of healthcare settings. Examples of these systems include the pulse oximeter of Masimo.com, the adhesive patch of Isansys.com, the electronic tattoo of mc10inc.com, or necklace of Tosense.com.

Several parameters can be analyzed such as: heart rate, heart rate variability, respiratory rate, skin temperature, stroke volume and cardiac output.

The information is transmitted to the Smartphone so that health professionals and/or patients can be informed quickly in case of clinical deterioration [61].

7.2 Remote monitoring of surgical wounds

Postoperatively, the Smartphone can be used as a tool for the monitoring and surveillance of postoperative infection sites. These infections can occur up to 30 days postoperatively. Monitoring can be done through sharing images of the surgical site and remote video conferencing [62, 63].

7.3 Monitoring of flap vitality

Some applications have also been developed in the field of plastic surgery to assess the vitality of grafted flaps through the communication of images postoperatively. Flap vitality assessment is done by comparison to a colorimetric scale, which reduces the time interval between the first notification of flap compromise and the start of re-exploration (4.0 vs. 1.4 hours).

8. Initial and continuing surgical education and information sharing

8.1 Access to medical information

Mobile phones facilitate access to medical information, particularly medicinal information, as they are more ergonomic and faster than consulting a paper book. The challenge for professionals is to identify validated applications that meet a real need and save time. Of the large number of applications available in the health sector, very few survive this triple filter.

Many specialists therefore stick to the applications proposed for their specialty, in addition to Vidal, which is appreciated by all.

Several learned societies and colleges of specialties offer specialized applications. This makes it possible to take advantage of reference systems and decision-making algorithms in just a few clicks.

8.2 Telemedicine, telemontoring, tele-expertise

The non-health-specific consumer platforms, Facebook (WhatsApp, Messenger and Instagram) and Google (Google Maps, YouTube and Google Play) largely dominate the mobile offer, but these applications do not allow the secure exchange of medical information.

TeamDoc has been proposed as a secure mobile application to replace WhatsApp, with features designed for healthcare professionals, which can be used in hospitals, clinics and private practices.

In the face of the coronavirus, many creative ideas and skills have led to the rapid launch of health applications [24].

A surgeon can now seek the expertise of a remote colleague at any time of the day through the transmission of images and videos. The use of social networking and instant messaging services is of real interest to developing countries because of its availability in remote and rural areas and its cost effectiveness [64].

With the new communication platforms, medical education has become more easily accessible.

The recording of an operation has become easy and reproducible with the Smartphone, thus allowing the creation of multimedia repertoires of great educational value.

Telementoring allows an experienced surgeon, located at a distance, to mentor a second operator in real time, thus boosting the dissemination of scholarly knowledge across borders and covering previously inaccessible geographical areas.

8.3 Simulation of surgical interventions by smartphone using virtual reality

Virtual Reality is being used to train and support healthcare professionals during initial and continuing training, during the simulation of surgical gestures and interventions, and during therapeutic treatments.

This directly therapeutic dimension of virtual reality is rare in the world of digital tools.

8.4 The advent of applications dedicated to learning

Several medical applications allow surgical trainees to become familiar with surgical interventions and to facilitate the learning of anatomy. Simulation is a validated method of medical learning. Simulations of certain surgical procedures have even become possible with several case scenarios [64].

8.5 Making laparoscopic Pelvi-trainers

It has become quite possible to create a laparoscopic surgery simulation box using a Smartphone. Improving skills through continuous practice is becoming an increasing priority in surgical training programs. It is an inexpensive, easily assembled, reproducible solution that is readily available as a useful tool for learning and improving laparoscopic techniques [65].

8.6 Touch surgery

The Touch Surgery mobile application is a mobile surgical training platform designed to simulate surgical procedures. As of October 2019, the Touch Surgery mobile app included surgical instructions for approximately 200 surgical procedures in 17 different specialties [66].

It is a useful tool for improving both technical skills and knowledge of the steps in the tendon repair procedure; however, its role may be limited to an additional tool as it does not improve theoretical knowledge. The TS has the potential to be implemented in an academic surgical program in low- and middle-income countries [66].

8.7 Other fields of application of the smartphone

Chat bots, or conversational agents, are used on many websites, mobile applications and consumer messengers.

An avatar greets the visitor and asks closed questions that lead the user through a tree structure. The concept originated in the medical world.

Many independent health mobile applications ask users questions about their symptoms to help them determine a pre-diagnosis or even guide them towards solutions.

9. Security of mobile health

Although mobile health represents a strong potential for innovation, it will have little future without a trusted environment. Its use requires a secure framework to guarantee the quality of care. The development of applications and connected health objects in an unregulated international framework presents several risks and raises ethical questions. These risks mainly concern:

- The reliability of technologies: malfunctioning of products and software, unreliable sensors.

- The protection of personal data: health data and confidentiality.

As a result, the establishment of a set of quality criteria for mobile health has proved necessary at the present time.

The French High Authority for Health has published a reference framework of good practices for manufacturers and assessors of connected applications or objects. The quality criteria adopted are divided into 5 areas (Haute Autorité de santé. Good practice guidelines on applications and connected objects (Mobile Health or mHealth) [66].

- Informing users: œ Description œ/Consent.

- Health content /œ Design of initial content /œ Standardization œ Generated content/œ Interpreted content.

- Technical content: œ Technical design œ/Data flow.

- Security/Reliability: œ Cybersecurity/œ Reliability/œ Confidentiality.

- Usability/use œ.

This standard was designed to ensure that an application or connected object is technically capable of delivering reliable and quality health information, protecting personal data and is easy to use.

In the US, the FDA has differentiated between medical and wellness applications, as well as between diagnostic and monitoring applications. It has applied regulatory oversight to the various internal or external sensors of the Smartphone as well as applications used to diagnose or monitor the health status of patients to ensure their safety [67]. To this effect, these different devices must provide evidence and undergo clinical trials that prove their reliability and safety [68]. Several mobile applications have received FDA approval. Examples include the KardiaMobile (AliveCor, Inc.) which provides electrocardiograms, the "Mobile MIM" diagnostic radiology application, the "BlueStar" for the management of type 2 diabetes... [69].

10. Conclusion

- Mobile telephony has profoundly transformed our lifestyles. The health sector has seized on these new technologies both on the side of health professionals, and on that of users.

- Mobile telephony via applications and connected objects make it possible to facilitate the pre-, per- and post-operative care of patients. This will allow better access to surgical care in developing countries and reduce healthcare costs in developed countries.

- These mobile systems will also facilitate data collection and transmission. This will allow better analysis of this data and will greatly pave the way for the introduction of artificial intelligence in medicine and surgery.

- The Smartphone can be used as an important tool for both diagnosis, care and surgical training. It can replace a whole column of operative endoscopy.

- Surgeons need to adapt their equipment according to local resources while respecting safety standards.

- Surgeons, policy makers and manufacturers need to work together to make more efforts in innovation to facilitate access to surgery in poor countries and reduce health care spending in rich countries.

- Covid-19 has put health systems around the world under severe strain. Policymakers are being forced to make adjustments. The long-vaunted digital health is becoming a reality and a necessity.

Author details

Sassi Boughizane[1,2*], Badra Bannour[1,2], Imen Bannour[1,2], Faten Hacheni[1,2], Imen Bannour[3], Marwa Masmoudi[1], Jalel Boughizane[4] and Sabri Youssef[5]

1 Department of Gynecology and Obstetrics, University Hospital Farhat Hached, Sousse, Tunisia

2 Faculty of Medicine Ibn Al Jazzar, University of Sousse, Sousse, Tunisia

3 Department of Anesthesiology-Intensive Care, University Hospital Farhat Hached, Sousse, Tunisia

4 The Higher Institute of Technological Studies in Sousse, University of Sousse, Tunisia

5 Department of Digestive Surgery, University Hospital Farhat Hached, Sousse, Tunisia

*Address all correspondence to: sassi.boughizane@laposte.net

References

[1] Shrime MG, Bickler SW, Alkire BC, Mock C. Global burden of surgicaldisease: an estimation from the provider perspective. LancetGlobHealth. 2015;3 (2):8-9DOI: 10.1016/S2214-109X(14)70384-5

[2] World Health Organization. World Health Statistics 2016: Monitoring Health for the Sustainable Development Goals. Geneva, Switzerland: WHO Press, 2016.

[3] Henry JA, Volk AS, Kariuki SK, Murungi K, Firmalo T, Masha RL et al. Ending Neglected Surgical Diseases (NSDs): Definitions, Strategies, and Goals for the Next Decade. Int J Health Policy Manag. 2020 , x(x), 1-8

[4] OCDE, Organisation mondiale de la Santé, World Bank Group. La qualité des services de santé : Un impératif mondial en vue de la couverture santé universelle. OECD; 2019. https://doi.org/10.1787/62f287af-fr.

[5] Statistiques de l'OCDE sur la santé 2020 - OCDE n.d. https://www.oecd.org/fr/els/systemes-sante/base-donnees-sante.htm (accessed March 26, 2021).

[6] Mukhopadhyay S, Ojomo K, Nyberger K, G. Meara J. Lancet Commission on Global Surgery, Iran J Pediatr. 2017 ; 27(4):e11273. doi: 10.5812/ijp.11273.

[7] WHO | Monitoring Progress towards Universal Health Coverage at Country and Global Levels: Framework, Measures and Targets n.d. https://www.who.int/healthinfo/universal_health_coverage/report/2014/en/ (accessed March 26, 2021)

[8] Reshadat, S., Zangeneh, A., Saeidi, S., Teimouri, R., Yigitcanlar, T.. Measures of spatial accessibility to health centers: Investigating urban and rural disparities in Kermanshah, Iran. Journal of Public Health 2019, 27(4), 519-529 DOI: 10.1007/s10389-018-0966-9

[9] Ng-Kamstra J, Raykar N, Meara JG, Shrime MG. Measuring Surgical Systems: A New Paradigm for Health Systems Strengthening. The Data Blog, 14 June 2016. Available at http://blogs.worldbank.org/opendata/measuring-surgical-systems-newparadigm healthsystems-strengthening (accessed 4 May 2018)

[10] Meara JG, Leather AJM, Hagander L, Alkire BC, Alonso N, Ameh EA, et al. Global surgery 2030: Evidence and solutions for achieving health, welfare, and economic development. Lancet Lond Engl 2015;386:569-624. https://doi.org/10.1016/S0140-6736(15)60160-X.

[11] Carte sanitaire année 2015. République Tunisienne Ministère de la Santé Direction des Etudes et de la Planification sous Direction des statistiques. Juin 2016. Availablefrom: http://www.santetunisie.rns.tn/images/docs/anis/stat/cartesanitaire2015.pdf.

[12] Chung, R. S., Ahmed, N.. The impact of minimally invasive surgery on residents' open operative experience: Analysis of two decades of national data. Annals of surgery 2010, 251(2), 205-212. DOI: 10.1097/SLA.0b013e3181c1b18e

[13] Fretland ÅA, Dagenborg VJ, Bjørnelv GMW, Kazaryan AM, Kristiansen R, Fagerland MW et al laparoscopic versus open resection for colorectal liver metastases: The OSLO-COMET randomized controlled trial. Ann Surg 2018;267(2):199-207 doi: 10.1097/SLA.0000000000002353

[14] Idrees JJ, Johnston FM, Canner JK, Dillhof M, Schmidt C, Haut ER et al .

Cost of major complications after liver resection in the United States: Are high-volume centers cost-efective? Ann Surg2019; 269(3):503-510 doi: 10.1097/SLA.0000000000002627

[15] Mboudou E., Frederick L.I., Pascal F., Sama J.D., Mbatsogo B.A.E., Minkande J.Z. Gynaecological laparoscopic surgery: Eight years experience in the Yaoundé Gynaeco-obstetric and Paediatric hospital. Cameroon. Trop. Doc. 2014;44(2):71-76 doi: 10.1177/0049475513517116

[16] Choy I, Kitto S, Adu-Aryee N., Okrainec A. Barriers to the uptake of laparoscopic surgery in a lower-middle-income country. Surg. Endosc 2013: 4009-4015. doi: 10.1007/s00464-013-3019-z

[17] Miller, C., Hoan, K., Minig, L., Chuang, L., &Shahabi, S.. A review of minimally invasive gynecologic surgery in developing nations. J Gynecol women's health 2017. 4(4), 555643. http://dx.doi.org/10.19080/jgwh.2017.04.555643

[18] Imran JB, Ochoa-Hernandez A, Herrejon J, Ortiz C, Mijangos B, Madni Tet al. Barriers to adoption of laparoscopic cholecystectomy in a county hospital in Guatemala. Surg Endosc. 2019 ;33(12):4128-4132. doi: 10.1007/s00464-019-06720-2.

[19] Boughizane S. May everyone develop his own simulator? Beyond Gynecologic Surgery. Clermont Ferrand 4,5 et 6 Avril 2018. Clermont Ferrand. France

[20] Boughizane S. Challenges for development of endoscopic surgery worldwide ? Beyond Gynecologic Surgery. Clermont Ferrand 4,5 et 6 Avril 2018. Clermont Ferrand. France

[21] Meara, JG, Leather, AJM, Hagander, L, Alkire, B.C., Alonso, N., Ameth, E.A.et al. Global surgery 2030: Evidence and solutions for achieving health, welfare, and economic development. Int. J. Obstet. Anesth. 2016; 25: 75-78 https://doi.org/10.1016/S0140-6736(15)60160-X

[22] Verguet S, Alkire BC, Bickler SW, Lauer JA, Uribe-Leitz T, Molina G et al. Timing and cost of scaling up surgical services in low-income and middle-income countries from 2012 to 2030: a modelling study. Lancet Glob Health. 2015 :27;3 (2):28-37. doi: 10.1016/S2214-109X(15)70086-0. PMID: 25926318.

[23] OMS : CINQUANTE-HUITIÈME ASSEMBLÉE MONDIALE DE LA SANTÉ [Internet]. [cited 2017 Oct 11]. Available from: http://www.who.int/ihr/training/laboratory_quality/cd_rom_ihr_revisions_58th_wha_pages_8-66_fr.pdf

[24] Silber D,Livre blanc : Le Praticien connecté. P8 Edimark 2020

[25] OMS.Santé mobile : utilisation des technologies mobiles sans fil pour la santé publique : rapport du Secrétariat. Conseil exécutif, 139. (2016). https://apps.who.int/iris/handle/10665/250884

[26] Park YR, Lee Y, Lee G, Lee JH, Shin SY. Smartphone applications with sensors used in a tertiary hospital-current status and future challenges. Sensors (Basel). 2015 : 27;15(5):9854-69. doi: 10.3390/s150509854. PMID: 25923933; PMCID: PMC4481990.

[27] Fernandes-Taylor, S., Gunter, R. L., Bennett, K. M., Awoyinka, L., Rahman, Set al. Feasibility of implementing a patient-centered postoperative wound monitoring program using smartphone images : a pilot protocol. JMIR research protocols 2017 ; 6(2):e26. DOI: 10.2196/resprot.6819

[28] Ríos Aguilar, S., Miguel Merino, J. L., Millan Sanchez, A., SanchezValdivieso, A. (2015). Variation

of the heartbeat and activity as an indicator of drowsiness at the wheel using a smartwatch. International Journal of Interactive Multimedia and Artificial Intelligence 2015 ;3(3):96-100 DOI: 10.9781/ijimai.2015.3313

[29] Arthur SURVILLE. Objets connectés et dispositifs médicaux connectés : Principaux outils disponibles à la pratique de la médecine générale en France en 2018. Thèse de doctorat en médecine. UNIVERSITÉ TOULOUSE III – Paul SABATIER FACULTÉ DE MÉDECINE, 2018

[30] Kelly, J.T. ; Campbell, K.L.; Gong, E.; Scuffham, P. The internet of things: Impact and implications for health care delivery. J. Med. Int. Res. 2020, 22 : e20135. doi: 10.2196/20135

[31] Pujari A, Mukhija R, Singh AB, Chawla R, Sharma N, Kumar A. Smartphone-based high definition anterior segment photography. Indian J Ophthalmol. 2018 ;66(9):1375-76. doi: 10.4103/ijo.IJO_544_18. PMID: 30127180; PMCID: PMC6113839.

[32] NihanGiderIşıkman et al. A Milestone in Film History: Smartphone Filmmaking. International Journal of Culture and History 2018 ;4(4) doi: 10.18178/ijch.2018.4.4.129

[33] Zhang, D.; Liu, Q. Biosensors and bioelectronics on smartphone for portable biochemical detection. Biosens. Bioelectron. 2016 ; 75, 273–284 https://doi.org/10.1016/j.bios.2015.08.037

[34] Chuchu N et al. Smartphone applications for triaging adults with skin lesions that are suspicious for melanoma (review). Cochrane Database of Systematic Reviews 2018 ;12(12): CD013192. doi: 10.1002/14651858.CD013192.

[35] Delores Jones, RDMS, RT(S), BDMS. Smartphone-compatible ultrasound probe. Journal of Diagnostic Medical Sonography 2014. 30(4) 200-204 DOI: 10.1177/8756479314534523

[36] Lumify transducers (probes) & accessories: Philips Healthcare. Philips. (Available at: https://www.usa.philips.com/healthcare/sites/lumify/products-accessories Date accessed: November 12, 2020

[37] Toscano, M., Szlachetka, K., Whaley, N., Thornburg, L. L. . Evaluating sensitivity and specificity of handheld point-of-care ultrasound testing for gynecologic pathology: A pilot study for use in low resource settings. BMC medical imaging 2020, 20(1), 1-15..doi: 10.1186/s12880-020-00518-8

[38] Sassolas, A., Marty, J. L.. Biocapteurs au service du diagnostic medical. Techniques de l'Ingénieur 2013 ; BIO7110.

[39] Nemcova, A., Jordanova, I., Varecka, M., Smisek, R., Marsanova, L., Smital, Let al .Monitoring of heart rate, blood oxygen saturation, and blood pressure using a smartphone. Biomedical Signal Processing and Control 2020 ; 59, 101928. https://doi.org/10.1016/j.bspc.2020.101928

[40] Zhang, G., Zhang, S., Dai, Y., Shi, B. Using rear smartphone cameras as sensors for measuring heart rate variability. IEEE Access 2021 ;(9): 20460-20468. https://doi.org/10.1109/ACCESS.2021.3054065

[41] Isakadze, N.; Martin, S. How useful is the smartwatch ECG? Trends Cardiovasc. Med. 2019, 30, 442-448 DOI: 10.1016/j.tcm.2019.10.010

[42] Chan PH, Wong CK, Poh YC, Pun L, Leung WWCet al. Diagnostic performance of a smartphone -based photoplethysmographic application for atrial fibrillation screening in a primary care setting.J Am Heart Assoc. 2016; 5:e003428

[43] C Chan , J A Inskip , A R Kirkham , J M Ansermino , G Dumont , L C Li et al A smartphone oximeter with a fingertip probe for use during exercise training: Usability, validity and reliability in individuals with chronic lung disease and healthy controls .Physiotherapy 2019 ; 105(3): 297-306 DOI: 10.1016/j.physio.2018.07.015

[44] EJ Wang, W Li, D Hawkins, T Gernsheimer,. C Norby-Slycord. HemaApp: noninvasive blood screening of hemoglobin using smartphone cameras. In Proceedings of the 2016 ACM International Joint Conference on Pervasive and Ubiquitous Computing. 2016: 593-604 https://doi.org/10.1145/2971648.2971653

[45] Lee, J., Song, J., Choi, J. H., Kim, S., Kim, U., Nguyen, V. Tet al. A Portable Smartphone-linked Device for Direct, Rapid and Chemical-Free Hemoglobin Assay. Scientific reports 2020. 10(1):1-10 | https://doi.org/10.1038/s41598-020-65607-8

[46] Kumar, R., Nixon, M., Alabsawy, E. I., Amin, A. A., Outlaw, F., Mookerjee, R. .A novel, smartphone-based scleral image capture technique accurately determines serum bilirubin level and can be used for home-based monitoring of patients discharged from hospital, after an episode of acute decompensation. Journal of Hepatology 2020 ; 73: S755-S756.

[47] Eko Core Stethoscope. Home page. Available at: https://www.ekohealth.com/. Accessed Mars 21, 2020

[48] asudevan, R. S., Horiuchi, Y., Torriani, F. J., Cotter, B., Maisel, S. M., Dadwal, S. Sat al .. Persistent value of the stethoscope in the age of COVID-19. The American Journal of Medicine 2020 ; 133(10): 1143-1150. doi: 10.1016/j.amjmed.2020.05.018

[49] Witvliet, M. P., Karregat, E. P., Himmelreich, J. C., de Jong, J. S., Lucassen, W. A., Harskamp, R. E. Usefulness, pitfalls and interpretation of handheld single-lead electrocardiograms. Journal of Electrocardiology 2021;66: 33-37 doi: 10.1016/j.jelectrocard.2021.02.011.

[50] Joshi AK, Kowey PR, Prystowsky EN, Benditt DG, Cannom DS, Pratt CM, et al. First experience with a Mobile cardiac outpatient telemetry (MCOT) system for the diagnosis and management of cardiac arrhythmia. Am J Cardiol. 2005;95(7):878-881 https://doi.org/10.1016/j.amjcard.2004.12.015

[51] Konig, G., Waters, J. H., Javidroozi, M., Philip, B., Ting, V., Abbi, G et al real-time evaluation of an image analysis system for monitoring surgical hemoglobin loss." Journal of clinical monitoring and computing 2018;32 (2): 303-310 https://doi.org/10.1007/s10877-017-0016-0

[52] Konig G, Holmes AA, Garcia R, Mendoza JM, Javidroozi M, Satish Set al. In vitro evaluation of a novel system for monitoring surgical hemoglobin loss. AnesthAnalg. 2014 ;119(3):595-600. doi: 10.1213/ANE.0000000000000198. PMID: 24806138; PMCID: PMC4139457.

[53] Konig, G., Waters, J. H., Javidroozi, M., Philip, B., Ting, V., Abbi, G et al real-time evaluation of an image analysis system for monitoring surgical hemoglobin loss." Journal of clinical monitoring and computing 2018;32 (2): 303-310 DOI: 10.1007/s10877-017-0016-0

[54] Hou, Y., Ma, L., Zhu, R., Chen, X., Zhang, J. A low-cost iPhone-assisted augmented reality solution for the localization of intracranial lesions. PloS one2016 ;25;11(7):e0159185. doi: 10.1371/journal.pone.0159185. eCollection 2016 https://doi.org/10.1371/journal.pone.0159185

[55] Chatzipapas, I., Kathopoulis, N., Protopapas, A., Loutradis, D. Using a

Mobile smartphone to perform laparoscopy. Journal of Minimally Invasive Gynecology 2018, 25(5), 912-915. doi:10.1016/j.jmig.2017.12.027

[56] Bae J, Vavilin A, You J, Kim H, Ryu S, Jang J et al. Smartphone-Based Endoscope System for Advanced Point-of-Care Diagnostics: Feasibility Study JMIR MhealthUhealth 2017;5(7):e99 https://doi.org/10.2196/mhealth.7232

[57] Lu, S., Cottone, C. M., Yoon, R., Jefferson, F. A., Sung, J. M., Okhunov, Zetal. Endockscope: A disruptive endoscopic technology. Journal of Endourology 2019. 33(11):960-965 ; doi:10.1089/end.2019.0252

[58] Sohn, W., Shreim, S., Yoon, R., Huynh, V. B., Dash, A., Clayman, R. et al .Endockscope: Using mobile technology to create global point of service endoscopy. Journal of endourology 2013; 27(9): 1154-1160 https://dx.doi.org/10.1089%2Fend.2013.0286

[59] Gheza, F., Oginni, F. O., Crivellaro, S., Masrur, M. A., Adisa, A. O.. Affordable laparoscopic camera system (ALCS) designed for low-and middle-income countries: A feasibility study. World journal of surgery 2018; 42(11):3501-3507 https://doi.org/10.1007/s00268-018-4657-z

[60] Tse C, Patel RM, Yoon R, Okhunov Z, Landman J, Clayman RV. The Endockscope using next generation smartphones: "a global opportunity". J Endourol. 2018;32(8):765-770. doi: 10.1089/end.2018.0275. Epub 2018 Jul 9. PMID: 29860870.

[61] Michard F. Smartphones and e-tablets in perioperative medicine. Korean J Anesthesiol. 2017 ;70(5):493-99. doi: 10.4097/kjae.2017.70.5.493. Epub 2017 Sep 28. PMID: 29046768; PMCID: PMC5645581.

[62] McLean, K. A., Mountain, K. E., Shaw, C. A., Drake, T. M., Ots, R., Knight, S. et al. Can a smartphone-delivered tool facilitate the assessment of surgical site infection and result in earlier treatment? Tracking wound infection with smartphone technology (TWIST): protocol for a randomised controlled trial in emergency surgery patients. BMJ open2019; 9(10):e029620. doi: 10.1136/bmjopen-2019-029620.

[63] Castillo, E., McIsaac, C., MacDougall, B., Wilson, D., Kohr, R. et al. Post-caesarean section surgical site infection surveillance using an online database and mobile phone technology. Journal of Obstetrics and Gynaecology Canada 2017; 39(8):645-651 https://doi.org/10.1016/j.jogc.2016.12.037

[64] Bunogerane, G. J., Taylor, K., Lin, Y., Costas-Chavarri, A.. Using touch surgery to improve surgical education in low-and middle-income settings: A randomized control trial. Journal of surgical education 2018; 75(1):231-237. DOI: 10.1016/j.jsurg.2017.06.016

[65] Lee, M., Savage, J., Dias, M., Bergersen, P., Winter, M.. Box, cable and smartphone: a simple laparoscopic trainer. The clinical teacher2015; 12(6):384-88

[66] Haute Autorité de Santé. Choix méthodologiques pour l'analyse de l'impact budgétaire à la HAS. https://www.has-sante.fr/upload/docs/application/pdf/2016-12/guide_methodologique__choix_methodologiques_pour_lanalyse_de_limpact_budgetaire_a_la_has_.pdf

[67] U.S. Department of Health and Human Services Food and Drug Administration. Mobile Medical Applications: Guidance for Industry and Food and Drug Administration Staff. 2015; Available online: https://www.fda.gov/media/80958/download

[68] Van Norman, G.A. Drugs and Devices. Comparison of European and U.S. Approval Processes. JACC Basic Transl. Sci. 2016, 1, 399-412 https://doi.org/10.1016/j.jacbts.2016.06.003

[69] Majumder, S.; Deen, M.J. Smartphone sensors for health monitoring and diagnosis. Sensors 2019; 19, 2164 DOI: 10.3390/s19092164

Chapter 15

Toward a Holistic Approach in Medical Education

Reema Safadi and Lubna Abushaikha

Abstract

In this chapter, we briefly present the case of medical practice and education as they evolved through history until modern times. The history of medical practice and education portrays a transformation from unstructured spiritual and apprenticeship practice of the older days transitioning toward the current biopsychosocial medical model that is based on scientific evidence-based methods and practice. Educational methods have also developed from didactic traditional pedagogies and passive learning to more interactive methods and technologies based on andragogy. A preview of theoretical frameworks sets the ground for a discussion about medical schools' curricula, values, and mission statements. The purpose of the frameworks is to illustrate the basic concepts on which a curriculum is constructed, and thus employ this in assessing whether these frameworks would fulfill the core values of medical practice as a holistic, bio-psychosocial science and practice; conceptual values that could address the communities' current needs and rights to care. The chapter concludes with an analysis of few examples of mission statements that reflect the existent medical schools' programs, values, and outcomes that are sought in future medical practitioners. A program that results in graduating competent, knowledgeable, and humanistic medical practitioners is the goal of all medical schools.

Keywords: Communication, cooperation and collaboration, medical education, research paradigms, transformative leadership

1. Introduction

This chapter is a discussion of medical schools' education curricula in preparing medical doctor practitioners to practice medicine in their countries and globally. The discussion will answer the questions about whether the worldwide medical schools' curricula are responding to the communities' needs with consideration of the most recent up-to-date evidence in the medical sciences and the psychosocial sciences combined. It will also answer the question of what kind of theoretical frameworks are being in use, and are these frameworks considering a comprehensive and holistic view of the beneficiaries of health care.

The idea of this discussion has emerged after a long-life career in health care as nurses working closely with doctors in primary, secondary, and tertiary care settings. Our long experience of over 30 years' duration as nurses and faculty members exposed us to practicing doctors as we were student nurses, as graduate nurses practicing nursing in multiple care settings, as academics (faculty members) teaching medical students some of their non-medical courses, and as colleagues working with medical doctors on research projects on different topic areas and research designs. This journey has enabled us to capture some crucial areas of strengths and weaknesses in the preparation of medical doctors that may benefit from using a critical lens that exposes issues of concern for the sake of the wider community and the beneficiaries of medical healthcare services. In this chapter, our aim is to elucidate these points by referring to the historical development of medical practice and education, to medical schools' curricula and mission statements in general without reference to any program or school in particular, and to explain the theoretical models of teaching and practice that have been in place over the last few decades at schools of medicine. This will be a critical eye of how medical education and medical practice have evolved (or not evolved) to meet the psycho-socio-cultural changes that occurred over time. What is presented in the following pages is not a definitive argument of medical education but rather a case that draws heavily on our observations that have long been echoed elsewhere.

2. A historical view of medical practice and education

2.1 Medicine in ancient times

The history of documented medical practice and medical education goes back to ancient times of great empires of China, Babylon, Egypt, and India [1]. The ancient history of medicine informs us of the culture and the conceptualization of health, disease and illness that were prevalent at those times. Ancient Egyptians (3300–525 BCE) used prayers as solutions to health problems, and had natural, practical remedies such as herbs to cure their ill people [2]. In traditional Chinese culture, medicine is traced back to 14 and 11th century BCE. Treatment of illnesses had no logical mechanism and they did not have a concept of medicine as distinct from other fields. Ancient Babylonians medicine and culture revolved around magic, supernaturalism and the absence of scientific methods. In India, medicine was known as Ayurveda [3, 4]. Ayurveda is a Sanskrit term in which Ayur means life and veda means science. Physicians used to prescribe individualized herbs, diet and exercise along with lifestyle recommendations. Ayuerveda physicians believed in environmental factors or forces such as weather, diet, work, society, the economy, and lifestyle as influencing one's health – the state of mind, body and soul. In one of the more recent times of ancient medicine, stories of the well acknowledged Greek physician Hippocrates (400 BCE) became familiar in the medical arena. His ethical Oath and code for practicing doctors was originated and taught then and remains until today as a code that is recited in graduation ceremonies in schools of medicine across the globe [5].

2.2 The middle ages

The Middle Ages have seen more formal recognition of medicine in Europe. Medicine was practiced as apprenticeship training in monasteries under the control of hospitals and churches. This period, 1220s, was the beginning of medical education where a medical school was established in Southern Italy and was followed by further expansion of medical education throughout Italy and Europe. Additionally, and during this period, medicine and medical education were growing in the Muslim world with more centers established in Baghdad, Cairo and Cordoba [6]. The Islamic Umayyad and Abbasid caliphate periods added further to western medicine by the translations of the works of Hippocrates and Galen. In fact, during the medical Islamic period (900 C.E.), the medieval Islamic doctors in their communities recognized the roles of causes of illness and possible treatments and cures. This period demonstrated the rise of known medical scientists such as Al-Razi, Ibn al-Nafis and Ibn Sina (Avicenna) [7].

2.3 Twelve to sixteenth centuries

The years between the 12th to 16th century demonstrated a great stride in the establishment of medical schools across Europe and other regions such as India and Egypt. Schools in hospitals and more medical schools at universities were established in the United Kingdom, Italy, Portugal, Germany, Czeck republic, Austria, Poland, Switzerland, Sweden, Denmark, and Spain. One of the earliest of these schools was established at the University of Oxford, UK [8]. In 1310, Dr. Gaddesden published *Rosa Anglica* the earliest surviving medical textbook in Britain. This period showed the rise of licensing and structured educational programs that involved years of study after the first degree of Master of Arts. The educational preparation of doctors involved studying for six years and undergoing practical training and lecturing for another two years once licensed. In 1421, the British Parliament petitioned the passing of a law that restricts medical practice to qualifications granted by university education only. In 1518, the first professional body, the Royal College of Physicians of London, was established as the oldest British professional membership body and medical college dedicated to improving the practice of medicine, and a medical society that regulates medical practice by licensing proficient and punishing pretending doctors [9].

2.4 Medical education between the seventeen and nineteen centuries in the United States

During the 17th to 19th century, and in the same line, the history of medical education took similar strides in the United States. The early 1750s saw informal classes in anatomy that were unstructured and run by doctors who traveled to Europe bringing back with them a series of anatomy lectures that were taught to gentlemen who could afford the fees of a reputable practitioner. The beginnings showed apprenticeship system where apprentices were trained in doctors' offices who had their private venture, in menial and pharmaceutical therapies. Although emulating the British medical system in practice and educational institutions, the American educational system remained unstructured and without formal legislation. The first theory and practice College of Philadelphia was founded by John Morgan in Philadelphia in 1765, and New York in 1768 [10]. Many more schools of medicine grew between 1810 and 1840 resulting in twenty-six new medical schools, and grew even more and doubled until 1876. Teaching at these institutions was at its beginning, and barely founded with some inexpensive anatomy benches and with little investment in teaching that was focused on didactic methods, except for the anatomy sessions. A school diploma was the license to practice after a brief, oral examination as no state boards were yet in place. During this period, teaching circumstances were not ideal with minimal clinical facilities and didactic teaching in badly lighted amphitheaters [10, 11].

In the United States, the beginnings of the 1800s showed the opening and merging of many medical schools including the medical department of King's College and the medical department of Harvard College. During the midst of the 19th century (1835), the American situation of unsuitable distorted mode of education endured protests from different medical education institutions in request of legislations and improved structured standards of education to earn a degree in medicine. These protests ended with the formation of the American Medical Association in 1847 that committed the profession to the requirement of suitable education and standards for the degree.

In the 1850s onward, the time for change was achieved by the dissolution of the preceptorship system where the medical schools of Harvard, Yale, Pennsylvania, became independent of the institutions with which they were legally united. At the time of commercial exploitation, schools were controlled by owners of these institutions and bestowed professorships by common agreement, segregating and dividing fees, along proprietary lines. These independent irresponsible conditions remained as such until the eighties. During this time, medical education was based within medical schools, using didactic methods of teaching that were focused on the chemical, biologic and physical sciences, and personal contact between teacher and student, and between student and patient were lost [12].

This time of medical institutions' wide spreading was associated with the new medical discoveries and the invention of the stethoscope in 1816, that came into fruition in the establishment of the first bachelor's degree at John Hopkins Medical School in 1893. This was the first school with adequate preparations of well-equipped laboratories run by modern faculty and hospital training for physicians. The school provided a standard for medical schools with a scientific curriculum [12].

The conditions of medical education were criticized calling for reforms of medical education. In 1910, Abraham Flexner, an educator, and not a physician, issued his report on the state of medical education after a comprehensive review of and visits to schools of medicine [13]. In his report, he declared that medical education in the USA and Canada must be an educational system by instituting standardized quality education that is university-based only and underpinned by a scientific foundation. Additionally, the report emphasized that students must be educated to be qualified and granted a degree in medicine [14]. This revolutionary report resulted in a decline in the number of commercial medical schools, and the establishment of the residency training and specialization and sub-specialization among American doctors by the 1930 and 1940s, and the foundation of four years' education that are completed with internship and residency programs and board examinations. The role of basic sciences flourished after the Flexner report (1910) which provided the grounds for designing undergraduate medical curriculum followed by clinical experiences and in academically oriented hospitals [15].

The publication of Flexner report was a turning point in medical education: the preclinical and clinical divide [10, 12, 14]. This divide of preclinical and clinical medical education that started in the 20th century showed another form of shortcomings in educational programs. With this polarity, the delivery of basic sciences teaching was more focused on scientific facts rather than the context of medical practice. Additionally, there were notions of poor retention of basic knowledge as students started clinical experiences as described by Pawlina [16].

By the 1960s and 1970s and after the transformative changes that were initiated by the Flexner report, medical education in schools has evolved from a haphazard, unstructured classes for interested gentlemen form to a scientific model of the late 20th century and early 21st century [12]. By the 1980s, education became more structured and clinical training was instituted and delivered by attending physicians in hospitals, ambulatory settings, and physicians' offices. However, training was not well served because physicians did not have enough time to train students and there were recommendations for more change in future doctors' education and training.

2.5 The twentieth century: the value of other than the scientific science in the curriculum

As medical education was established in universities with emphasis on a scientific base, there were critiques about the intensity of the focus on the biosciences and the absence of subjects such as the history of medicine and social ethics as part of the curriculum. Rajan [17] argues that in the first two years, medical students sit in lecture rooms learning about DNA replication while it is more important to learn the interpersonal skills to be a good doctor. The medical historian Eugene Cordell, in a speech at the State of Maryland, in 1913, criticized the lack of any formal teaching on the history of medicine [18] and emphasized the importance of this knowledge throughout all stages of the educational program. A century later, and in support of Dr. Cordell presidential speech, Yarnall [18] emphasized the importance of studying the history of medicine because we learn from our successes and failures and many time scientists' names are associated with disease discoveries such as Cushing disease and Boerhaave syndrome. Yarnall quotes Maxmilien Littre as, "There is nothing in the most advanced contemporary medicine whose embryo cannot be found in the medicine of the past".

Besides history, El-Moamly [19] emphasized the importance of integrating medical humanities in medical curriculum and the use of the psychosocial-biological approach in understanding health, illness, life and death. To address the global new trends in medical practice, Irby and Wilkerson [20] suggested reforms in many directions. One of these areas involve the integration of multiple disciplines to be congruent with the current change in the meaning of human health and disease. The authors presented six core competencies that are necessary for practicing physicians: patient care, knowledge, practice-based learning and improvement, interpersonal communication skills, professionalism, and system-based practice. Need for reforms became imperative because of the new science of learning and technology, the changing communities' needs, and required skills in managing new patterns of health problems, examples of which are the recent COVID-19 pandemic, chronic diseases, pain management, and complementary medicine that is expanding widely recently. To conclude this section, a paradigm shift is now required as we quote from Gwee et al.: *"From students receiving intensive instruction of in-depth scientific facts derived from disciplinary courses, to student acquisition of scientific competencies required for the development of the desired habits of mind, behavior and action for medical practice in the 21st century"* [14].

In light of the worldwide historical evolvement of medical education with its ups and downs, the Association of Faculties of Medicine in Canada [21] has published its vision of undergraduate education in the collective report of the future of medical education in Canada (FMEC). The 10 recommendations address aspects of: "1. Address Individual and Community Needs 2. Enhance Admissions Processes 3. Build on the Scientific Basis of Medicine 4. Promote Prevention and Public Health 5. Address the Hidden Curriculum 6. Diversify Learning Contexts 7. Value Generalism 8. Advance Inter- and Intra-Professional Practice 9. Adopt a Competency-Based and Flexible Approach 10. Foster Medical Leadership". In this view, questions are raised as to how should the medical curriculum be redesigned to serve the scientific foundations of medicine in the 21st century [14].

3. Health and the biomedical model

As preceded in outlining the historical development of medicine and medical education, it is observed that medical education has transitioned from being unstructured and designed by individual endeavors, known as healers in offering holistic health services [22], to become more structured, institutionally-based and regulated by members of professional medical practice. In other words, the transition emphasized the biomedical model, as the sole path to improving health in the community.

The biomedical model is the most prevalent in medical practice and educational institutions in the western countries and other parts of the world [14, 23]. Cockerham [24] revealed that ignoring the social role in studies of health and illness is a sign for the pervasiveness of the biomedical model in conceptualizing sickness. According to Cockerham, this model is based on the concepts of pathogens as causes of disease that are prevented or controlled by medical interventions such as medical procedures and medications. In an argument to dispel the current prevalent role of the biomedical model, Roy Porter [25] argued that "Basic research, clinical science and technology working with one another have characterized the cutting edge of modern medicine" (in Cockerham, 2021, p.10). In a counterargument of the benefit of the biomedical model, Cockerham argued that the biomedical model was useful when infectious diseases were most prevalent as it provided the right drugs to treat these infections. However, in the recent days, with the changing patterns of disease outbreaks as in the most recent Corona Virus pandemic, and the emergence of chronic diseases, such as heart diseases and cancer as a result of the increasing life span of the population, there are new factors to consider. Globalization, modernization of life styles, economy, and the quality of working environment which also have influenced the kind of diseases and health problems that people suffer from, imply the need to revisit medical treatment management strategies, schools' curricula and instructional methods.

Understanding the past control of infectious diseases (i.e., small pox and poliomyelitis), the recent emergence of viral infections, concerns about chronic diseases, and the increased life span of the people, together with modern life and environmental and work conditions change call for an alteration in medical approaches to treat health problems. A more holistic approach of care that deals with the whole person became more eminent. In this regard, the biomedical model which dealt with microorganisms, pathology and biochemistry falls short of providing care based on humanistic modes of care, and suggestions of a replacement model with new strategies for treatment should emerge to meet this change in the healthcare needs.

4. Current medical education and adult learning theories

Medical education has undergone significant transformations reflecting the changes that have occurred in global healthcare as well as educational systems [26]. One of the most significant changes is the shift from passive learning to active learning using a variety of teaching and learning strategies. These strategies include case-based learning, experiential learning, peer problem solving, and project-based learning [26]. However, many challenges were associated with this shift that are related to the organization, resources, staff, and students [27]. The traditional medical model focused on passive learning and emphasized biological aspects of diseases and disorders with total disregard to psychological, social, behavioral, and spiritual aspects and responses [28, 29], while active learning focused on the implementation of adult learning theories.

Adult learning theories based in "andragogy", provide a guiding framework for all types of higher educational programs, including programs for healthcare professionals. Andragogy focuses on viewing the "adult learner" as a partner in the teaching-learning process who possesses the ability to determine his/her learning needs based on various experiential backgrounds, skills, and motivations. Educational programs for healthcare professionals usually stem from different philosophical and theoretical frameworks that provide curricular guidance in the formulation of educational programs and their contents. There are several adult learning theories based on a constructivist philosophy which entails building new knowledge on previously existing knowledge and is congruent with the views presented in andragogy which was established by Alexander Kapp in 1833 and revived and modified by Malcolm Knowles in the 1980s. Modern andragogy is based on five assumptions which are self-concept, experience, readiness to learn, orientation to learning, and motivation to learn [30]. Adult learning theories include instrumental, humanistic, transformative, social, motivational, reflective, and constructivist theories.

Instrumental theories include behavioral theories, cognitivism, and experiential learning [31]. Behavioral theories stipulate that learning happens as a result of the influence of environmental stimuli on the individual which manifests in behavioral changes. Cognitivism focuses on the cognitive processes such as perception, memory, and reflection that are precursors to knowledge acquisition and retainment. In experiential learning, knowledge is constructed through interactions and active experiences with the individual's environment. Humanistic theories focus on viewing the learner through a humanistic lens that emphasizes student-centered, self-directed learning and views educators as facilitators. Transformative theories focus on empowering the learner to evaluate and reflect on previously held assumptions and meanings to transform to a new level of knowledge. Social theories focus on acquiring knowledge and learning through social interactions. The main premise in motivational theories stipulates that motivation and reflection are precursors to learning. Reflective theories are based on two types of reflection: reflection-on-action and reflection-in-action which help the learner to test knowledge and learn from experience and practice. Constructivist theories focus on the sociohistorical and situated dimension of learning. The learner acquires new knowledge through social interactions with their peers and instructors and builds upon previously acquired skills.

The use of varied adult learning theories, which have both strengths and shortcomings, in medical education programs around the world has led to varied instructional methods employed by faculty and ultimately varied levels of achievement of learning outcomes.

5. Current medical education and communication skills

In the traditional medical model, effective and proper clinical communication was not valued nor was it included in the curriculum of many medical programs. The paradigm shift occurred during the eighties when consumerism in health care became a prevalent phenomenon. During this shift, consumers of health care became partners in the health care industry and the dynamics between health care providers and "clients" witnessed significant changes from the traditional medical model where "paternalistic" physicians were in control of all aspects of health care delivery including health-related decisions, and health-care recipients had very minimal roles and input, if any. The focus on including effective communication skills in medical curricula has emphasized the need for fostering positive physician-patient dyads in different clinical settings and contexts which results in the professional confidence and satisfaction of physicians [32–34]. Effective communication skills (e.g., empathy, breaking bad news, theater, and drama-based educational methods) in medical education should be taught, modeled, and re-demonstrated [33, 34]. However, even if communication skills such as interview skills and non-verbal behavior are taught and practiced, retention of these skills over time has been shown to fluctuate when physicians start practicing in the "real world" [34]. Relevant literature indicates that undergraduate medical students attain clinical communications skills along with other medical skills, but these skills are not fully maintained or retained when transitioning from medical student to practicing physician, or from the preclinical to clinical years of study, or even when transitioning from one course to another, [16, 34, 35].

6. Current medical education and research

In medical education, up-to-date research evidence informs and directs medical science and clinical practice. As in other disciplines, medicine struggles with finding a research culture that enhances the medical profession as well as academia. Moreover, ethical approval, adequate funding, publishing, authorship, plagiarism, redundant publication, ethical conduct in research, and conflict of interests remain extant issues for both novice and expert researchers in medicine [36]. Historically, physicians from all subspecialities have had access to patients in clinical settings. There is a non-spoken norm that a physician's patients are automatically considered his/her research "subjects" and are under his/her will when recruiting patients in different research studies as well as granting or denying others (e.g., other health care team members such as nurses, pharmacists, dentists) access to these subjects.

Traditionally, research in medicine has been mostly quantitative designs, such as observational and cross-sectional studies [37]. The most common new trends of medical education research topics reported in the literature have been curriculum and teaching issues, skills and attitudes relevant to the structure of the profession, individual characteristics of medical students, and the evaluation of students and residents [36, 38, 39].

A fairly recent trend in medical research has been shifting to qualitative research methodology and employing different qualitative research designs stemming from a social sciences framework and interpretive paradigm. Physicians and educators in medicine have come to appreciate the richness and holistic viewpoint innate in qualitative research especially in investigating and comprehending complex phenomena such as health, illness, and team-based care [40]. Qualitative methodologies have also helped medical educators to gain insight and understand the experiences of medical students, teamwork dynamics among different health professionals as well as between students and faculty, and identify appropriate instructional methods in medical education [40].

7. Current medical education and leadership

In medical education, a sense of leadership and what it entails is first acquired, appraised, and evaluated in many forms during undergraduate studies. These forms include group academic and clinical assignments with an assigned leader, the leadership of faculty in their respective courses, the leadership of the school administrative team, the leadership of professional medical associations, and the local, regional, and/or international leadership of the medical profession.

Leaders initiate and sustain change and direction in individuals and organizations. Leaders, as opposed to managers who run the day-to-day administrative activities and functions of an organization, inspire, motivate, set direction, and focus on achieving organizational goals and aspirations [41]. In clinical practice, medical leaders focus their efforts toward achieving positive patient outcomes as well an organizational autonomy, accountability, and sustainability. The new trends in leadership in healthcare are now known as "transactional" and "transformative" leadership. Transactional leadership establishes a more authoritative relationship between leader and followers to achieve specific goals. The downfall of transactional leadership includes lack of innovation, incentive, and motivation has given rise to the adoption of "transformative leadership" in healthcare disciplines.

Transformative leadership focuses on influencing and "transforming" individuals in an effort to achieve organizational goals. The most recent trend in leadership is "team leadership" or "shared governance" in which the focus has shifted from the leader to the team. In this type of leadership, roles and responsibilities are shared by interdependent team members [41]. Thus, team collaboration is the main tool that can be used to achieve expected and desired outcomes. New leadership styles fit with the concept of "teamwork" since physicians realistically do not work in isolation of the other members of a health team including nurses, pharmacists, nutritionists, anesthetists. Etc.

8. Current medical education, simulation, and technology

After medical students acquire basic knowledge in the first few years of medical school, they begin to acquire clinical skills through the different clinical rotations either in simulation labs or actual clinical settings (e.g., hospitals, clinics, private offices). The use of simulation and clinical focus have been used to meet arising societal and global needs [42]. For example, in the past 15–16 months of the COVID-19 pandemic, healthcare professional schools, including medical schools, have somewhat altered their rotation schedules and have used new and creative venues to meet the clinical training needs of their students, while keeping them safe and sound. This included online instruction and online clinical simulation using available technologies such as Microsoft Teams, Google Meet, and Zoom. So basically, the whole world was united in higher education teaching methods during the global pandemic. The new trend now, is to move away from traditional in-class instruction to more hybrid strategies such as blended learning and flipped learning methods in both theoretical and clinical courses at the university level, across the globe, where it may be available. However, simulation and new technologies are still considered poor substitutes to actual live, face-to-face, doctor-patient interactions in which communication and practical skills are applied and refined.

9. Current medical education, ethical and legal issues

During the course of their study, medical students become aware of a wide array of ethical and legal issues which present learning opportunities on how to manage once they become licensed practitioners. In the literature, authors report that medical schools and residency programs expose medical students to common ethical issues that they may encounter in their future professional life [42]. However, schools and programs do not prepare graduates to adequately understand and deal with the legal or regulatory aspects of medical practice [43]. Some of the challenging, complex, and multidimensional ethical and legal issues in medical practice are how to understand and deal with insurance companies' modes of action, malpractice, patient safety, organ transplant, prescribing controlled substances, and licensure [43, 44]. Some authors have concluded that the current state of medical education does not prepare graduates to tactfully tackle ethical and legal issues that are prevalent in current medical practice and need to include courses that explore these issues in more details [45, 46].

10. Medical schools' curricula: mission and core values

A curriculum is a universally acknowledged course of study or training of an educational program [47]. All educational programs must have a set curriculum plan. In an introduction to highlight the importance of writing a curriculum in educational programs, Parkay, Anktil, and Hass [48] as cited in Iwasiw [47] offered a very relevant curriculum definition to the context of this chapter. This definition emphasizes a written plan that considers the theoretical and research aspects of the courses besides the social context such as the classroom experiences. "The curriculum is all of the educational experiences learners have in an educational program, the purpose of which is to achieve broad goals and related specific objectives that have been developed within a framework of theory and research, past and present professional practice, and the changing needs of society [47]. According to Simiao Li-Sauerwine and Andrew King [49], a curriculum is a map that can help both educators and learners to be oriented to the key elements of a curriculum and the role of each during the learning process [49].

A curriculum is composed of essential components that reflect its construction, purposes and outcomes. The principle component of the curriculum is a strategic plan that consists of a mission statement and a vision statement [50–53]. Campbell [54] defined a mission statement as a reflection of the institution's purpose, values, strategy and standards and behaviors. A mission statement is also described as defining the organization's scope of business operations/activities, provides a common purpose/direction, promotes a sense of shared expectations, and guides leadership styles [55].

A vision statement is a visual statement that describes where the organization wants to be in the future or what it hopes to achieve. Vision statements are broad and do not provide specific targets [56, 57].

The values statement, also called the code of ethics, provides a moral direction for the organization that guides decision making and establishes a standard for assessing actions. A value can act as an ultimate control system when there is a need for control [58, 59]. Although it is essential to have a vision and a value statement in a curriculum, we decided to exclude these components as they do little contribution to the aim of this discussion.

Having introduced the meanings and definitions of the core concepts in a curriculum plan, herein we discuss examples of mission statements of some medical schools as our guide to understand the current medical schools' programs and the focus of the educational programs run by some medical institutions.

In one statement, it is stated that the school's mission is "to improve the health of the community through a set of medical education, research and clinical care". The statement continues to put more focus on the provision of patient-centered 'medicine' that aims at preventing, diagnosing and treating illness. On the positive side, this statement includes 'the health of the community' and to 'preventing, diagnosing and treating illness' as elements of care that are parts of today's emphasis on primary health care, and it uses the concept of illness rather than disease in recognition of the subjective dimension of human's wellbeing. However, this statement falls short of recognizing the social contextual factors that perceives health as a 'whole' and places more emphasis on diagnosing and treating illnesses. Although community was the target of care management, the community or social structure were not recognized as factors contributing to illnesses and should be considered in preventing and diagnosing illnesses. Socio-cultural factors, economy, lifestyle, individual responses, and social support as contributing to illnesses were kept implicit in this statement.

In a second mission statement that aims "to improve human health through ..., and the delivery of outstanding patient-centered care", it is noted that human health is distinct for its social context, and the effect of the environment or the external influences. This is also emphasized when it singles out care as patient-centered ignoring the role of the community as a factor in influencing health and illness. In other words, there is no recognition of the clients as being a family, a larger community, and probably not having a disease, but having a social and psychological issue that needs to be tackled to prevent an illness as in primary care services.

In a third example of a medical school, the mission statement specifies clearly its graduate preparation by stating: "to educate health science professionals in biomedical and social sciences, and model the best practices in clinical care and public health". In this statement, we see the recognition and inclusion of social sciences and public health as part of the learning content material and context of care.

A fourth example of a stated medical school mission is from another region of the world. The mission has stated its aim as: "providing the society with qualified physicians that are capable of delivering quality healthcare services" at more than one level, that is the national, regional and international". In this statement, it has ignored the kind of service and the targeted people of this service, i.e., the individual client and the community. The focus of this mission is to prepare scientists that are specialized in higher studies and engaged in scientific research, and interacting with the world medical community". This mission statement is limited in identifying its target group, in its instructional strategies, and the kind of service provided by its graduates (bio-psycho-social). Many questions would be raised regarding the complexity and diversity of meeting the national, regional and the global needs in one single program. A major goal of the curriculum reformers is to produce physicians who can deliver an individualized plan of care that reflects the physician's mastery of basic anatomy and physiology, awareness of the best current evidence, skillful patient communication, and shared decision-making [43, 44].

A final and more comprehensive and holistic mission statement was that which stated, "nurturing a diverse, inclusive community that is dedicated to alleviating suffering and improving health and well-being for all through excellence in teaching and learning, discovery and scholarship, and service and leadership". In this statement, we captured more than one concept that recognized a more holistic and advanced meaning in the type of service and pedagogy in the program and the program's graduates. The statement recognizes "nurturing", "alleviate suffering", (and not treating disease), "improving health and well-being" (Well-being as more of a subjective nature of a definition of the health status). It also acknowledges a more active role of learners by identifying teaching and 'learning' excellence, besides adding other than the biomedical clinical skills by including discovery, scholarship and leadership.

With this analysis of a few examples of mission statements, although not many to make conclusions from, we think it is appropriate to reflect on the theoretical frames of the caring sciences explained earlier in this chapter. These frameworks set the floor for a more holistic caring approach that considers both the learners as active participants, and the teachers employing the most recent andragogy and sources of online, interactive, and blended learning strategies in the learning process. It is also central in today's medical caring professions to be more considerate of the bio-psycho-social aspects of care by the judicious use of the modern technological advancement of sciences within a contextual and global aspects of care.

11. Conclusion

Modern medical education has witnessed significant changes and developments throughout the past 30 years while retaining the core values and identity of the medical profession. These changes have taken on many forms represented in the shift from pedagogy to andragogy, as well as keeping up with the latest discoveries in medical sciences and technology and their applications. The rapid leaps in sciences, technology, and medical practice must not divert our track away from the humanistic sense of the profession in caring for patients, their families, and the community at large. Adopting and utilizing various educational philosophies; applying diverse learning theories and frameworks; establishing distinct mission and vision statements congruent with the relatively novel biopsychosocial medical model; and creating educational programs that focus on producing graduates that become practitioners who are guided by a holistic, interdisciplinary, and humanistic framework is the responsibility of the medical profession. Maintaining up-to-date status that is congruent with the everchanging world of sciences and technology in both medical education and practice remain a big challenge for many schools of medicine around the world.

Author details

Reema Safadi* and Lubna Abushaikha
Maternal and Child Health Department, School of Nursing, The University of Jordan, Jordan

*Address all correspondence to: r.safadi@ju.edu.jo

References

[1] History of medicine. [Internet]. Available from https://timelines.issarice.com/wiki/Timeline_of_medical_education#cite_note-History_of_Medicine-1 [Accessed: 2021-06-20]

[2] Brazier, Y. What was ancient Egyptian medicine like? MedicalNewsToday [Internet]. 2018. Available from: https://www.medicalnewstoday.com/articles/323633 [Accessed:2021-06-18]

[3] Miller, K. What is Ayurveda? 2021. Available from: https://www.webmd.com/balance/guide/ayurvedic-treatments. WebMD [Accessed: 2021-06-18]

[4] Lad, V. A brief introduction and guide. Available from: https://www.ayurveda.com/resources/articles/ayurveda-a-brief-introduction-and-guide [Accessed: 2021-06-28]

[5] Scarborough, Harold, Turner, Edward Lewis and Gregg, Alan. "Medical education". Encyclopedia Britannica, Available from: https://www.britannica.com/science/medical-education. [Accessed 2021-07-1]

[6] The Golden age of Islam. Khan Academy. Available from: https://www.khanacademy.org/humanities/world-history/medieval-times/cross-cultural-diffusion-of-knowledge/a/the-golden-age-of-islam [Accessed: 2021-07-07]

[7] Brazier, Yvette. November 9, 2018. Why was medieval Islamic medicine important? Available from: https://www.medicalnewstoday.com/articles/323612 [Accessed: 2021-06-28]

[8] Best medical degrees: "30 of the oldest medical schools in the world". *Available from:* https://www.bestmedicaldegrees.com/30-of-the-oldest-medical-schools-in-the-world/ Accessed: 2021-07-02]

[9] Clark, G. History Of The Royal College Of Physicians Of London. The British Medical Journal. 1965;1(5427), 79-82. Available from http://www.jstor.org/stable/25401681 [Accessed: 2021-07-14]

[10] Flexner, A. Medical Education in the United States and Canada: A Report to the Carnegie Foundation for the Advancement of Teaching. New York: Carnegie Foundation for the Advancement of Teaching; 1910.

[11] Slosar-Cheah, M. History in Medical Education and the Roots of Knowledge. 2016. Available from: HTTPS://WWW.THEATLANTIC.COM/MAGAZINE/ARCHIVE/1910/06/MEDICAL-EDUCATION-IN-AMERICA/306088/ [Accessed:2021-06-27]

[12] Alton, G. (nd). The history of medical education. Available from: https://www.theclassroom.com/history-american-medical-education-6292307.html

[13] Medical education in the United States and Canada: A report to the Carnegie Foundation for the Advancement of teaching, Bulletin Number four 1910 reproduced in 1972. Available from: https://centerforinquiry.org/wpcontent/uploads/sites/33/quackwatch/flexner_1910.pdf

[14] Gwee MCE, Samarasekera D, Chay-Hoon T. Role of Basic Sciences in 21st Century Medical Education: An Asian Perspective. International Association of Medical Science educations. 2010; 20(3) 299-306.

[15] Cooke M, Irby DM, Sullivan W, Ludmerer KM. American medical education 100 years after the Flexner report. New England Journal of Medicine. 2006; 28; 355(13):1339-44. DOI: 10.1056/NEJMra055445.

[16] Pawlina W. Basic Sciences in Medical Education: Why? How? When? Where? Medical Teacher 2009; 31: 787-789.

[17] Rajan TV. Making Medical Education Relevant. The Chronicle of Higher Education. 2006; 52:20 Available from: https://www.chronicle.com/article/making-medical-education-relevant/

[18] Yarnall R. The Value of an Education in the History of Medicine. In-training, the Agora of the medical student community. 2017. Available from: https://in-training.org/value-education-history-medicine-14177

[19] El-Moamly A.A. Medical Humanities in Education: Definition, History, Benefits, Challenges, Debates and Experiences of Medical Schools Around the World (Education in a Competitive and Globalizing World). 2007. Nova Science Publisher.

[20] Irby DM, Wilkerson L. Educational innovations in academic medicine and environmental trends. Journal of General Internal Medicine. 2003; 18(5):370-376. DOI: 10.1046/j.1525-1497.2003.21049.x.

[21] An AFMC project: The Association of faculties of Medicine of Canada. The Future of Medical Education in Canada: A Collective Vision for MD Education, An AFMC Project. 2009. Available from: https://www.afmc.ca/sites/default/files/pdf/2010-FMEC-MD_EN.pdf

[22] Riska E, Vinten-Johansen P. The involvement of the behavioral sciences in American Medicine: A historical perspective. International Journal of Health Services, 1981; 11 (4)583-595. DOI: 10.2190/W1P9-3HR6-U9E3-4JCW

[23] White, K. The Sage dictionary of health and society. London: Sage, 2006 ISBN: 9780761941163

[24] Cockerham W.C. 2021 The Social causes of health and diseases. 3rd ed. Cambridge: Polity; 2011.

[25] Porter R. The greatest benefit to mankind: a medical history of humanity. 1999. New York: Norton.

[26] McCoy L, Pettit RK, Kellar C, Morgan C. Tracking active learning in the medical school curriculum: A learning-centered approach. J Med Edu Curric Dev. 2018; 5:1-9. doi:10.1177/2382120518765135

[27] Jambi S, Khalifah AM, Fadel HT. Shifting from traditional lecturing to interactive learning in Saudi dental schools: How important is staff development? J Taibah Univ Medical Sci. 2015; 10(1):45-49. https://doi.org/10.1016/j.jtumed.2015.01.004

[28] Engel G. The clinical application of the biopsychosocial model. Am J Psychiatry. 1980; 137 (5), 535-544.

[29] Farre A, Rapley T. The new old (and old new) medical model: Four decades navigating the biomedical and psychosocial understandings of health and illness. Healthcare (Basel). 2017;5(4):88. doi: 10.3390/healthcare5040088.

[30] Smith MK. (1996, 1999, 2010) 'Andragogy', *the encyclopedia of informal* education. https://infed.org/mobi/andragogy-what-is-it-and-does-it-help-thinking-about-adult-learning/ [Accessed: 2021-07-16]

[31] Mukhalalati BA, Taylor A. Adult learning theories in context: A quick guide for healthcare professional educators. J Med Educ Curric Dev. 2019; 6:2382120519840332. doi: 10.1177/2382120519840332.

[32] Koponen J, Pyörälä E, Isotalus P. Communication skills for medical students: Results from three experiential methods. Simul. Gaming. 2014;

45(2):235-254. doi:10.1177/1046878114538915

[33] Ranjan P, Kumari A, Chakrawarty A. How can doctors improve their communication skills? JCDR. 2015;9 (3):JE01-JE04. DOI: 10.7860/jcdr/2015/12072.5712.

[34] Taveira-Gomes I, Mota-Cardoso R, Figueiredo-Braga M. Communication skills in medical students – An exploratory study before and after clerkships. Porto Biomed. 2016; 1(5), 173-180. https://doi.org/10.1016/j.pbj.2016.08.002.

[35] Ratelle JT, Sawatsky AP, Kashiwagi DT, Schouten WM, Erwin PJ, Gonzalo JD, Beckman TJ, West CP. Implementing bedside rounds to improve patient-centred outcomes: a systematic review. BMJ Qual Saf. 2019;28(4):317-326. doi: 10.1136/bmjqs-2017-007778.

[36] Todres M, Stephenson A, Jones R. Medical education research remains the poor relation. BMJ. 2007; 18:335(7615):333-5. doi: 10.1136/bmj.

[37] Ng CJ. Common ethical issues in research and publication. MFP. 2006;1(2&3):74-76.

[38] Abramson EL, Paul CR, Petershack J, Serwint J, Fischel JE, Rocha M, Treitz M, McPhillips H, Lockspeiser T, Hicks P, Tewksbury L, Vasquez M, Tancredi DJ, Li ST. Conducting Quantitative Medical Education Research: From Design to Dissemination. Acad Pediatr. 2018;18(2):129-139. doi: 10.1016/j.acap.2017.10.008.

[39] Sawatsky AP, Ratelle JT, Beckman TJ. Qualitative research methods in Medical Education. Anesthesiology. 2019;131(1):14-22. doi:10.1097/ALN.0000000000002728.

[40] van Diggele, C., Burgess, A., Roberts, C. *et al.* Leadership in healthcare education. BMC Med Educ. 2020; 20**:** 456. https://doi.org/10.1186/s12909-020-02288-x

[41] Kimura T, Kojo K, Shiga M, Chihara I, Ikeda A, Kandori S, Kojima T, Haruta J, Nishiyama H. Impact of early exposure to simulation program on undergraduate medical students' interest in urology. J Med Educ Curric Dev. 2021; 31:8:23821205211020750. doi: 10.1177/23821205211020750.

[42] Nandi PL, Chan JNF, Chan CPK, Chan P, Chan LPK. Undergraduate medical education: comparison of problem-based learning and conventional teaching. HKMJ. 2000; 6:301-306.

[43] Buja L.M. Medical education today: all that glitters is not gold. BMC Medical Education. 2019; 19, 110. https://doi.org/10.1186/s12909-019-1535-9

[44] Shelton PG, Corral I, Kyle B. Advancements in undergraduate medical education: meeting the challenges of an evolving world of education, healthcare and technology. Psychiatric Quarterly. 2016; 88: 225-234. DOI 10.1007/s11126-016-9471-x

[45] Shah N.D. The teaching of law in medical education. AMA J Ethics, 2008;10(5):332-337. doi: 10.1001/virtualmentor.2008.10.5.oped1-0805.

[46] Kadivar M, Manookian A, Asghari F, Niknafs N, Okazi A, Zarvani A. Ethical and legal aspects of patient's safety: a clinical case report. J Med Ethics Hist Med. 2017; 10:15.

[47] Iwasiw C.L, AndrusysZyn M, Goldenberg D. Curriculum development in nursing education. 4thed. Massachusetts: Jones and Bartlett; 2020.

[48] Parkay F.W, Anctil E.J, Hass G. Curriculum leadership: readings for developing quality educational

programs. 10^{th}ed. Upper Saddle River, NJ: Prentice Hall; 2014.

[49] Li-Sauerwine S, King A. Curriculum Development: Foundations and Modern Advances in Graduate Medical Education. DOI: 10.5772/intechopen.

[50] Bart C. Exploring the application of mission statements on the World Wide Web. Internet Research, 2001; 11(4), 360-369. https://doi.org/10.1108/10662240110402812

[51] Cady S.H, Wheeler J.V, Brodke M, De Wolf J.J. Mission, Vision, and Values: What Do They Say? Organization Development Journal. 2011; 29(1): 63-78.

[52] Meacham J. Gaff J. Learning Goals in Mission Statements: Implications for Educational Leadership. Liberal Education. 2006; 92(1) 6-13.

[53] Niall C. Hegarty, N.C, Silliman B.R. How to approach teaching philosophy statements as career mission statements. Journal of Business and Educational Leadership. 2016; 6(1): 103-114.

[54] Campbell A. Does your organization need a mission? Leadership & Organization Development Journal. 1989; 10(3): 3-9. https://doi.org/10.1108/EUM0000000001134

[55] Baetz M.C, Bart C.K. Developing Mission Statements Which Work. Long Range Planning. 1996; 29(4): 526-533. https://doi.org/10.1016/0024-6301(96)00044-1

[56] Cortés-Sánchez J.D. Mission statements of universities worldwide -Text mining and visualization Intangible Capital IC. 2018; 14(4): 584-603 https://doi.org/10.3926/ic.1258

[57] Principles of Management (Lumen), LibreTexts, State University of New York OER Services Principles of management; Mission, vision and values, 2018: (https://courses.lumenlearning.com/wm-principlesofmanagement/chapter/reading-mission-vision-and-values/)

[58] Poorchangizi B, Borhani F, Abbaszadeh A. et al. The importance of professional values from nursing students' perspective. BMC Nursing. 2019; 18:26. https://doi.org/10.1186/s12912-019-0351-1

[59] Verma H. V. Mission statements: A study of intent and influence. Journal of Services Research. 2009; 9(2): 153-172.

Chapter 16

Learning through Art in Medical Education

Vincenza Ferrara

Abstract

Medical Humanities approach is becoming an important action in the health curriculum. Art can play a central role in the training of care staff for the development of skills and for the humanization of the therapeutic path. The application of art as a tool for learning and its historical relationship with medicine can be a valid support for the development of skills such as observation, active listening, problem solving and empathy, useful for improving the profession and the relationship with the patient. It is possible to rediscover the link between art, medicine, and care to help health professionals to improve their activities and resilience. Particular methods such as that of the Visual Thinking Strategies (VTS) can help health students and professionals to become better actors in the care context.

Keywords: medical humanities, skills, visual art, resilience, health curriculum

1. Introduction

This contribution introduces the Medical Humanities approach to the health sector. Medical Humanities constitute an approach to care using the "human sciences" as a tool to improve skills and abilities and to limit the stress of care professionals and operators.

A useful discipline in this context is related to cultural heritage, as all artistic objects can be "places" of observation and "mirror" of one's knowledge and skills, becoming tools for learning and well-being. In particular, we will refer to experiences in the medical education sector that uses visual art.

Going deeper into the topic, we can realize, for example, how art and medicine have been integrated for centuries. It is enough to go far back in time to find examples transmitted by artistic objects to understand, as a whole, the importance of the solid relationship between medicine and the visual arts.

Art can therefore lead us, through its observation, to understand the anatomy represented or the reality of the cure, in fact, over the centuries, it has become a witness to illness, death, and healing activities. In the care sector, there are many references to art as therapy and many studies that show psycho-physiological evidence of the positive effects that artistic practice and its use can have on the person for the promotion of well-being and health.

For some years, the humanities and in particular, arts have also been used for the development of skills in learning environments. One of these sectors is that of basic and permanent training in the area of care (medicine, health professions) and more generally in the area of health in which Human Sciences have been introduced for the application of innovative models for the development of useful skills. This approach is referred to as Medical Humanities.

We will therefore try to describe the opportunity that the visual arts and pedagogical methodologies can offer to the field of medical education for the development of skills and abilities to improve the work of health professionals, increase resilience, and promote their well-being.

2. Art and medicine

As a result of reading history, we can be aware of how much art and medicine have remained integrated for centuries. It is enough to go far back in time to find examples transmitted by artistic objects to understand, as a whole, the importance of the solid relationship between medicine and visual arts starting from when in ancient Greece, which can be considered the cradle of our modern culture, the anatomists asked the artists for help to understand the human body. In fact, at that time, dissection was practiced on the bodies of animals, while it was forbidden to explore human anatomy for social and religious reasons.

Respect for the body of the deceased on the one hand and the consideration of the corpse as a source of impurity on the other had meant that the conditions were not created for carrying out this type of investigation. Even after 1241, the year of the edict of Frederick II which authorized, and indeed stimulated, the use of dissection of corpses, the anatomical investigation was accompanied throughout its path by the activity of artists who have put their skills at the service of scientific studies and of the representation of the human body, which needed scientific investigation to be able to fully express itself.

The practice of observation and the in-depth study of shapes allowed them to reproduce the muscles in a way that exactly correspond to anatomical science and often in the sculptures we can look at muscle groups portrayed in the act of participating in the movement of the body as a whole.

Art can therefore lead us, through its observation, to understand the anatomy represented or the reality of the cure; in fact, over the centuries, it has become a witness to illness, death, and healing activities. Through art it is possible to have evidence of missing pathologies and diseases useful for study, as the Italian doctor, G. Franceschini already wrote about it in 1906, who suggested that "Even the saddest and most painful sides of human life... have been... subject of study by artists, and how even the most pitiful and repulsive sciences of medicine have snatched from the creative brush of the passionate craftsman, pulsating works of life, truth, sentiment. And since beauty is the splendor of truth, it can be said that even the crudest truths of human pathology, clothed in the splendors of art from a skillful hand of craftsman, contributed to the creation of beauty, with sublime works of painting and sculpture" [1].

Art is also a representation of reality and can present itself as a "mirror" for the viewer who can understand emotions and knowledge of activities and meanings related to their personal experiences. Art, as experience, has often guided the pedagogical studies to be used as a tool to develop innovative educational methods [2].

The cognitive reaction to the processes of creation and use of the artistic image can determine knowledge. Starting from this concept, we can understand, first of all, why the observation of art can stimulate us to consider more than one interpretation and therefore more than one possible solution to a single question. Important in this area is the research of R. Arnheim. It explains the connection between visual perception and thought. "Identifying what we see is an act of knowledge," Arnheim tells us according to the psychology of perception [3]. When we look at something, mechanisms of understanding are rapidly implemented to recognize and grasp the sense of what is placed before our eyes. Furthermore, thanks to visual stimuli, thoughts and skills to solve problems are automatically set in motion. The careful observation of a work of art activates, in an almost instinctive way, multiple reasoning capable to achieve logical and analytical solutions, thanks to the multiple intelligences useful for cognitive development, including, mostly, the visual-spatial one [4].

In the care sector, there are many references to art as therapy and many studies that show psycho-physiological evidence of the positive effects that artistic practice and its use can have on the person for the promotion of well-being and health.

The role of visual arts and their usefulness, both for therapy and for the promotion of well-being and for the development of clinical skills, is highlighted by the report of the European section of the World Health Organization [5]. Furthermore, exposure to arts or exercising artistic activities can be "therapeutic," lowering cortisol levels and therefore limiting stress [6, 7].

3. Learning through art

For some years, the humanities, specially the arts, have also been used for the development of skills in learning environments. One of these sectors is that of basic and continuing medical education in the area of care (medicine, health professions) and more generally of the health sector in which for several years the Human Sciences have been introduced. These disciplines have been applied in innovative learning models for the development of skills useful to the care profession for building a Medical Humanities approach. Recent studies have shown how activities related to the arts can help; for example, medical students have benefitted from such activities to develop a certain type of skills and, moreover, to limit the risk of stress and burnout during the years of clinical practice [8].

It should be noted that already in 1948, the Constitution of the World Health Organization gave an alternative definition of health to that considered by the biomedical model: "A state of complete physical, social and mental well-being, and not only the 'absence of disease or infirmity..." [9], and subsequently describing health promotion in the Ottawa charter: "Health is considered not so much an abstract condition as a means aimed at an objective which, in operational terms, can be considered a resource that allows people to lead a productive life on an individual, social and economic level. Health is a resource for daily life and not the purpose of existence. It is a positive concept that enhances social and personal resources, as well as physical abilities" [10].

This holistic vision of health led to the research and definition of a new bio-psycho-social approach applied to the medical and health area with the assumption that every health condition or disease is the consequence of the interaction between biological, psychological, and social. In addition, the basic methodological triad for the clinical trial is defined consisting of observation (external vision), introspection (internal vision), and dialog (interview) and these ultimately render the patient's data as scientific [11].

We can therefore talk to extend the concept of health about "global well-being."

This approach places the patient at the center of the treatment process and solicits the doctor or health professional to review his preparation in order to face the knowledge of the disease in a holistic context trying to improve "The medical gaze", the so-called clinical eye considered the "semiological ability to use the senses to produce the diagnosis of a disease." The skills and abilities useful in this context are therefore linked to soft skills, teamwork, understanding the other through empathy and self-care of the health worker to limit the stress that this type of activity can feed. Among the activities useful for the development of skills we also find pedagogical methods that use the arts and in particular the visual arts. Regarding the adoption of these methods in medical and health education, a lot of scientific literature can be found indicating growing evidence that traits associated with empathy, for example, can be cultivated and taught through guided observation of works of visual art [12]. In addition, visual arts help in the development of clinical skills, including the observation, analysis, and communication of visual information. Representational art allows students to focus on identifying recognizable shapes and contextual information, while abstract art encourages the development of pattern recognition skills and greater tolerance of ambiguity with the freedom to follow one's imagination and emotion. Also in Italy, the introduction of pedagogical methods that use visual art as a tool for improving certain skills and abilities in the field of Medical Education is being experimented with positive results [13].

An important element in this context is training for all those who work to improve the relations between professional care and patients. Important skills are those related to collaborative work, communication, and empathy. Being empathetic, patient-centered, compassionate, humble, and respectful is essential for healthcare professionals to deliver holistic care. Another important activity to practice is to facilitate useful strategies for limiting stress and burnout in operators with a decrease in empathy and observation and analysis skills starting from basic training to continuing education. Furthermore, an important skill is that related to critical thinking to keep an open mind, self-awareness and respect and appreciation of different points of view that make each situation and patient experience unique [14].

4. Art practice and medical education

The art works represent the moods, the relational dynamics, and the emotions that can be learned and recognized through exercise. Some collaborative activities related to the observation of a work of art can also help to change the approach with the other and therefore with the patient and his family.

One of the methods that use artistic images and which has been applied for years in the United States and experimented in Italy for basic and continuing training in the medical and health area is Visual Thinking Strategies (VTS). VTS originated in 1988 from the integration of the research of the cognitive psychologist Abigail Housen and Philip Yenawine educator at the Museum of Modern Art in New York [15, 16].

This structured method for involving museum visitors becomes an important tool for learning in school and an important activity in the medical and health education sector [17]. The practice of VTS takes place in small groups, in front of a work of art, considered equal for basic knowledge and culture. An experienced facilitator will use only three questions to lead the discussion. It is important to listen to the opinions of others, as everyone will be able to enrich their point of view, creating a collective consciousness.

The questions are as follows: What is going on in this picture? What do you see that makes you say that? What else can you find?

It is therefore important that the observations and opinions of the participants are always substantiated by visual elements. This apparently simple step activates cognitive mechanisms for recognizing reality on the basis of one's previous experiences.

The experience of observing the image with the VTS method stimulates the awareness of how perception works: at the beginning, we have an overview, we identify details that, based on our knowledge and experience, lead us to an elaboration of the information perceived by assigning a certain meaning, the subsequent observation and listening to other possible interpretations, based on new details or the same decoded in a different way, lead us to a further elaboration and assignment of meaning, thus activating a problem-solving process. This experience also suggests that we need to take time in front of an image to understand its meaning. This exercise makes us reflect on the multiple interpretations that the same image can suggest; in fact, if we are based on previous knowledge and experiences, the same image can be understood and therefore described differently by each participant, thus learning to accept the ambiguity of the perception related to our knowledge and that of others. This exercise helps us to develop divergent thinking at the basis of creativity. Group discussion also allows to improve communication and listening skills.

In summary, we can list a series of objectives and purposes that have emerged in the various studies conducted on VTS related to the medical and health profession:

a. Improve observation and clinical reasoning skills, or better understand the clinical scenario (patient and social context).

b. Improve communication skills, fundamental skills in the work of the doctor and nurse and more generally of the health professional, both in the relationship with the patient and family members, and with colleagues.

c. Encourage critical thinking and problem solving, which in clinical practice translate into a guide to choose the best solution for the patient.

d. Promote empathy, which is fundamental in the relationship of care with the patient.

e. Express oneself freely; this is especially important for students, as it improves the quality of learning.

f. Improve the tolerance of ambiguity, that is, get used to the diversity of the individual and the individuality of responses to treatment.

g. Improve interpersonal skills and therefore group work.

An interesting analogy that we can focus on is that between the modality of discussion in small groups that the VTS stimulates in front of a work of art and the visits or meetings organized with the care team during which doctors present, discuss, and plan for patient health with students' request for hypothesis with experts acting as mentors and facilitators to guide discussion and formulate a care plan [18].

These activities with art can be very useful for improving the skills such as observation, problem solving, and critical thinking. In this context, the clinical observation, which includes the identification of data, the recognition of patterns in the collected data, and the interpretation and re-reading of the same, is the basis of the complex decision-making process of the doctor, through which he collects data, achieves the conclusions and chooses the most suitable therapy.

The skills of problem solving and critical thinking are also considered key and fundamental skills in the care sector, and art can help in their development. This arrangement is linked to the essence of the artistic artifact: the work of art can be defined as a "text" open to multiple levels of reading and the information it offers can be correlated with each other even if with a different meaning, as they can be represented as conceptual nodes of a hypertext that is configured while the perception continues to be applied with the identification of new details and therefore with the elaboration of new contents starting from the attributed meanings. In relation to the development of Critical Thinking, we find an interesting example that represents a useful collaboration between the cultural sector and medicine. Ohio State University College of Medicine (OSUCOM), in partnership with the Columbus Museum of Art (CMA), during the 2010–2011 academic year conducted an innovative experience for medical students who applied the analysis of works of art using observation supported by a column on critical thinking combined with a group discussion called "Art of Analysis." The critical thinking column is called "ODIP", an acronym for "observe, describe, interpret, and demonstrate." The goals of the Art of Analysis (AoA) are to encourage critical thinking skills, generate empathy, create a foundation for cooperative outcomes, increase students' tolerance for ambiguity, and improve the observation skills of junior doctors. This activity includes a form that suggests activating an observation, a description, an interpretation and a test, stimulating the students to learn to collect information objectively, to identify different possible interpretations to choose the best one based on evidence and therefore to implement a problem solving and critical thinking process [19]. Another fundamental skill for doctors and care staff is empathy. The term empathy derives from the Greek word "εμπαθεία" (> en and patheo, that is "inside" and "feel" = "feel inside", "put yourself in the other's shoes"); it indicated the emotional relationship of participation that bound the author-cantor to his audience. The term "empathy" has been equated with the German "Einfühlung", coined by the philosopher Robert Vischer at the end of the nineteenth century and only later it was translated into the English term "empathy." Vischer also defined for the first time the specific meaning of esthetic sympathy, or the feeling, not otherwise definable, that one feels in front of a work of art.

Vischer conceived this term as the ability to feel inside and to allow, that is, to perceive the external nature, as internal, belonging to our own body. It therefore represents the ability to project feelings from us to others and to the things we perceive [20].

In the human sciences, empathy designates an attitude toward others characterized by a commitment to understanding the other, excluding any personal affective attitude (sympathy, antipathy) and any moral judgment. Fundamental in this context was the discovery of mirror neurons by the research group of Prof. G. Rizzolatti. It is a particular class of cells that are activated both when a person performs an action and when he sees him doing, thus allowing us to understand what others are doing or feeling. It is therefore a fundamental mechanism not only for learning through imitation, but also to make the observer participates in the emotions of others or rather recognize the state of the other [21]. It is now clear that we cannot ignore taking care of the whole person to treat his illness and therefore empathy is considered essential for a good doctor-patient relationship. Also, for this type of ability, the work of art can be a valid tool for understanding the complexity of human nature. In particular, courses based on the observation of art have been shown to help students be more aware of emotions, their role in medicine, and to express empathy.

An interesting example concerns the program of the course for medical students of the Weill Cornell Medical College in collaboration with the Frick Collection art museum of New York published in 2001. The program included the examination of the portraits of the museum by students with the help of experts of art and by doctors according to indications that they had to replicate with photographs of the faces of patients. This activity is useful not only to improve observation skills but also to learn to understand the different states mood and the different emotions of the faces developing a greater emotional awareness [22].

A capacity whose concept was defined not so long ago is the Tolerance of Ambiguity.

Intolerance to ambiguity, or aversion to ambiguity, was first identified more than 50 years ago. It has been described as a personality trait in which "new, complex or insoluble" situations are perceived as "sources of threat." Given that the field of medicine and healthcare can be characterized by novelty, complexity, and sometimes insolubility, it is extremely important to understand how clinicians, and others, react to such circumstances. In general, individuals with high tolerance for ambiguity are attracted or fascinated by the unknown. Conversely, those with low tolerance tend to deny, avoid, or minimize ambiguity and experience significant stress on account of it. In medical practice, low tolerance of ambiguity is associated with the biomedical model rather than a bio-psycho-social vision of care [23].

The increase in the intolerance of ambiguity can be associated with stress [24]. Yet studies indicate that medical students or healthcare staff may feel uncomfortable with ambiguity. The use of Medical Humanities and in particular art can help improve this ability.

Another important practice that uses art is icono-diagnosis, which can help in learning a correct diagnosis process. The concept of icono-diagnosis was introduced in 1983 by A. Pontius, a psychiatrist at Harvard University, committed to demonstrate the ancient presence of Crouzon syndrome in the Cook archipelago, examining the features of the statues found in these islands [25]. In recent years, several doctors such as V. Franco, pathologist of the University of Palermo [26] or F.J. Barbado bring their students to the Prado Museum for a "medical examination" to the artworks exposed [27]. The enormous talent of the great masters of painting allows only by looking at a portrait to imagine the thoughts of this person and his state of mind. With our didactic activity, however, we can go further, and by observing carefully, know more intimate details such as; a disease that may have plagued the person, their past history and their wishes. For example, always with careful observation, a spot on the skin, a knot in the neck or a strange formation in the fingers can show signs of specific pathologies. These can be traced back to the models that have been immortalized and confirm our theoires with other historical sources. Thus, through this practice, it is possible to "train" the clinical eye. It allows also to rewrite the history of the people portrayed or of the artists. An Italian study published in the Journal of the Royal Society of Medicine analyzed three portraits of Michelangelo, arguing that the joints of the artist's left hand were almost certainly affected by arthrosis, a disease that would have affected Michelangelo at the end of the seventh decade of his life. In the details of the portraits, we can see the nodules precisely, the typical deformities of arthrosis, the diagnosis of which offers a plausible explanation for Michelangelo's loss of dexterity in old age and also underlines his victory over the disease. The continuous and intense work would have helped the artist to maintain the use of his hands as long as possible [28]. There are several studies that are represented in the scientific literature and that give us an idea of how to use a multidisciplinary team for research on particular pathologies and offer students suggestions for the development of clinical skills [29–31].

This brief description can give an idea of how art and medicine have a lot in common and how one can support the other. As you will see, art can promote the development of skills useful to doctors and medicine can help in understanding the history of the characters and communities represented but also be able to rewrite the history of art by suggesting other visions.

The experimentation of art as a tool in medical education is being carried out in many different countries. In Italy, at the Sapienza University of Rome, a special course that applies art practice was introduced in the curriculum of medicine and nursing. From the 2014–2015 academic year, a Sapienza research group began experimenting this type of activities and currently the Laboratory of Art and Medical Humanities has been developed to coordinate art courses for the training of physicians and nursing and healthcare operators and continues in the context of study and research in this sector. The results were very interesting; even the activities organized in distance learning in the pandemic period were effective [32]. These courses are acquiring a curricular character with positive qualitative and quantitative results in line with those presented by the international literature of the sector.

These experiences also led to the validation of a useful grid to measure the improvement of some of the skills previously mentioned after participating in the proposed discussion and art production activities [33]. Other experiences in other countries reported the positive results obtained by adopting this useful evaluation system [34].

Other experiences in the field of continuing education, always in the health sector, have found a positive welcome by the attendants. In the United States, the use of works of art has become an approach used in the care sector by many universities to involve medical students, residents, doctors, and nurses in an innovative learning process. Medical schools are expanding their educational programs by collaborating with local art museums [35]. In Italy too, an experimentation linked to the activities applied in the United States is underway.

The last notation that is considered important to report is the one that is linked to these experiences carried out at a distance in period of COVID pandemic with extremely positive results in the various areas in which they have been applied—university environment, groups connected to palliative care, patients in psychotherapy, in distance teaching.

These experiences have helped to raise awareness of how much arts, and in this case visual art, can be a valuable tool for developing to upgrade useful skills and abilities in the care sector and improve the state of well-being of professionals in the medicine and healthcare field.

Author details

Vincenza Ferrara
Faculty of Pharmacy and Medicine, Sapienza University, Rome, Italy

*Address all correspondence to: vincenza.ferrara@uniroma1.it

References

[1] Franceschini G. La Patologia umana nell'arte. EMPORIUM. 1906;**24**(144): 424-448

[2] Dewey J. In: Boydston JA, editor. Art as Experience in Later Works of John Dewey, 1925-1953. Vol. 10. Carbondale: Southern Illinois University Press; 1987

[3] Arnheim R. Visual Thinking. Berkeley: University of California Press; 1969

[4] Gardner H. Frames of Mind. The Theory of Multiple Intelligences. New York: Basic Books; 2011

[5] Report 67. What is the evidence on the role of the arts in improving health and well-being? A scoping review (2019). World Health Organization, WHO Regional Office for Europe, WHO Europe. 2019. Available from: https://apps.who.int/iris/bitstream/handle/10665/329834/9789289054553-eng.pdf [Accessed: 17 May 2021]

[6] Grossi E, Tavano Blessi G, Sacco PL. Magic moments: Determinants of stress relief and subjective wellbeing from visiting a cultural heritage site. Culture, Medicine and Psychiatry. 2019;**43**(1): 4-24. DOI: 10.1007/s11013-018-9593-8

[7] Bolwerk A, Mack-Andrick J, Lang FR, Dörfler A, Maihöfner C. How art changes your brain: Differential effects of visual art production and cognitive art evaluation on functional brain connectivity. PLOS One. 2014;**9**(7):e101035

[8] Mangione S, Chakraborti C, Staltari G, Harrison R, Tunkel AR, Liou KT, Cerceo E, Voeller M, Bedwell WL, Fletcher K, et al., Medical students' exposure to the humanities correlates with positive personal qualities and reduced burnout: A multi-institutional U.S. survey. J Journal of General Internal Medicine. 2018;**33**:628-634.

[9] Constitution of the World Health Organization. Available from: https://www.who.int/about/governance/constitution [Accessed: 17 May 2021]

[10] Ottawa Charter. 1986. Available from: https://www.who.int/teams/health-promotion/enhanced-wellbeing/first-global-conference [Accessed: 17 May 2021]

[11] Engel GL. The need for a new medical model (a challenge for biomedicine). Science. 1977; **196**:129-136

[12] Mukunda N, Moghbeli N, Rizzo A, Niepold S, Bassett B, Delisser HM. Visual art instruction in medical education: A narrative review. Medical Education Online. 2019;**24**:1558657. DOI: 10.1080/10872981.2018.1558657

[13] Ferrara V, De Santis S, Manicone F, Martinino A, Consorti F. The visual art as a lerning tool in medical education. Senses and Sciences. 2020;**7**(2): 1028-1040

[14] Zazulak J, Halgren C, Tan M, Grierson LE. The impact of an arts-based programme on the affective and cognitive components of empathic development. Medical Humanities. 2015;**41**:69-74

[15] Housen A. Aesthetic thought, critical thinking and transfer. Arts Learn Res J. 2001;**18**(1):99-132.

[16] Yenawine, P. *Visual thinking strategies: Using art to deepen thinking across school disciplines*. Cambridge, MA: Harvard Education Press; 2013.

[17] Agarwal GG, McNulty M, Santiago KM, Torrents H, Caban-Martinez AJ. Impact of visual thinking strategies (VTS) on the analysis of

clinical images: A pre-post study of VTS in first-year medical students. The Journal of Medical Humanities. 2020; **41**(4):561-572. DOI: 10.1007/s10912-020-09652-4

[18] Polianski IJ, Fangerau H. Toward harder medical humanities: Moving beyond the two cultures dichotomy. Academic Medicine. 2012;**87**:121-126

[19] Jacques A, Trinkley R, Stone L, Tang R, Hudson WA, Khandelwal S. Art of analysis: A cooperative program between a museum and medicine. Journal for Learning through the Arts. 2012;**8**:1-10. Available from: http://www.escholarship.org/uc/item/36n2t2w9

[20] Vischer R. Über das optische Formgefühl. Ein Beitrag zur Ästhetik. Leipzig: Herman Credner [English edition: On the Optical Sense of Form: a Contribution to Aesthetics. In: Mallgrave, HF, Ikonomou E, editors. Empathy, form, and space: Problems in german aesthetics. 1873-1893. Santa Monica, California: Getty Center for the History of Art and the Humanities; 1994. pp 89-123.

[21] Iacoboni M, Molnar-Szakacs I, Gallese V, Buccino G, Mazziotta JC, Rizzolatti G. Grasping the intentions of others with one's own mirror neuron system. PLOS Biology. 2005;**3**(3):e79

[22] Bardes CL, Gillers D, Herman AE. Learning to look: Developing clinical observation skills at an art museum. Medical Education. 2001;**35**:1157-1161

[23] Geller G. Tolerance for ambiguity: An ethics based criterion for medical student selection. Academic Medicine. 1990;**88**(5):581-584

[24] Iannello P, Mottini A, Tirelli S, Riva S, Antonietti A. Ambiguity and uncertainty tolerance, need for cognition, and their association with stress. A study among Italian practicing physicians. Medical Education Online. 2017;**22**(1):1-10

[25] Pontius A. Icono-diagnosis: A medical humanistic approach, detecting Crouzon's malformation in Cook Islands' prehistoric art. Perspectives in Biology and Medicine. 1983;**27**:107-120

[26] Franco V. Icono-diagnosis: A challenge between medicine and art. Senses and Sciences. 2019;**6**(2):747-752

[27] Barbado Hernández FJ. Una visita médica a Las Meninas. El dentista del siglo XXI. 2015;**5**:30-34

[28] Lazzeri D, Castello MF, Matucci-Cerinic M, Lippi D, Weisz GM. Osteoarthritis in the hands of Michelangelo Buonarroti. Journal of the Royal Society of Medicine. 2016; **109**(5):180-183

[29] Sterpetti AV, Fiori E, De Cesare A. Goiter in the Art of Renaissance Europe. Am J Med. 2016 Aug;**129**(8):892-895. DOI: 10.1016/j.amjmed.2016.04.015. Epub 2016 May 3. PMID: 27154774.

[30] Ruggieri M, Gentile AE, Ferrara V, Papi M, Praticò AD, Mudry A, et al. Neurocutaneous syndromes in art and antiquities. American Journal of Medical Genetics. Part C; 2021;**187**(2): 224-234. DOI: 10.1002/ajmg.c.31917

[31] Toriello H. Literature review: Genetic conditions or anomalies in artworks. American Journal of Medical Genetics. Part C; 2021;**187**(2):111-121. DOI: 10.1002/ajmg.c.31886

[32] Ferrara V. L'arte come strumento per la formazione in area medica e sanitaria. 2020. Roma, Aracne

[33] Ferrara V, De Santis S, MelchioriI FM. Art for improving skills in medical education: The validation of a scale for measuring the visual thinking strategies method. La Clinica Terapeutica. 2020;**171**(3):e253-e259. ISSN 1972-6007

[34] Agarwal GG, McNulty M. Santiago impact of visual thinking strategies

(VTS) on the analysis of clinical images: A pre-post study of VTS in first-year medical students. The Journal of Medical Humanities. 2020;**41**:561-572

[35] Art and medicine resources. UT Dallas University. Available from https://arthistory.utdallas.edu/medicine/ [Accessed: 17 May 2021]

Chapter 17

Contemporary Medical Education: Revolution versus Evolution

Louis Maximilian Buja

Abstract

Contemporary and traditional approaches to undergraduate medical education (UME) and graduate medical education (GME) are compared and differences are highlighted. A case is made that the contemporary medical education system is being subject to the downside of disruptive innovation with unintended and potentially detrimental long-term outcomes for academic medicine and clinical practice. The impact on various constituencies is discussed. Proposed solutions are presented. The challenges for education of the best possible physicians are daunting but must be met to honor the social contract between medicine and society.

Keywords: medical education, basic science, pathology, integrated curriculum, traditional curriculum

1. Introduction

The standard medical educational system during most of the twentieth century was developed in response to the 1910 Flexner report and has served as a successful template for the development of generations of physicians [1]. Yet the new millennium has ushered in major changes that have constituted a revolution in undergraduate medical education (UME) and graduate medical education (GME) [2–4]. Measured change has been supplanted by disruptive innovation with the risk of unintended consequences and potentially detrimental long-term outcomes for academic medicine and clinical practice [1, 5]. This critique is based on the author's experiences over a long career as a physician-scientist engaged in medical education, translational research and clinical practice of autopsy and cardiovascular pathology, and as an academician who also has held several academic leadership positions.

2. The past century in medical education

Traditional medical education has been shaped by guiding principles formulated by Abraham Flexner and William Osler early in the twentieth century. In his seminal 1910 report, Flexner stated that medical schools should be university based, have minimum admission requirements, implement a rigorous curriculum with applied laboratory and clinical science content, and have faculty actively engaged in research. Osler developed a system of bedside teaching which emphasized medical students learning clinical medicine from direct encounters with patients under the guidance of faculty clinicians. The insights of Flexner and

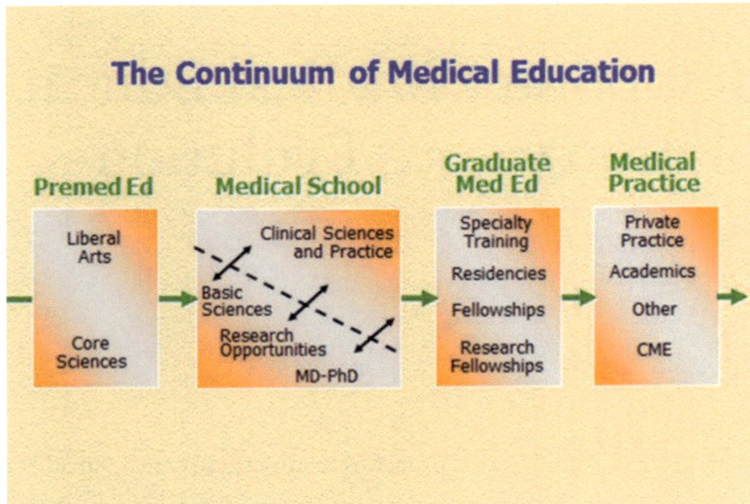

Figure 1.
Diagram presenting the continuum of medical education including a traditional approach to undergraduate medical education modified to provide progressive integration of basic biomedical sciences and clinical disciplines.

Osler resulted in the establishment of a model of medical education with two key components or pillars, namely, the basic or foundational sciences and the clinical sciences [1]. The two-pillar model of medical education served as the basis for a four-year UME curriculum comprising biomedical science courses in the pre-clinical years and clinical clerkships in the clinical years. Over the years, thoughtful analysis has brought about modifications to promote integration of the two components (**Figure 1**). Medical schools utilizing this construct produced scientifically grounded and clinically skilled physicians as well as a subset who pursued successful careers as physician-scientists and academicians.

3. The new curriculum and competency-based education

Yet, in response to criticisms of the traditional system and changes in the health-care landscape, sweeping changes have been launched in UME and GME with the goal of producing physicians "fit for the twenty-first century" who are adept in functioning in ever changing health care delivery systems [2–4]. The post-Flexnerian UME is based on the so-called fully integrated spiral curriculum encompassing both horizontal and vertical integration across time and across disciplines (**Figure 2**) [6].

The fully integrated UME curriculum resulting from the redesign eliminates a distinct focus on the critically important pre-clinical, basic medical sciences as a foundation for the clinical clerkships. Health Systems Science encompassing diverse topics including population health and interdisciplinary care now is included as a co-equal to basic and clinical sciences. The emphasis is on developing skills in modern clinical reasoning and decision-making and on the demonstration of "competencies" rather than cognitive knowledge. The result of these initiatives has been a loss of a significant amount of time and emphasis on the basic biomedical sciences in the curriculum. The new post-Flexnerian paradigm fits the definition of disruptive innovation. Innovation is a driver of progress, but disruptive innovation is prone to risks and unintended consequences [5].

In the United States, standards for UME and GME are set by the Liaison Committee for Medical Education (LCME), and its sponsoring institutions, the

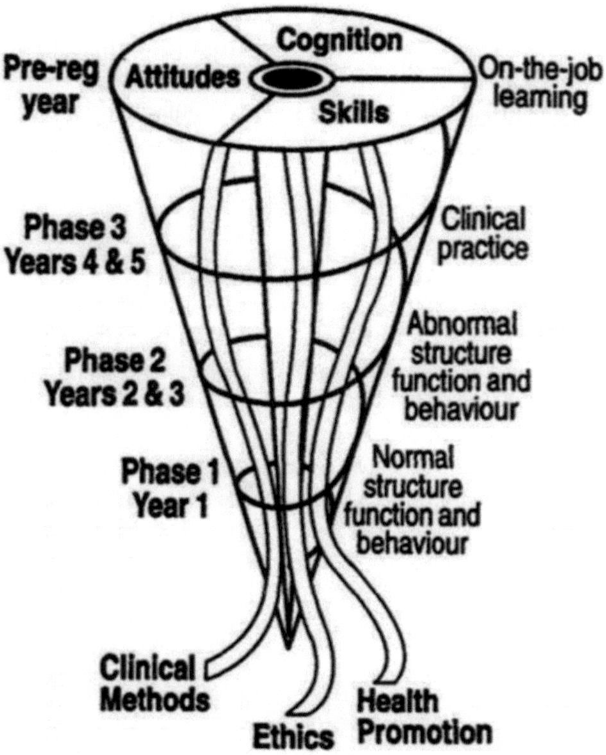

Figure 2.
Diagram presenting the concept of a fully or spirally integrated curriculum including simultaneous vertical and horizontal integration. The complexities in realizing this model are considerable, as reflected in the diagram.

American Association of Medical Colleges (AAMC) and the American Medical Association (AMA), and the Accreditation Council for Graduate Medical Education (ACGME). Regulatory bodies in other countries have had similar roles. Curriculum reformers have used actual and perceived expectations of the LCME and ACGME to drive curriculum revision.

The movement toward outcomes and competency-based education in UME follows innovations in GME, which the Accreditation Council for Graduate Medical Education (ACGME) to implement the six competencies as key elements in residency training programs [3, 4]. These competencies relate to patient care, medical knowledge, interpersonal and communication skills, professionalism and practice-based learning and improvement. The ACGME has moved further along the path of competency-based training with the introduction of milestones as a focus of the new accreditation system (NAS). Competencies also have been linked to Entrustable Professional Activities (EPA). Other concepts under discussion include an accelerated three-year UME program and/or time variable criteria for the granting of the medical degree as well as certification in medical specialties following a period of graduate training.

4. Critique

4.1 Paradoxes

The fully integrated, competency focused curriculum for UME and GME is promoted as the optimal approach to produce physicians with skills in modern clinical reasoning and diagnostic and therapeutic decision making. Yet, the solid grounding in the basic biomedical sciences required for high level clinical reasoning and decision making has been diminished. Also, deterioration in history taking and physical examination skills of medical trainees has occurred over the last twenty years contemporaneously with the implementation of the new curriculum [7].

4.2 Unintended consequences and downsides

The paradigm shift in medical education is based on the premise that changes in the healthcare system and in medical practice in the clinic and hospital have outpaced those in the classroom, resulting in a declining relevance of the traditional curriculum [2]. The claim is that reduction and revamping of the basic science content is readily achieved by elimination of perceived redundancy in the old curriculum. But the reality is that biomedical science, both in terms of curriculum time and emphasis, has been diminished in the new curriculum. Further negative pressure on the basic sciences is coming from the initiative to incorporate Health Systems Science into the curriculum with the associated need to develop faculty with skills in teaching this material. Furthermore, transitioning from a few basic scientists lecturing entire classes from the podium to numerous small groups often tutored by clinical faculty dramatically increases the teaching demands on all faculty and especially faculty clinicians.

Implementation of the new curriculum has required trade-offs, with certain topics such as clinical decision-making, comparative effectiveness and other Health Systems Science topics given priority over the depth of basic science content presented in traditional courses. The justification given for this major revamping and truncation of basic science in the curriculum is perceived excessive and unnecessary detail of course content as well as major overlap and repetition among traditional basic science courses. While strong emphasis is placed on integrating basic science courses and providing clinical experiences early in the curriculum, the extension of basic science content into the clinical years has been a major challenge and a major shortcoming of the integrated curriculum [1].

4.3 Impact on medical educators

The reconstruction of the content of the UME curriculum as well as pedagogical methods geared to the learning styles of contemporary students requires a major increase in commitment of faculty and staff for the delivery of content in smaller groups than in a lecture format [8]. The lecturer now is being reprogrammed as a learning facilitator, creating stress for many faculty members [9].

Medical educators, including basic biomedical science educators and clinician educators, are faced with adapting to major changes in the curriculum. Many medical educators have experienced significant challenges in the implementation of the new curriculum. A curriculum heavily geared to small group teaching places considerable additional demand on faculty who have to meet multiple competing demands. A significant inverse relationship has been found between faculty members' readiness to change teaching approaches and their severity of burnout [10].

While attempting to cope with major revision of the curriculum, faculty also have special challenges in educating the current generation of medical students [8]. Certainly, faculty educators need to be cognizant of the characteristics of today's students and how they approach leading in the Information Age. However, faculty educators still need to set expectations regarding standards of performance. Pedagogical approaches can be modified to meet the learning pattern of today's medical students, for example, by blending lecture and non-lecture formats.

Nevertheless, faculty educators must continue to set standards for content and learning without compromise on the material that must be learned.

4.4 Impact on pathology

As both a medical science and a clinical discipline, pathology is seminally important in linking the basic biomedical sciences to clinical medicine and providing an understanding of the pathobiological basis of disease [1]. Since a solid understanding of pathology is core to the practice of medicine in any specialty, all medical students must learn the basic mechanisms of disease, their manifestations in major organ systems, and how to apply that knowledge to clinical practice for diagnosis and management of patients. However, the place given to the pathobiological basis of disease and pathophysiology of mechanisms of disease in the new curriculum models is undervalued.

Although a traditional curriculum includes a formal pathology course, students generally have little exposure to pathology or pathologists in the professionally formative clerkship years. In the new curriculum, the goal of grounding medical students in principles of pathology, including pathogenesis and pathophysiology of disease, has been made considerably more difficult. The resultant discontinuance of pathology courses and their replacement by elements of pathology scattered episodically in the pre-clinical years likely has resulted in the dilution of core scientific principles and a decreased appreciation of pathophysiology.

The assessment of pathology educators is that the new LCME-driven curriculum is producing a medical graduate who is being taught to think differently, but is deficient in subject-specific knowledge for a variety of medical specialties [11]. Pathology educators are striving to adapt pathology teaching to changes brought about by the new curriculum and compounded by the disruption caused by the COVID-19 pandemic [12]. While these approaches cannot fully substitute for the coherent presentation of the pathobiological basis of disease in a pathology course, it is imperative that pathology educators make this effort.

5. Solutions

5.1 Restore a focus on the scientific basis of medical practice

The first two years of the UME curriculum is the time when the fundamentals of biomedical science and the clinical skills of taking a history and physical examination are to be formally taught and learned. A combination of factual knowledge and relationships among facts is crucial for developing clinical skills, critical thinking and evidence-based medical decision-making. Clinical skill and judgment are gained from the integration of conceptual knowledge (facts, "what" information), strategic knowledge ("how" information) and conditional knowledge ("why" information) [13]. The learning experience of the core material in the pre-clinical years should not be diluted by substituting other topics that are best learned after a foundation is laid for clinical practice.

There are more effective ways to achieve the objective of integration in the curriculum without sacrificing the foundations of a good medical education. An overarching priority is the repositioning of medical science in the medical education curriculum to reflect its unchanging and continued importance. While restoration of subject-based foundational courses is unlikely to happen, the integrity and cohesion of the foundational disciplines should be maintained. This is especially true for pathology which fulfills the essential functions of linking basic biomedical science to clinical medicine and providing an understanding of the pathological basis of disease. Studies have repeatedly shown that factual knowledge of biomedical science is essential for the development of clinical skills [1]. The deemphasis on biomedical science also cannot be good for the development of future physician-scientists, a small and already endangered group [1].

There is general agreement that medical education should be focused on developing competent physicians. However, application of competency-based curriculum adapted from lower-level occupations to highly skilled professions including medicine is controversial [14]. The logistics of implementing such programs are daunting and represent another major draw on faculty time to provide evaluation of the set of competencies and entrustable professional activities (EPAs) expected of the learners. A more feasible approach would be to maintain fixed time programs but allow accelerated advancement coupled with opportunities for dual degrees, pursuit of research, and other projects.

It is also important to counter the undue influence of the United States Medical Licensing Exam (USMLE) Step 1, as the sole objective evaluator of medical students' cognitive achievement. This has created an adverse "Step 1 climate" in the preclinical years [15]. The recent decision of the National Board of Medical Examiners to make the USMLE a pass/fail exam without reported numerical score is well intended. However, the most residency program directors have raised concerns and are seeking alternatives for objective assessment of residency candidates [16]. A definitive solution requires a return to providing meaningful grades for courses and an overall rigorous summative evaluation for the four years of medical school.

5.2 Promote a culture of professionalism

A major goal of the new curriculum is the development of holistic, ethical physicians who manifest empathy and compassion for patients. These ideals of the medical profession are time-honored and intrinsic to its code of ethics. A long-standing consensus holds that professionalism and professional identity formation need to be key elements of medical education. However, there is not a unifying theoretical or practical model to integrate the teaching of professionalism into the medical curriculum. Nevertheless, there is recognition that the most effective techniques for developing professionalism involve role modeling and personal reflections guided by faculty rather than blocks of time devoted to didactic exercises. A practical approach to dealing with differing expectations and to effectively instill professionalism is to provide students, residents and staff with a written list of expected behaviors coupled with teaching and role modeling, assessment and remediation [17].

Clinician educators have crucially important roles in developing clinical skills in trainees as well as serving as role models of professionalism and excellence in medical practice [18]. Medical schools need to address barriers to the professional development of clinician educators and provide appropriate incentives to foster their ongoing educational activities. Similar recognition should be given to a cadre of basic science educators. The Academy movement has developed to meet the need to recognize and support medical educators [19].

5.3 Focus on the physician as medical expert

There is a broad consensus that the good doctor manifests a combination of humanistic and scientific attributes and capabilities. Seven key roles of the ideal doctor have been identified as communicator, collaborator, manager, health advocate, scholar, professional, and the integrating role of medical expert [20].

Importantly all the roles overlap equally to create the 'Medical Expert'. Maturation from novice to master in (medical expert) needs to be built on a solid foundation in biomedical science and the pathobiology of disease. The time and place to inculcate the core of this foundation is the first two years of the UME. A solid foundation in biomedical science is essential for perfecting clinical skills and practicing evidence-based medicine. A byproduct of a restoration of a strong medical science curriculum will be a boost to the development of future generations of physician-scientists. Conversely, the combination of educational deficiencies coupled with lifestyle preferences carries the risk of diminishing the status of future physicians.

6. Conclusion

Whereas there is merit in the goal of the new curricula to produce holistic physicians, educational revisions must avoid producing graduates who do not have the level of expected clinical expertise because they do not have a sufficient grounding in biomedical science or a deep understanding of the pathological basis of disease. Enthusiasm for reform needs to be tempered by a more cautious and realistic approach to avoid unintended consequences.

Unless there is further modification, the new curriculum is at risk of producing graduates who are lacking in the characteristics which have set physicians apart from other healthcare professionals, namely superior clinical expertise based on a deep grounding in biomedical science and understanding of the pathobiology of disease. Physicians need to remain the preeminent medical experts who have understanding of basic pathophysiological mechanisms, particularly in dealing with difficult cases. The challenges for education of the best possible physicians are great but the benefits for medicine and society are enormous.

Author details

Louis Maximilian Buja
Department of Pathology and Laboratory Medicine, McGovern Medical School, The University of Texas Health Science Center at Houston, Houston, TX, USA

*Address all correspondence to: l.maximilian.buja@uth.tmc.edu

References

[1] Buja LM. Medical education today: all that glitters is not gold. BMC Med Educ. 2019 Apr 16;19(1):110. DOI:10.1186/s12909-019-1535-9.

[2] Irby DM, Cooke M, O'Brien BC. Calls for reform of medical education by the Carnegie Foundation for the Advancement of Teaching: 1910 and 2010. Acad Med. 2010 Feb;85(2):220-7. DOI:10.1097/ACM.0b013e3181c88449.

[3] Carraccio C, Englander R, Van Melle E, ten Cate O, Lockyer J, Chan MK, Frank JR, Snell LS, on behalf of the International Competency-Based Medical Education Collaborators. Advancing competency-based medical education: A charter for clinician-educators. Acad Med. 2016;91:645-649. DOI:10.1097/ACM.00000000000 01048.

[4] Powell DE, Carraccio C. Toward Competency-Based Medical Education. N Engl J Med. 2018 Jan 4;378(1):3-5. DOI:10.1056/nejmp1712900.

[5] Neem J. The downside of innovation and disruption. Inside Higher Ed. https://www.insidehighered.com/views/2017/03/16/downside-innovation-and-disruption-essay. Accessed 15 May 2021.

[6] Brauer DG, Ferguson KJ. The integrated curriculum in medical education: AMEE Guide No. 96. Med Teach. 2015 Apr;37(4):312-22. DOI:10.31 09/0142159X.2014.970998.

[7] Faustinella F, Jacobs RJ. The decline of clinical skills: a challenge for medical schools. Internatl J Med Ed. 2018;9:195-197. DOI:10.5116/ijme.5b3f.9fb3.

[8] Twenge JM. Generational changes and their impact in the classroom: teaching Generation Me. Med Educ. 2009 May;43(5):398-405. DOI:10.1111/j.1365-2923.2009.03310.x.

[9] Pylman S, Ward A. When did "teaching" become a taboo word for clinician educators? Med Teacher. 202;42:233-234. DOI:10.1080/01421 59X.2019.1620199.

[10] Arvandi Z, Emami A, Zarghi N, Alavinia SM, Shirazi M, Parikh SV. Linking medical faculty stress/burnout to willingness to implement medical school curriculum change: A preliminary investigation. J Eval Clin Prac. 2016;22:86-92. DOI:10.1111/jep.12439.

[11] Naritoku WY, Vasovic L, Steinberg JJ, Prystowsky MB, Powell SZ. Anatomic and clinical pathology boot camps: filling pathology-specific gaps in undergraduate medical education. Arch Pathol Lab Med. 2014 Mar;138(3):316-21. DOI:10.5858/arpa.2013-0356-SA.

[12] Krasowski MD, Blau JL, Chen SJ, Jones KA, Schmidt TJ, Bruch LA. Teaching pathology in an integrated preclinical medical school curriculum and adaptations to COVID-19 restrictions. Acad Pathol. 2021; Volume 8. DOI:10.1177/23742895211015337

[13] Schmidmaier R, Eiber S, Ebersbach R, Schiller M, Hege I, Holzer M, Fischer MR. Learning the facts in medical school is not enough: which factors predict successful application of procedural knowledge in a laboratory setting? BMC Med Educ. 2013 Feb 22;13:28. DOI:10.1186/1472-6920-13-28.

[14] Malone K, Supri S. A critical time for medical education: the perils of competence-based reform of the curriculum. Adv Health Sci Educ Theory Pract. 2012 May;17(2):241-6. DOI:10.1007/s10459-010-9247-2.

[15] Chen DR, Priest KC, Batten JN, Fragoso LE, Reinfeld BI, Laitman BM. Student Perspectives on the "Step 1

Climate" in Preclinical Medical Education. Acad Med. 2019 Mar;94(3):302-304. DOI:10.1097/ ACM.0000000000002565.

[16] Makhoul AT, Pontell ME, Ganesh Kumar N, Drolet BC. Objective measures needed – program directors' perspectives on a pass/fail USMLE Step 1. N Engl J Med. 2020 Jun 18;382(25): 2389-2392. DOI:10.1056/NEJMp 2006148.

[17] Kirk LM. Professionalism in medicine: definitions and considerations for teaching. Proc (Bayl Univ Med Cent). 2007 Jan;20(1):13-6. DOI:10.1080/ 08998280.2007.11928225

[18] Cofrancesco Jr J, Ziegelstein RC, Hellmann DB. Developing foundational principles for teaching and education for a school of medicine. The Pharos/ Spring 2018, pp. 43-46.

[19] Buja LM, Cox SM, Lieberman SA, MacClements J, Williams JF, Esterl RM Jr, Shine KI. A university system's approach to enhancing the educational mission of health science schools and institutions: the University of Texas Academy of Health Science Education. Med Ed Online. 2013;18:1,20540. DOI:10.3402/meo.v18i0.20540.

[20] CanMEDS 2000: Extract from the CanMEDS 2000 Project Societal Needs Working Group Report. Med Teach. 2000;22(6):549-54. DOI:10.1080/ 01421590050175505.